Clinical Examination of
OPHTHALMIC CASES

History | Investigations | Features | Management

THIRD EDITION

W0234561

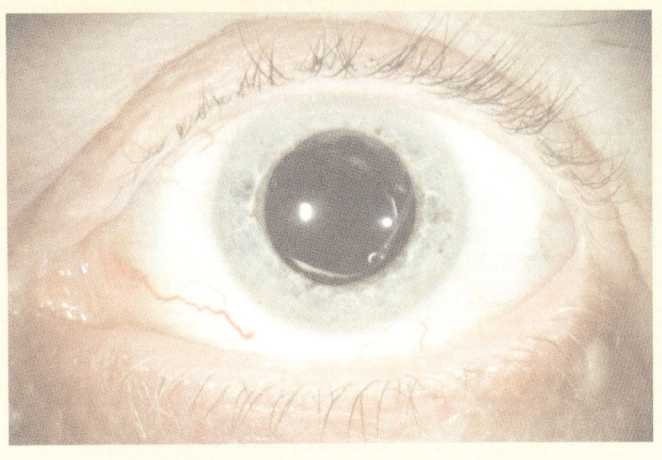

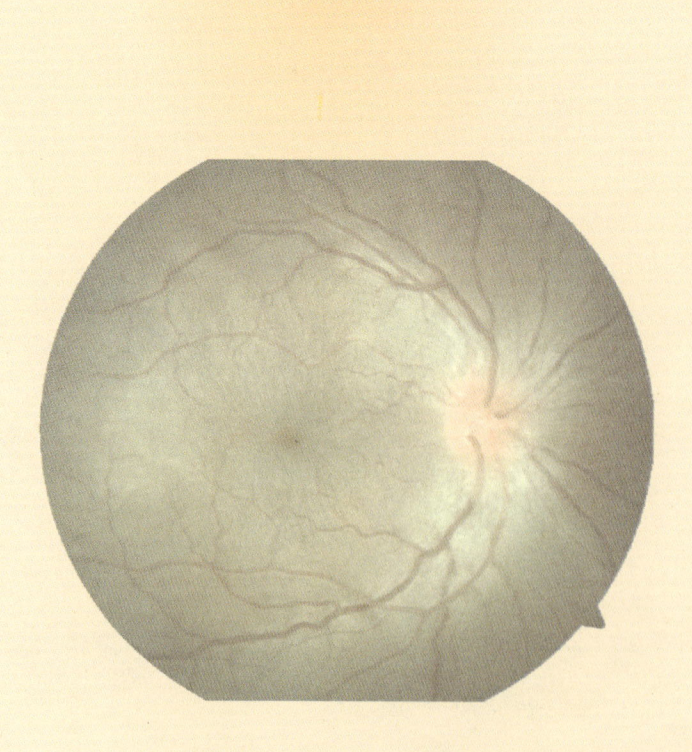

Clinical Examination of
OPHTHALMIC CASES

History | Investigations | Features | Management

THIRD EDITION

ML Agarwal MS
Professor Emeritus—Ophthalmology
GR Medical College
Gwalior, MP

Sanjeev Agarwal MS
Professor of Ophthalmology
Regional Institute of Ophthalmology
Gandhi Medical College
Bhopal, MP

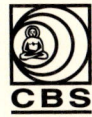

CBS

CBS Publishers & Distributors Pvt Ltd

New Delhi • Bengaluru • Chennai • Kochi • Kolkata • Mumbai
Hyderabad • Jharkhand • Nagpur • Patna • Pune • Uttarakhand

Clinical Examination of
OPHTHALMIC CASES History | Investigations | Features | Management
Third Edition

ISBN: 978-81-239-2056-6

Copyright © Authors and Publisher

Third Edition: 2012
Reprint: 2016, 2022
First Edition: 1992
Second Edition: 1996

Published by Satish Kumar Jain and produced by Varun Jain for

CBS Publishers & Distributors Pvt Ltd
4819/XI Prahlad Street, 24 Ansari Road, Daryaganj, New Delhi 110 002, India.
Ph: 011-23289259, 23266861, 23266867   Website: www.cbspd.com
Fax: 011-23243014   e-mail: delhi@cbspd.com;
                                                 cbspubs@airtelmail.in.

Corporate Office: 204 FIE, Industrial Area, Patparganj, Delhi 110 092
Ph: 011-4934 4934   Fax: 011-4934 4935   e-mail: publishing@cbspd.com;
                                                     publicity@cbspd.com

Branches

- **Bengaluru:** Seema House 2975, 17th Cross, K.R. Road, Banasankari 2nd Stage, Bengaluru 560 070, Karnataka
  Ph: +91-80-26771678/79   Fax: +91-80-26771680   e-mail: bangalore@cbspd.com
- **Chennai:** 7, Subbaraya Street, Shenoy Nagar, Chennai 600 030, Tamil Nadu
  Ph: +91-44-26680620, 26681266   Fax: +91-44-42032115   e-mail: chennai@cbspd.com
- **Kochi:** 42/1325, 1326, Power House Road, Opp KSEB, Power House, Ernakulum Kochi 682 018, Kerala, India
  Ph: +91-484-4059061-65,67   Fax: +91-484-4059065   e-mail: kochi@cbspd.com
- **Kolkata:** 147, Hind Ceramics Compound, 1st Floor, Nilgunj Road, Belghoria, Kolkata-700056, India
  Ph: +91-9096713055/7798394118, 9836841399   e-mail: kolkata@cbspd.com
- **Mumbai:** PWD Shed, Gala no 25/26, Ramchandra Bhatt Marg, Next to JJ Hospital Gate no. 2, Opp. Union Bank of India, Noorbaug, Mumbai-400009, Maharashtra, India
  Ph: 022-66661880/89   Mob: +0-8424005858   e-mail: mumbai@cbspd.com

Representatives

• Hyderabad	0-9885175004	• Jharkhand	0-9811541605	• Nagpur	0-9421945513
• Patna	0-9334159340	• Pune	0-9623451994	• Uttarakhand	0-9716462459

Printed at HT Media Ltd., Greater Noida, UP, India

Sri Krishna

with blessings

from our family members

and friends

postgraduate students,

young ophthalmologists

and the publisher

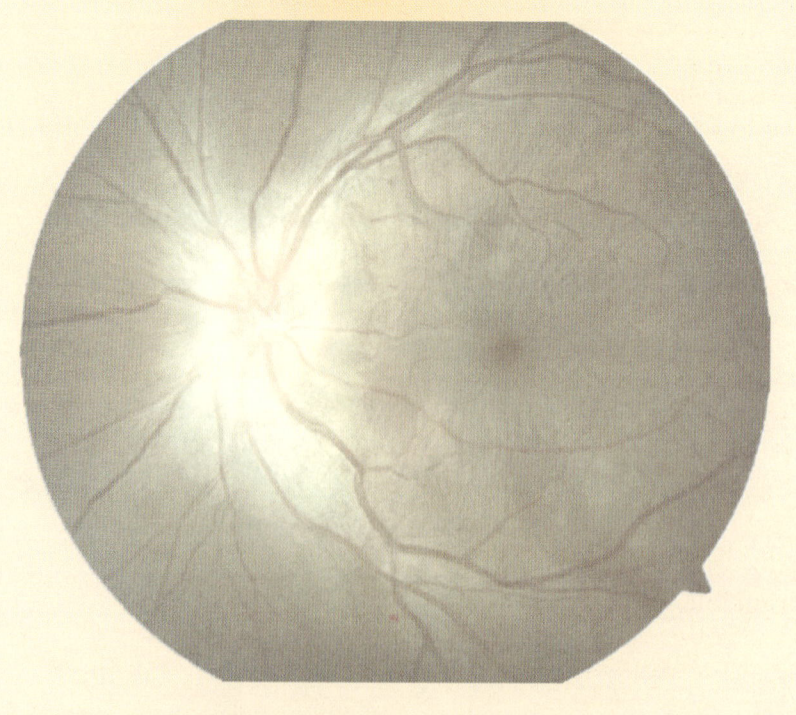

Preface to the Third Edition

Even as postgraduate students we felt the need of a book that deals with the clinical examination of ophthalmic cases especially for postgraduates. Every postgraduate student is allotted a clinical case for presentation to the entire faculty as a part of the clinical training. He/she prepares the case in its totality and then presents to the faculty along with the other colleagues. The faculty desires to expose the postgraduates to all types of cases so as to prepare them for theory and practical examination and their clinical practice after awarding the degree.

Sometimes the student gets a few days or at times may have to present the case at a short notice. If a postgraduate student can prepare the case allotted to him/her in its total depth then we find no reason for anyone to fail at any stage in the examinations or thereafter in private profession or service. Each postgraduate student will prepare and present more than 60–100 ophthalmic cases during the tenure of three years covering almost all types of clinical maladies that he/she faces day-to-day in outpatient, examination, job and clinic. Keeping this fact in our mind alive for years, we have ultimately brought out this book based on clinical examination of ophthalmic cases covering more than 90% ocular maladies that postgraduate students, residents and consultants come to see, examine and treat during their clinical postings of three years, and later for the rest of their lives.

We have presented clinical examination of the ophthalmic cases in a clear and simple format that would be suitable for postgraduate students during their study and later when they enter the profession independently. This book is like a guide and a ready-reckoner. The reader can flip through the pages for immediate reference during the training period prior to presentation and later as a consultant during clinical practice. The moment any student comes to face a presentable case, he can refer the case to faculty and offer to present the case. Every case presented by students during the clinical presentation is a step forward to their envisaged goal to earn postgraduate degree with grace.

This book shall help all postgraduate students to strive to present the cases and to show their capability to faculty members and colleagues — a sure-shot strategy to pass in the very first attempt with pride.

The third edition of the book has been thoroughly revised and updated. Ten chapters have been added to make up for the deficiencies in the previous edition. The last three chapters cover many congenital defects, many difficult and rare topics and syndromes with notes which should prove very useful for practical examination.

With the use of computers and cameras, including mobile phones with camera facility, postgraduate students can work up and prepare files for themselves taking keen interest in their patients. The record of cases presented during three years shall help them to correlate the cases in their examination with the cases they had studied. The knowledge and information gained from this book will help them to transcend the case and its presentation to the examiner with confidence and ease.

We have made sincere effort in presenting verified text material for its correctness, yet there could be a few inaccuracies or ambiguities left due to human error which is unavoidable.

ML Agarwal
E-mail: mlapla@rediffmail.com

Sanjeev Agarwal
sanjnino2122@yahoo.com

Preface to the First Edition

There was a long-felt need of a book which may help postgraduate students in clinical examination of ophthalmic cases.

We have tried to cover every common eye ailment for which patient comes to a doctor in our country. To make small book more effective, investigations, differential diagnosis and management of ophthalmic conditions with operation steps have been included. We hope that the book will prove useful to the ophthalmologists in practice serving the society.

To a great extent credit of bringing out the book in this form goes to Dr. Sanjeev Agarwal from Bhopal.

Healthy suggestions are welcome.

ML Agarwal
LC Gupta

Introduction

Keeping in view the present need of the postgraduate students, this thoroughly revised and updated edition of the book has been brought out in full colour using a poetic format that is most suitable for clinical examination and presentation of a case during the three-year tenure wherein they have to present cases to the faculty and colleagues.

Each chapter begins with a brief history followed by comprehensive clinical examination, investigations and clinical features with management of ocular maladies in relation to the chapter. In fact this book is a ready-reckoner for the reader, whether a postgraduate student, a faculty member or a practising ophthalmologist. The poetic format of the book helps the postgraduate student to understand, imbibe, retain and reproduce the facts easily, anytime and anywhere, especially in a practical examination while presenting a case to the examiners who are keen to evaluate critically the analytical presentation of the case in hand.

The clinical workup for a medical professional, especially an ophthalmologist, starts with an elaborate case history recording. Emphatic case history with keen inspection and receptiveness will increase patient's confidence and usually rewards with clues about the disease with which the patient is suffering. The present complaint, past, personal, family and social history helps to arrive at provisional diagnosis. Clinical workup for ocular and systemic examination further points out the diagnosis. Laboratory and other specialized tests usually confirm the diagnosis.

This clinical workup provides a real good chance for a postgraduate student to show his/ her clinical aptitude, mindset, intelligence, as well as confidence to handle not only an ophthalmic case but personal life and life style. The impression created during the presentation is very helpful for the self and the faculty. This self-earned self-esteem helps the students to cross over the unstable bridge and earn postgraduate degree to earn and live affluent materialistic life with least amount of stress. It is advisable for the postgraduate students to follow a definite scheme of case examination so that nothing is missed. Later, depending on personal experience and maturity, everyone evolves one's own scheme of case examination and management.

Sanjeev Agarwal
sanjnino2122@yahoo.com

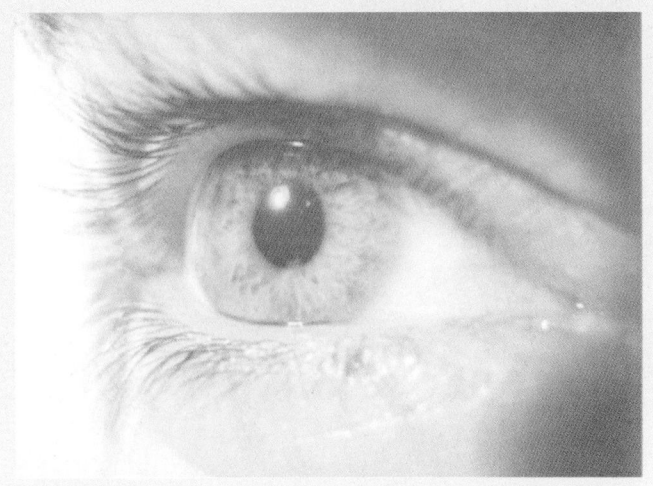

Contents

1

A Case with Proptosis

A case of proptosis is a riddle for an ophthalmologist and the patient. The most common cause for unilateral or bilateral proptosis is Graves' disease. If this has been excluded then the case needs a thorough clinical inspection, examination and investigation to clinch the diagnosis. The proptosis is a passive protrusion of the eyeball. In contrast to it, the exophthalmos is an active process causing protrusion of the eyeball. There are various types of proptosis. Proptosis can be unilateral or bilateral. These can be associated with variety of factors: developmental, endocrine, inflammatory, neoplastic, cysts, vascular or trauma. Proptosis can be acute, intermittent, pulsating or even pseudo. Thus a case of proptosis needs thorough, careful and deep clinical examination, investigations and management to solve the puzzle faced by an ophthalmologist.

History

Record the history with reference to the following:
- Course and duration of proptosis.
- Any loss of vision. If yes then it was sudden or gradual.
- Any associated pain, tenderness, diplopia or squint.
- Any association with coughing or straining.
- Any associated known systemic disease.
- Any history of trauma.
- Any positive family history.
- Any change in the direction and protrusion.

CLINICAL EXAMINATION

Visual Acuity and Fields of Vision

Recording of visual acuity and fields of vision is essential to know and assess the progress of the malady. Patient is much more concerned with his vision than the protrusion of the eyeball. A consistent fall in the visual acuity and increase in the visual fields defect indicates affection of the optic nerve though the fundus appears normal.

Pupillary Reaction

Observe the reaction to light-direct and consensual in both the eyes.

Intraocular Pressure

Record the intraocular pressure of both the eyes.

Slit Lamp Biomicroscopy

Examine anterior and posterior segment using fundus contact lens if necessary.

Ophthalmoscopy

The fundus may be normal. There may be papilledema, optic atrophy or folds in the retina. Normal fundus indicates no pressure on the optic nerve or eyeball. Optic atrophy, papilledema or venous engorgement indicates involvement of the optic nerve by the orbital mass. Presence of folds or striae in the retina indicates indentation of the globe by orbital mass.

SYSTEMIC MEDICAL EXAMINATION

Graves' disease is the most common cause for proptosis. Refer the case to endocrinologist to exclude thyrotoxicosis. Orbit is a common site for metastatic carcinoma from lungs in males and breast in females. Metastatic neuroblastoma occurs in orbit due to adrenal tumor. Consult neurologist and otorhinologist to exclude intracranial and nasopharyngeal lesion invading the orbit. Role of a hematologist cannot be ignored to exclude leukemia.

OCULAR AND ORBITAL EXAMINATION

Inspection

- Assess the age, built, weight, any skeletal deformity of the skull, asymmetry of face, swelling in the thyroid region and general appearance especially for a frightened and stare look.
- Proptosis is unilateral or bilateral.
- Direction of the displacement of the globe.
- Presence of swelling, chemosis, congestion, lid retraction and lagophthalmos.

Palpation

Palpate the orbital margin and lids for any tenderness and swelling.

Insert the little finger between the orbital margin and the eyeball to feel for a mass which might have grown to reach forward. Feel for the consistency. A vascular tumor gives a soft feeling and all other tumors a hard feeling.

Retropulsion

Ask the patient to close the lids. Apply light pressure on the closed lids by the palm of your hand. The proptosis may reduce on pressure. The consultant feels the reducibility of the globe. Proptosis reappears on releasing the pressure. The proptosis is reducible in early stage of Graves' disease and vascular lesions like hemangioma, lymphangioma and orbital varix.

Pulsation

The pulsation may be visible on inspection or felt on palpation for reducibility. A pulsating proptosis occurs in arteriovenous communication, the most common being the caroticocavernous communication.

Auscultation

Detection of a bruit over the eyeball or the bone indicates the transmission of the arterial pulse in the carotid or ophthalmic artery to the orbital contents through an arteriovenous communication.

Bending Forward and Coughing

Ask the patient to bend forward and also to cough so as to produce strain. Proptosis may be induced in a case of orbital varix after a latent period of five seconds simply by bending the head forwards. Proptosis due to orbital varix is always unilateral and usually left sided due to narrowness of the jugular foramen on the left side. This will help to diagnose or exclude orbital varix as the cause of proptosis.

Valsalva's Maneuver

Ask the patient to make an attempted forceful expiration after closing the mouth and nostrils by the hand. Proptosis may be induced in a case of orbital varix. In few cases of orbital varix, the proptosis may be induced even by lifting heavy weight, stooping, wearing a tight collar, coughing, deep inspiration, holding the breath and applying pressure on jugular vein.

Direction and Displacement of the Eyeball

a. *Axial displacement:* The proptosis is axial in Graves' disease and lesion in the muscle cone or apex of the orbit like glioma of the optic nerve, meningioma and hemangioma.
b. *Down and outward displacement:* The eyeball is displaced down and outwards by a lesion in the upper and inner quadrant of the orbit like dermoid, dermolipoma or from an invading lesion

or mucocele from the ethmoid and frontal sinus.

c. *Down and inward displacement:* The eyeball is displaced down and inwards in the lacrimal gland tumor and dermoid at the outer orbital margin.

d. *Upward displacement:* A carcinoma of the maxillary antrum is the most common cause for the upward displacement of the eyeball.

e. *Outward displacement:* The eyeball is displaced outwards in the lesion of the anterior ethmoid sinus and naso-pharyngeal tumor.

f. *Downward displacement:* The eyeball is displaced downwards in the lesion at roof of the orbit.

Ocular Motility

Test the eye movements in all the cardinal direction. The eyeball movements remain free and normal in proptosis due to a lesion in the muscle cone and in Graves' disease for a long time. An early restriction of movement indicates a malignant growth which is growing fast causing proptosis. Defective ocular movements may result due to stretching of the extrinsic ocular muscles, displacement of the globe, infiltration of the muscles, myositis, myopathy, myasthenia gravis and neurogenic paresis.

Exophthalmometry

An exophthalmometer measures in an antero-posterior plane the distance between the apex of the cornea and the deepest portion of the lateral orbital margin of the orbit. The normal distance between the apex of the cornea and orbital rim is usually less than 20 mm. A reading of 21 mm or more is taken as abnormal. The result of the measurement of proptosis can be compared with a known normal value or compared on the two eyes. In comparing the two eyes, a difference of over 2 mm, is taken as abnormal and the patient should be further investigated and watched.

The amount of proptosis is measured with a Hertel exophthalmometer or a plastic rule placed at the lateral orbital rim. The extent of vertical or horizontal displacement of the eye is measured by perspex ruler.

Hertel Exophthalmometer

Ask the patient to stand up with his back against the wall. The observer fits the concave parts of the exophthalmometer against the lateral orbital margin and the bar reading is noted. This reading represents the distance between the lateral orbital walls. Ask the patient to fix his right eye on the examiner's left eye. The examiner then views the cornea of the patient's right eye in the mirror and takes a reading on the scale. The left eye is observed in the same way with patient fixing his left eye on the examiner's right eye. Both, the bar reading and the degree of proptosis are recorded in millimeters. The normal range is 12 to 20 mm.

A typical reading is recorded as: Bar reading of 98 mm; right eye 24 mm; left eye 20 mm. The reading indicates right eye proptosis.

For the follow up keep the same bar reading to judge the course of proptosis in that patient.

Perspex Ruler

Perspex ruler is used to measure a non-axial displacement of the eyeball. In this method the upper edge of the ruler is kept in level with both outer canthi to measure the vertical deviation. For the measurement of any horizontal deviation, the measurement is taken from the centre of the bridge of the nose to the nasal limbus.

Laboratory Investigation

* Complete blood picture and ESR.
* Blood sugar-fasting and postprandial.
* Urine examination-routine, microscopic and culture with sensitivity.
* Stool examination for cysts and ova.
* Lipid, renal and liver profile.
* Thyroid profile for thyroid ophthalmopathy.
* Casoni's test to confirm or rule out hydatid cyst.
* Angiotensin converting enzyme for sarcoidosis.

- Antinuclear cytoplasmic antibody for Wegener's granulomatosis
- Immunology screening for lupus erythematosus

Orbital Imaging

- Plain X-ray of the orbit.
- Ultrasonography (USG).
- Computerized tomography scanning (CT scan).
- Magnetic resonance imaging (MRI).
- Magnetic resonance angiography (MRA).

Plain X-ray of Orbit

The plain X-ray of the orbit may show the enlargement of the orbit, sphenoid fissure or optic foramen, bone destruction, hyperostosis, calcification, soft tissue changes and orbital emphysema.

a. *Enlargement of the orbit:* A localized enlargement of the orbit is seen commonly in the lacrimal gland tumor.

A generalized enlargement of the orbit occurs in children with long-standing space occupying lesions of the orbit causing raised intraorbital pressure seen in hemangioma, lymphangioma or rhabdomyosarcoma.

b. *Enlargement of the sphenoidal fissure:* It is seen in cases with aneurysm, meningioma, corticocavernous communication and extrasellar extension of a pituitary tumor.

c. *Enlargement of the optic foramen:* A uniform enlargement of the optic foramen is seen in children with glioma of the optic nerve or due to metastasis of retinoblastoma.

d. *Bone destruction:* Localized bone destruction with clear cut margin is seen in cases with dermoid or epidermoid tumors in the orbit.

e. *Hyperostosis:* Hyperostosis denotes increase in the bone density. It is seen in cases with chronic periostitis, malignant tumor of the lacrimal gland, Paget's disease, leontiasis and meningioma of the sphenoid ridge.

f. *Calcification:* It may occur in the orbital mass or in the eyeball. It is associated with infections, neoplasia, parasitic infestation, mucoceles, hematoma, meningioma of optic nerve sheath and neurofibroma.

g. *Soft tissue changes:* Paranasal sinuses may show clouding due to infection or a growth.

h. *Orbital emphysema:* Emphysema indicates leakage of air from sinuses in the orbit. The most common cause is the fracture of the medial wall of the orbit.

Ultrasonography

Ultrasonography is complimentary to CT scan in the diagnosis of proptosis due to orbital lesions. It is helpful as an initial procedure. It is very helpful in the cases of thyroid ophthalmopathy wherein the ultrasonography may demonstrate the extra large lateral and medial rectus muscle.

Computerized Tomography Scan (CT Scan)

For an ophthalmologist, the CT scan is very helpful to visualize the lesions in the orbit, optic nerve and ocular muscles. The orbit is outlined clearly showing the optic nerve within the muscle cone. The globe can also be seen clearly with the crystalline lens. The lateral and medial rectus muscles are outlined showing its thickness thus useful in the thyroid exophthalmos (Fig. 1.1).

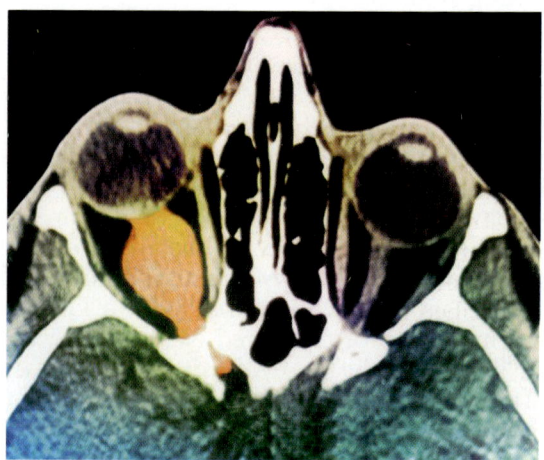

Fig. 1.1: Color CT scan in axial section showing optic nerve glioma.

Magnetic Resonance Imaging (MRI)

Magnetic resonance imaging (MRI) is a major advance among the various techniques available for visualization. The technique produces tomographic images which are superficially very similar to CT scan but rely on entirely different physical principles for their production. There is no ionizing radiation and no need for contrast injection. There is no evidence of any hazard from exposure to magnetic waves. It is very sensitive for detecting differences between normal and abnormal tissue. It has better image resolution. It is not indicated in pregnancy, case with epileptic fits, patients with metallic implants especially cardiac pace maker and patients with surgical clips. It is all due to use of a strong static magnetic field.

Magnetic Resonance Angiography (MRA)

It is a non-invasive procedure in certain vascular disorders of orbit. There is neither exposure to ionizing radiation nor any use of contrast medium. When using arterial phase the vascular lesions like aneurysms of ophthalmic artery and cavernous sinus lesions greater than 4 mm can be visualized. When using venous phase the arteriovenous malformations, superior ophthalmic vein enlargement or venous thrombosis can be visualized.

Histopathological Studies

- **Fine needle aspiration biopsy:** It is an easy technique for cytodiagnosis. It is useful in cases wherein there is strong suspicion of orbital metastases. CT scan and ultrasound shall be helpful in guiding the location for aspiration.
- **Incisional biopsy:** For malignant or inflammatory lesions.
- **Excisional biopsy:** For well circumscribed benign lesions.

Clinical Provisional Diagnosis

The following observation if put together shall help to arrive at provisional diagnosis
- Age.
- Proptosis is pseudo, acute, intermittent, or pulsating.

- Proptosis is unilateral or bilateral.
- Proptosis is reducible or non-reducible.
- Direction of the displacement of the globe.
- Eyeball movements are normal or restricted.
- Any ocular or systemic signs of thyrotoxicosis.
- Any inflammatory signs.
- Any other associated clinical finding.
- Any changes in the fundus.
- Any deformity.

Differential Diagnosis

It shall be of great help to discuss the various causes and types of proptosis and its occurrence in different age group to arrive at a diagnosis.

TYPES OF PROPTOSIS AND ITS COMMON CAUSE

Pseudoproptosis

In pseudoproptosis there is no real axial displacement of the eyeball yet the patient gives an appearance of protrusion of the globe.
- Cranial dysostosis.
- Facial asymmetry (Romberg's syndrome).
- High axial myopia.
- Buphthalmos.
- Congenital cystic eyeball.
- Staphyloma.
- Microblepharon.

The most common cause for pseudo-proptosis is high axial myopia and Graves' disease. In high axial myopia of 20 diopter, there is an increase of 6 mm in the length of the eyeball resulting in appearance of pseudoproptosis. In the early stage of Graves' disease there is lid retraction but no exophthalmos.

Acute Proptosis

- Orbital emphysema.
- Orbital hemorrhage.

The most usual cause for an acute proptosis is orbital emphysema owing to the fracture of the medial wall of the orbit due to fragile ethmoid bone. It may also occur spontaneously in a normal person even after blowing the nose.

Orbital hemorrhage is a rare cause. Orbital hemorrhage has been seen following retrobulbar injection.

Intermittent or Transitory Proptosis

- Orbital varix.
- Orbital vascular tumors.

In 90% of cases the cause is the orbital varix. Sometimes vascular tumors can also cause an intermittent proptosis.

Pulsating Proptosis

In a case of pulsating proptosis, there is pulsation which may be vascular or cerebral in its origin such as meningocele or meningo-encephalocele.

- A carotico-cavernous communication is the most common cause covering 90% of all the cases.
- Rarely a communication between ophthalmic artery and orbital vein can produce a pulsating proptosis.

Painful Proptosis

- Pseudotumor.
- Tolosa-Hunt syndrome.
- Nasopharyngeal tumor.
- Intracavernous carotid aneurysm.
- Tuberculoma.
- Orbital abscess or cellulitis.
- Orbital periostitis.
- Acute dacryoadenitis (Fig. 1.2).

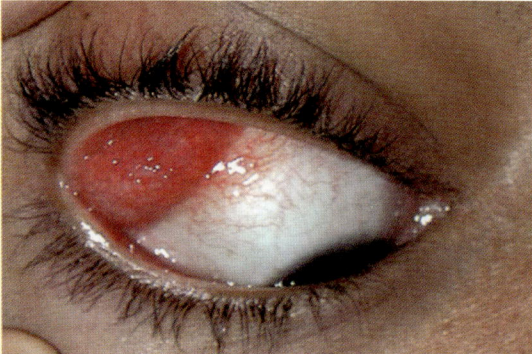

Fig. 1.2: Painful proptosis due to Acute Dacryoadenitis

Reducible Proptosis

- Proptosis.
- Early stage of Graves' disease.
- Hemangioma.
- Lymphangioma.
- Orbital varix.

Unreducible Proptosis

- Late stage of Graves' disease
- Optic nerve glioma
- Meningioma of optic nerve.
- Pseudotumor.

Axial Proptosis

- Graves' disease.
- Optic nerve glioma and meningioma.
- Hemangioma.

Proptosis—down and out (Fig. 1.3)

- Dermoid.
- Dermolipoma.
- Carcinoma of ethmoid.
- Carcinoma of frontal sinus.

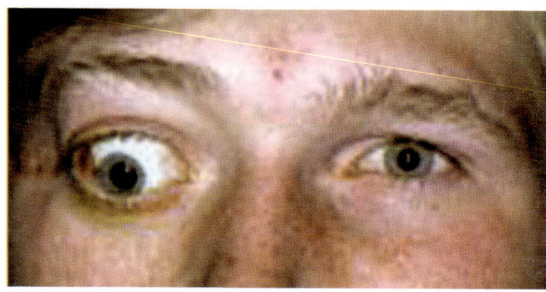

Fig. 1.3: Proptosis—down and out

Proptosis—down and in

- Dermoid.
- Dermolipoma.
- Benign mixed tumor of lacrimal gland.
- Malignant tumor of lacrimal gland.

Proptosis—upwards

- Carcinoma of maxillary antrum.
- Nasopharyngeal tumor.

Proptosis—outwards

- Carcinoma of ethmoid.
- Nasopharyngeal tumor.

Unilateral Proptosis

Developmental
- Cranial dysostosis.
- Asymmetry of the face.

Endocrine
- Graves' disease.

Inflammatory
- Orbital cellulitis.
- Cavernous sinus thrombophlebitis.
- Pseudotumor.
- Tuberculoma of the orbit.
- Dacryoadenitis.
- Osteoperiostitis.

Neoplastic
- Primary orbital tumors.
- Hemangioma.
- Optic nerve glioma.
- Meningioma.
- Rhabdomyosarcoma.
- Lacrimal gland tumor.
- Metastatic orbital tumors.
- Tumors invading from the sinuses, nasopharynx and cranium.

Cysts
- Dermoid cyst.
- Hydatid cyst.

General disease
- Leukemia.
- Xanthomatosis.
- Thyrotoxicosis.

Trauma
- Hemorrhage.
- Emphysema.

Bilateral Proptosis

Developmental
- Cranial dysostosis.

Endocrine
- Graves' disease.

Inflammatory
- Orbital cellulitis.
- Cavernous sinus thrombophlebitis.
- Pseudotumors.

Neoplastic
- Symmetrical lymphoma or lymphosarcoma.
- Chloroma.
- Multiple myeloma.
- Nasopharyngeal tumor.
- Metastatic neuroblastoma.

General disease
- Leukemia.
- Xanthomatosis.
- Thyrotoxicosis.

Proptosis In Infancy and Childhood

- Cranial dysostosis.
- Capillary hemangioma.
- Metastatic neuroblastoma.
- Metastatic orbital retinoblastoma.
- Dermoid cyst.
- Orbital varix.
- Neurofibromatosis.
- Rhabdomyosarcoma.
- Leukemia.
- Glioma of the optic nerve.
- Hydatid cyst.

Proptosis In Adults

- Graves' disease.
- Pseudotumor.
- Cavernous hemangioma.
- Meningioma.
- Carotico-cavernous communication.
- Carcinoma from sinuses.
- Nasopharyngeal carcinoma.
- Lacrimal gland tumor.

Congenital Proptosis

- Craniofacial dysostosis.
- Congenital cystic eyeball.
- Dermoid of the orbit.
- Teratoma.
- Angioma.

Proptosis due to Primary Orbital Tumors

- Dermoids, epidermoids, lipodermoids.
- Capillary hemangioma, cavernous hemangioma, lymphangioma.
- Rhabdomyosarcoma.
- Optic nerve glioma.

- Meningiomas.
- Lymphomas.

Proptosis due to Secondary Orbital Tumors

- Carcinoma from the sinuses.
- Nasopharyngeal carcinoma.
- Intracranial meningioma and glioma.
- Retinoblastoma and melanoma from the eyeball.

Proptosis due To Metastatic Orbital Tumors

- Neuroblastoma from the adrenal medulla
- Retinoblastoma
- Carcinoma from the breast in females.
- Carcinoma from the lungs and prostate in males.

CLINICAL FEATURES AND MANAGEMENT

1. Cranial dysostosis.
2. Congenital cystic eyeball.
3. Metastatic neuroblastoma.
4. Orbital retinoblastoma.
5. Dermoid cyst.
6. Orbital varix.
7. Carotid cavernous fistula.
8. Neurofibromatosis.
9. Rhabdomyosarcoma.
10. Leukemia.
11. Glioma of the optic nerve.
12. Meningioma of optic nerve sheath
13. Hydatid cyst.
14. Capillary hemangioma.
15. Cavernous hemangioma.
16. Intracranial meningioma invading orbit.
17. Carcinoma from sinuses invading orbit.
18. Nasopharyngeal tumor.
19. Metastatic carcinoma of the orbit.
20. Benign mixed tumor of the lacrimal gland.
21. Malignant mixed tumor of the lacrimal gland.

Cranial Dysostosis

It is a congenital condition of premature closure of the cranial sutures and becomes conspicuous during the first year of life. The ophthalmic complications are invariably associated with coronal stenosis rather than sagittal stenosis. The ophthalmic complications are as follows:

- Proptosis.
- Papilledema.

- Optic atrophy.
- Squint.

The proptosis is due to presence of a normal eyeball within a reduced size of orbit. The papilledema and optic atrophy can result due to increased intracranial pressure. The squint occurs due to reduced vision. The proptosis being a pseudo-proptosis it needs no treatment. The squint can be corrected by surgery.

Congenital Cystic Eyeball

A defect in the closure of the fetal fissure results in formation of a cystic eyeball. The cyst is apparent at birth. It occupies the inferior part of the orbit and produces a bulge in the lower lid. The cyst along with the diminutive eye can be removed surgically without any complications.

Metastatic Neuroblastoma

Neuroblastoma is one of the common malignant tumor of the infancy and the childhood. Neuroblastoma is a tumor of embryonic neuroblastic tissue and usually arises in the adrenal medula. It commonly metastasizes to both the orbits. The presence of a bilateral hemorrhagic proptosis with facial masses in an infant or a child is pathognomonic for metastatic neuroblastoma. Radiography shows osseous lesions. There is an increased catecholamines in the urine.

Orbital Retinoblastoma

The incidence of the orbital retinoblastoma has decreased due to early detection and treatment of retinoblastoma. The orbital retinoblastoma occurs due to extension of the retinoblastoma in the orbit through the choroidal emissary or optic nerve.

Dermoid Cyst

It is congenital in origin. Because of its small size it remains undetected during early years of life. Gradually it enlarges in a smooth painless swelling in the upper temporal or nasal quadrant of the orbit. The cyst is usually free. It may be attached to the orbital bones.

Sometimes it is connected to the orbital bones. Sometimes it is connected to the intracranial dura through a stalk-like extension of the cyst passing through an opening between the orbital bones. It can be easily removed surgically without any complications.

Orbital Varix

The most prominent symptom of orbital varix is the transient or intermittent proptosis. The condition is rare.

Etiology

- Primary varices are due to congenital venous anomaly in the orbit. It is usually seen soon after birth.
- Secondary varices are caused by the arteriovenous fistula in the orbit or intracranially. In these cases a pulsating intermittent proptosis may be seen.

Clinical Features

- Transient proptosis is always unilateral and usually left sided. It can be induced even by bending the head forward, pressure on the jugular veins, stooping, coughing and lifting up heavy weight.
- Occasionally case may show pulsation.
- Some cases may be symptomless with proptosis while others may have severe pain.
- Few cases may have dim vision.
- Some cases report about the visual black-out.
- Rise in the intraocular pressure is unusual.

Differential Diagnosis

Transient or intermittent proptosis occurs due to orbital varix, emphysema of the orbit and in periodic orbital edema. The eyeball returns to normal during remissions of the varix and not in other conditions.

In some cases pulsation may be present. In such cases the presence of the bruit and relief obtained by compressing the carotid artery shall help to differentiate orbital varix with pulsation from a case of arteriovenous aneurysm.

Management

The prognosis is good. The surgery is indicated in a case with marked proptosis associated with severe pain. Advise patient to avoid venous congestion and to lie supine if there is a crisis.

Carotid Cavernous Fistula

The arteriovenous aneurysm in the cavernous sinus is the most common cause of pulsating proptosis. The carotid cavernous fistula or communication can occur spontaneously or due to trauma.

Spontaneous cases: It occurs due to bursting of an aneurysm in the cavernous sinus most likely due to inherent weakness of the vessel wall. It accounts for few familial cases. The associated condition of atheroma, arteriosclerosis and hypertension favors rupture of aneurysm. It is common in females, the basis not known. The strain is not a common predisposing factor.

Traumatic cases: Trauma is the most common cause in males. It is common with fracture of the base of skull. A trauma may result in a saccular aneurysm which later on gives way and results in fistula.

Clinical Features

Unilateral pulsating proptosis: The onset is sudden following head injury or without any apparent cause. There is a pulsating proptosis with swishing noise in the head, pain and dim vision. The onset may be gradual in a post-traumatic case where in a saccular aneurysm has formed which later on gives way. The Proptosis is axial with pulsation.

Bruit: The bruit can be heard with the stethoscope over the temple or directly over the eye. The patient may describe the noise like rushing of water or rumble of a mill or a roaring sound of a passing train.

Thrill: The palpation of the globe or lids shall reveal the thrill.

Associated symptoms: The eyes are chemosed with dilated veins. The cranial nerves may be involved.

Management: The course and prognosis is not good. In some cases there is spontaneous cure through the thrombosis in the aneurysm spreading towards the orbit.

Neurofibromatosis

The neurofibromatous proliferations extend anteriorly causing deformation of the lids. On palpation of the eyelids, it gives a feeling of cord like masses. This feeling is pathognomonic for neurofibrosis. A neurofibroma is due to proliferation of all the various components of the peripheral nerves.

Rhabdomyosarcoma

The proptosis is unilateral, rapidly growing and of sudden onset in a child. The proptosis is marked with lid swelling and chemosis. The symptoms are minimal. It is a highly malignant tumor.

Leukemia

The patient with acute lymphocytic leukemia usually gets involvement of the orbit resulting in proptosis. The blood picture reveals the presence of acute lymphocytic leukemia.

Glioma of the Optic Nerve

Primary tumors of the optic nerve are divided into three groups
- *Glioma:* Ectodermal tumors of the optic nerve.
- *Meningioma:* Mesodermal tumors of the nerve sheath.
- *Melanoma:* Neuroectodermal tumors of optic nerve.

Gliomas are the most common primary tumors of the optic nerve. These tumors are usually unilateral and occur in children, the peak incidence is 2 to 6 years of age. These grow very slowly over years and extend intracranially by direct extension along the nerve and invades chiasma and then to hypothalamus. Glioma is a solitary tumor, non-neoplasmic and self limiting. It may appear as a solitary spindle mass or may be spherical around the optic nerve. Though it extends along the nerve yet it does not penetrate the dura. It presents as a hypertrophic capsulated mass without invading the surrounding structures. It usually extends centripetally but it may extend towards the optic disk to retina appearing as a cyst on ophthalmoscopy.

The proptosis is unilateral, axial, irreducible, non-pulsatile, painless and slowly progressive. There is early visual loss that may precede proptosis by years. Ocular movements are normal for long time until it occupies the posterior orbit.

X-ray of the optic foramen may show erosion and enlargement of the optic foramen.

Fundus is normal in early stage. With growth, the pressure on the globe may manifest as retinal striae, retinal hemorrhages, venous thrombosis, exudates and star at macula. Some cases may show papilledema and later optic atrophy.

Unilateral axial proptosis which is irreducible, non-pulsatile, painless, slowly growing in a child is enough to clinch the diagnosis. Early visual loss with optic atrophy and normal ocular movements favors glioma. X-ray shall demonstrate eroded and enlarged optic foramen. CT scan demonstrates the clear cut mass around the optic nerve.

Surgical removal of the tumor in the orbit is safe and rewarding.

Meningioma of Optic Nerve Sheath

It arises from the meninges of the optic nerve. It causes early visual loss. Ophthalmoscopy shows papilledema or optic atrophy. Its clinical features resemble to those of optic nerve glioma. The proptosis is unilateral, axial, irreducible, non-pulsatile and slowly growing.

Hydatid Cyst (Echinococcosis)

Hydatid cyst is due to parasitic infestation with taenia echinococcus. The natural host for this tapeworm is the intestines of the dog. Hydatid cyst occurs due to ingestion of egg in the dog feces or ingestion of poorly cooked meat containing the encysted form of the larvae.

Hydatid cysts in the orbit are uncommon. The onset of symptoms may be insidious or rapid. Trauma acts as a trigger. In a typical case, the classical signs are unilateral proptosis, tumor and pain. The proptosis is irreducible and not characteristic. The pain may vary from dull ache to acute neuralgia. The ideal treatment is surgical excision.

Capillary Hemangioma

The capillary hemangioma is the most common orbital tumor (Fig. 1.4). It occurs as an ill-defined bluish mass usually in the upper nasal quadrant of the orbit. It becomes more prominent when the infant cries. It is compressible. It has a tendency for a spontaneous regression. Irradiation and steroids have been used to induce early and rapid regression. The complications of the therapy must be kept in mind.

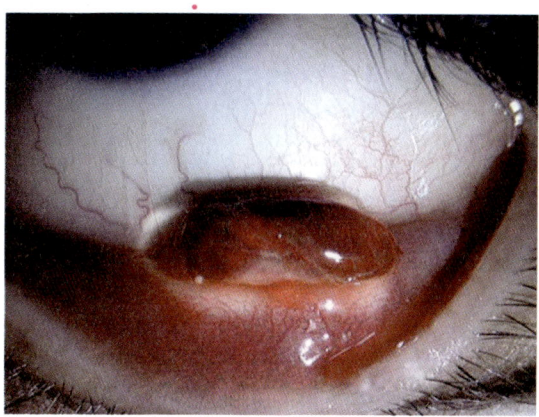

Fig. 1.4: Hemangioma conjunctiva

Cavernous Hemangioma

Cavernous hemangioma is the most common orbital lesion after thyroid exophthalmos and pseudotumor. It occurs in muscle cone. It is well encapsulated reddish or bluish in color without large feeding vessels. The proptosis is unilateral, slowly progressive and axial. It can be removed surgically with gratifying results without hemorrhagic complications.

Intracranial Meningioma Invading Orbit

The meningioma arising from the sphenoid ridge invades the orbit. In these cases the proptosis is due to hyperostosis and osteoblastic destruction of the sphenoid bone with compression of the venous return from the orbit and less commonly by the actual orbital invasion. The proptosis is marked with lid edema and shows bilateral ocular findings. It is to be managed by a neurosurgeon.

Carcinoma from Sinuses Invading Orbit

The most common carcinoma invading the orbit is from the maxillary antrum. It displaces the eye upwards and anteriorly. The cheek is swollen. The patient complains of watering of the eye with pain. The prognosis is poor due to wide spread metastasis. A carcinoma arising in the ethmoidal sinus shall displace the eye outwards. It is less common than the maxillary carcinoma. The frontal and sphenoidal carcinomas occur rarely.

Nasopharyngeal Tumor

A nasopharyngeal carcinoma invades the orbit through the inferior orbital fissure. The proptosis occurs late. There is an early involvement of the fifth and sixth cranial nerves which results in trigeminal neuralgia and paresis of the lateral rectus muscle. The patient develops a conduction type of hearing loss due to blockage of the eustachian tube. It has early metastasis. The prognosis is poor.

Metastatic Carcinoma of the Orbit

Metastatic carcinoma occurs most frequently in the age group of 40 to 70. The left orbit is more commonly involved. The proptosis develops rapidly with pain, diplopia, lid swelling, ptosis and visual loss. Lung carcinoma is the most common metastatic orbital tumor in males. Other common sites are kidney, pancreas, thyroid, stomach, testis and prostate. Breast carcinoma is the most common tumor which gets metastatic into the orbit in females.

Benign Mixed Tumor of the Lacrimal Gland
(Pleomorphic Adenoma)

There is a painless swelling in the lacrimal gland region growing slowly and pushing the eye downwards and medially. The patient complains of watering of the eye and diplopia.

It is a unilateral tumor of slow evolution with no symptoms of pain or any discomfort. There is a long history of slowly increasing proptosis. The tumor appears as a palpable mass in the upper and outer quadrant of the orbit. On palpation, the mass may appear to be soft or hard nodular mass under the orbital rim. It is slightly mobile. There is proptosis with downward and inward displacement of the eyeball. There is limitation of the ocular movement in the upper and outer side. Patient complains of diplopia and slow protrusion of the eyeball.

Manage the case with surgical removal of the tumor. It is safe and gratifying.

Malignant Mixed Tumor of the Lacrimal gland
(Pleomorphic Adenocarcinoma)

A malignant mixed tumor of the lacrimal gland is rare. It is a fast growing tumor of the lacrimal gland. Patient presents with proptosis and diplopia with some discomfort. There is tenderness on palpation of the mass. The proptosis is downwards and medially. It extends to the lower temporal quadrant of the orbit. Tumor may remain encapsulated for a long time. It has a tendency to invade the surrounding tissue particularly in the bony orbit. There is metastasis in the regional lymph nodes. The prognosis is poor due to recurrences and metastasis. Manage by surgical removal with radiotherapy.

GENERAL MANAGEMENT OF PROPTOSIS

- Intensive medical therapy.
- Radiotherapy.
- Chemotherapy.
- Decompression of the orbit.
- Surgical excision of the orbital mass by orbitotomy.
- Orbital surgery.
    1. Anterior orbitotomy.
    2. Lateral orbitotomy.
    3. Transfrontal orbitotomy.
    4. Temporofrontal orbitotomy.

The lateral orbitotomy provides an adequate exposure to the orbital contents especially for retrobulbar lesions. The classical technique of lateral orbitotomy with S-shaped brow skin incision is known as Kronlein's operation.

2

A Case with Orbital Inflammatory Lesions

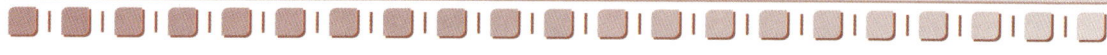

History

Record the history with reference to the following:
- Any recent history of acute sinusitis, dental abscess, boils on the face, lips, and body.
- Any history of recent furuncle in nose.
- Any recent history of flu, influenza, viral or non specific fever.
- Any trauma, direct or indirect.
- Any surgical interference followed by fever.
- A complain of pain and tenderness always favors an inflammatory cause.

CLINICAL EXAMINATION

Inspection

- Some cases may show boils on face, lips or body.
- Some cases may show a furuncle.
- All the signs and symptoms of flu or influenza.
- The conjunctiva appears congested with chemosis.
- The lid is swollen with dilated veins.
- The eyeball may appear proptosed.

Ocular Examination

- The lids are swollen and may show few dilated veins over it.
- The eyeball shows proptosis usually down and out.
- The proptosis is irreducible with pain and tenderness on touch even with slight pressure.

- The ocular motility is reduced with tenderness on the movement of the eyes.

Pupillary Reaction

- The pupils may be normal.
- There may be an abnormal reaction to light due to involvement of the optic nerve.

Ophthalmoscopy

The fundus may be normal or there may be signs of papillitis or papilledema.

Systemic Examination

Complete systemic examination to exclude any septic focus in the oropharynx, nose, teeth, and genitourinary tract.

Investigations

- Complete blood picture.
- Culture-blood, nasal and conjunctival swab.
- Blood sugar fasting and postprandial.
- X-ray paranasal sinus to exclude sinusitis.
- X-ray for any dental abscess or dental caries.
- CT scan and MRI are useful to diagnose abscess, pseudotumor or any inflammatory mass behind the eyeball.
- Ultrasonography: It is useful in detecting an abscess or any mass behind the eyeball.

Clinical features and management

1. Orbital cellulitis.
2. Orbital thrombophlebitis.
3. Osteoperiostitis of the apex of orbit.
4. Collier's sphenoidal palsy.
5. Tenonitis.
6. Chronic orbital myositis.
7. Pseudotumor.

ORBITAL CELLULITIS

Orbital cellulitis is an inflammation of the soft tissue in the orbit posterior to orbital septum (Fig. 2.1).

Etiology

- Infection from neighboring structures via venous stream from sinuses, nose, boils on face, lips, dental abscess or caries.
- Hematogenous seeding from systemic inflammatory diseases.
- Penetrating trauma.

Clinical Features

- General symptoms of fever, malaise, pain and nausea.
- Swollen lids, woody hard with few dilated veins. The upper lid might overhang over the lower.
- Intense conjunctival congestion with chemosis.
- Proptosis, which is irreducible and usually out and down.
- Limitation of ocular movements.
- The pulse may be slow though the temperature is high. This can be due to oculocardiac reflex.
- Fundus examination may show papillitis or papilledema.

Complications

- Loss of vision, diplopia.
- Exposure keratitis.
- Optic neuritis.
- Central retinal artery occlusion.
- Endophthalmitis.
- Orbital venous thrombophlebitis.
- Cavernous sinus thrombosis.
- Meningitis.
- Septicemia.
- Subperiosteal abscess.
- Orbital abscess.

Treatment

- Intensive systemic and local antibiotic therapy.
- Analgesics and antiinflammatory drugs to alleviate pain and fever.

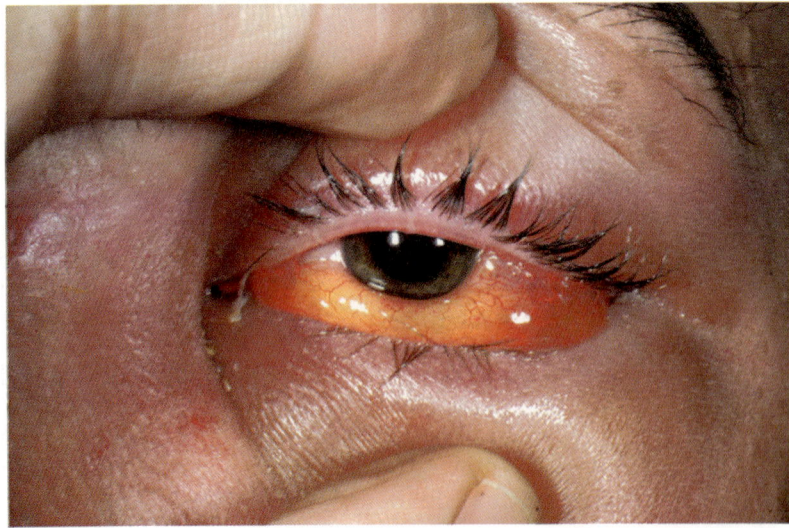

Fig. 2.1: Orbital cellulitis—edema and chemosis

- Surgical intervention to drain the abscess if and when indicated.

ORBITAL THROMBOPHLEBITIS

Clinical Features

- The infection may spread via veins, from the infection of sinuses, face, lids, nasal fossa, teeth, and throat.
- The infection may spread forward from the infection of cavernous sinus.
- The lids are swollen.
- The conjunctiva is hyperemic with chemosis.
- The eyeball shows proptosis.
- There is disturbance of ocular motility.

Complications are same as in orbital cellulitis.

Treat by intensive systemic and local antibiotic therapy and analgesics.

OSTEOPERIOSTIITIS OF APEX OF ORBIT
(Syndrome of Orbital Apex)

Syndrome of orbital apex occurs due to inflammation, tumor or trauma in the region of orbital apex. There is axial proptosis, edema of the lids and conjunctival chemosis which are the common signs of any acute orbital inflammation.

The syndrome of apex of orbit is associated with the triad of sensory-motor ophthalmoplegia:

   i. An immobile globe with internal ophthalmoplegia, i.e. total ophthalmoplegia due to involvement of the oculomotor, trochlear and abducens nerves.

  ii. Anesthesia often associated with neuralgic pains in the area of distribution of the first and second division of the trigeminal nerve.

 iii. Amaurosis due to post neuritic or post papilledematous optic atrophy.

COLLIER'S SPHENOIDAL PALSY

It can occur any time after puberty. It occurs due to periosteal inflammation and therefore is comparable to Bell's palsy. It may arise from exposure to cold, sinusitis or without any obvious causative factor. All the cases recover in a course of time varying from few weeks to few months. It is associated with:

   i. Slight proptosis with pain in the orbit.

  ii. Progressive involvement of the cranial nerves passing through the superior sphenoid fissure in the order of the VI, the IVth, the first division of Vth, the third and the second division of the Vth nerve.

There may be involvement of only VIth nerve alone or more than one nerve or manifestation of typical sensory-motor syndrome of the sphenoidal fissure.

The syndrome of the sphenoidal fissure is associated with:

   i. Total ophthalmoplegia.

  ii. Anesthesia and neuralgia along the distribution of first and second division of the trigeminal nerve.

Superior sphenoidal fissure lies between the roof and lateral wall of the orbit. It is a fissure between the small and great wings of the sphenoid bone. The fissure is narrow in the outer part and wider in the medial part. It is about 22 mm long and provides largest communication between the orbit and the middle cranial fossa. The structures passing through the superior sphenoid fissure above the annulus are the fourth, frontal and lacrimal nerves, the superior ophthalmic vein and the recurrent lacrimal artery. The structures passing through the annulus are the superior division of the IIIrd nerve, the nasociliary and sympathetic root of the ciliary ganglion, the inferior division of the IIIrd nerve, the VIth nerve, and the inferior ophthalmic vein, in this order from above downwards. Nothing passes through the narrow portion of the fissure (Fig. 2.2).

Annulus of Zinn appears as an oval area on cross-section. It encloses the optic foramen and a part of the medial portion of the superior sphenoid fissure. The four recti muscles arise from the annulus of Zinn. The lower tendon of annulus gives origin to part of medial and lateral rectus muscle and inferior rectus muscle. The upper tendon of annulus gives

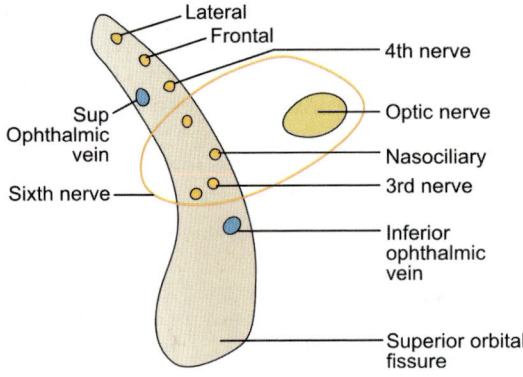

Fig. 2.2: Structure passing through orbital fissure

origin to part of medial and lateral rectus muscle and superior rectus muscle. All the recti muscles are inserted into the sclera at different distances from the limbus of the cornea.

TENONITIS

Serous Tenonitis

- It is a disease with vague etiology. Most cases are angioneurotic in nature.
- The most common cause is rheumatic.
- The other causes are allergic, acute fevers due to measles, mumps and influenza and after operation on extraocular muscles.
- It has a tendency for a sudden onset and relapses are common.
- The early symptom is the paresis of one extraocular muscle.
- Later the clinical picture becomes characteristic with signs of slight proptosis, limitation of movement of the eyeball, mild serous chemosis, tenderness of the eyeball and pain especially on movement of the eyeball. There is no congestion, redness or any secretion. The vision is usually normal.
- Steroids are effective in treating the malady.

Purulent tenonitis is rare and is due to formation of an abscess within Tenon's capsule. The usual cause is trauma or postoperative following an operation on extraocular muscles. The pus points through the conjunctive at the site of insertion of either lateral or medial rectus muscle. With the discharge of the pus and proper antibiotic therapy the disease shows a favorable response and early resolution.

CHRONIC ORBITAL MYOSITIS

Chronic orbital myositis has a varied etiology. It can occur due to rheumatoid diseases, tuberculosis and in association with orbital cellulitis, orbital phlebitis and pseudotumor. The clinical picture resembles to that seen in unilateral endocrine exophthalmos. In a case of myositis, there is ptosis, while in a case endocrine exophthalmos, there is a lid retraction. Clinically, there is edema of lids, limitation of the movement of the eyeball depending on whether one or more muscles are involved. There is mild conjunctival congestion and tenderness on the movement of the eyeball. There are remissions and exacerbations which may last for a long time. Steroids have been effective.

PSEUDOTUMOR (Idiopathic Orbital Inflammatory Disease)

The term *pseudotumor* embraces all those conditions of the orbit which clinically present as tumors but histopathologically proved to be a mass of chronic inflammation. Now, this term has been replaced by *idiopathic orbital inflammatory disease (IOID)* an inflammatory mass mainly consisting of lymphocytic infiltration with polymorphonuclear cellular response coupled with fibrovascular tissue reaction graced with variable self-limiting course.

Clinical Features

Pseudotumor affects people at any age usually between 20 and 60 years. There is no preference for sex and bilaterality is rare. A pseudotumor can present as asymptomatic condition or may show all the signs and symptoms of inflammation like pain, proptosis, ptosis, chemosis, congestion, restriction of the ocular movements, diplopia and marked visual loss. The proptosis is irreducible and on palpation a mass may be felt displacing the globe without signs of acute inflammation. Proptosis deve-lops rapidly than in a case of orbital neoplasm. It may resolve and may have episodes of acute activity. Chronic inflammation often leads to fibrosis of the orbital tissue resulting in *frozen orbit*–an absolute immobility of the eyeball with visual loss and ptosis.

CT scan shows enlargement of the extra-ocular muscles and thickening of the sclera.

Ultrasonography demonstrates sono-leucency (edema) posterior to the globe. The area behind the globe appears in the form of a square rather than the usual W-shaped optic nerve area. There is thickness of extraocular muscles.

Differential Diagnosis

- Thyroid ophthalmopathy.
- Orbital cellulitis.
- Orbital myositis.
- Tolosa-Hunt syndrome.

Thyroid Ophthalmopathy

It is of a gradual onset, unassociated with pain and typical features, which cannot be mistaken.

Orbital Cellulitis

It is an acute condition, usually affects children.

Orbital Myositis

Usually one muscle is involved. There is pain and redness over one muscle. The movement towards the involved muscle is restricted. The patient responds well to topical and systemic steroids. It seems an immunological induced inflammation.

Tolosa-Hunt Syndrome

It is characterized by
- Unilateral ocular cranial nerve palsies.
- Pain which may be periorbital or hemi-cranial.
- Sensory loss along the first division of trigeminal nerve.
- Pupil may show abnormal reaction.
- It responds to systemic steroids.
- It is to be differentiated from orbital apex syndrome, superior orbital fissure syn-drome and inflammatory process of cavernous sinus.

Management

Clinically pseudotumor-idiopathic orbital inflammatory disease is diagnosed by exclusion of other causative factors.

A thorough systemic examination to exclude any infective process may help. Fine-needle aspiration biopsy may help to confirm the diagnosis. It is a self-limiting malady. A course of systemic steroids is advisable for the diagnostic and therapeutic purpose for a long time. Most of the cases show a positive response to steroids. Start with 60–80 mg of prednisolone per day in three divided doses for a week and then taper steroids gradually to a maintenance dose of about 10 mg daily for a long time.

History

Record the history with reference to the following
- Any feeling of fast heart beats (tachycardia).
- Any feeling of tremors in hand.
- Any change in the look of a patient.
- Any difficulty in reading and writing due to weakness of the convergence.
- Any difference in the level of two eyes.
- Any complain of lacrimation, pain and photophobia.
- Any loss of weight.
- Feeling of nervousness.
- Any increase in appetite.
- Any symptom of double vision. Diplopia is due to restriction of ocular movements.
- Dim vision.

CLINICAL EXAMINATION

Inspection

Patient is usually of thin built and shows prominent eyes with wide palpebral aperture with staring and frightened look.

Palpation

The proptosis is reducible in early stage. Later in the infiltrative stage of orbitopathy the proptosis is irreducible.

Ocular Movement

There is partial or complete ophthalmoplegia. There is weakness of convergence. In early stage there is restriction of movement in the extreme lateral gaze. In late stage there is fixation of globe. Patient complains of diplopia and eye strain for near work as reading and writing.

Pupillary Reaction

The pupil reacts normally. Later due to involvement of the optic nerve the papillary reaction becomes sluggish.

Ophthalmoscopy

The fundus may appear normal or show varying degree of papilledema or atrophy of the optic nerve.

Visual Fields

It may show a central, paracentral, or arcuate defect.

Color Vision

The color vision is impaired if there is an involvement of optic nerve.

CLINICAL INVESTIGATION

Ultrasonography

It shows enlargement of extraocular muscles.

CT Scan

It shows proptosis, enlargement of lateral and medial rectus muscles, thickening of the optic nerve and anterior prolapse of the orbital septum (Fig. 3.1).

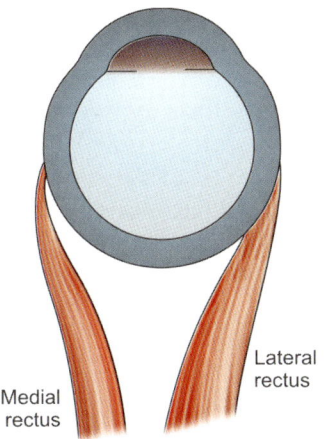

Fig. 3.1: Enlarged rectus muscle in thyroid orbitopathy

Magnetic Resonance Imaging

It is more sensitive than CT scan. It is helpful in detecting difference between the normal and abnormal tissues.

Exophthalmometry

A reading of 21 mm or more indicates proptosis. It helps to keep a watch on proptosis and prognosis.

Thyroid Profile with Antibody Test

Thyroid profile is the best guide to adjust the doses to control thyrotoxicosis.

THYROID ORBITOPATHY

Thyroid orbitopathy is one of the most puzzling malady in the domain of ophthalmic cases.

Thyroid orbitopathy denotes an ocular malady that presents with lid retraction, lid lag and proptosis. This malady is usually associated with hyperthyroidism, goiter and ocular signs of lid retraction, lid lag and proptosis. It may be associated with hypothyroidism or even euthyroidism.

Types of Thyroid Orbitopathy

1. Thyrotoxic exophthalmos.
2. Thyrotropic exophthalmos.

From clinical point of view thyroid orbitopthy has been differentiated in two types depending on the ocular signs and symptoms.

Thyrotoxic Orbitopathy

Thyrotoxic exophthalmos is a kind of non-infiltrative Graves' ophthalmopathy. It occurs more commonly in females with peak incidence in third to fifth decade of life while in males the peak incidence is in fourth to sixth decade of life. The onset of thyrotoxicosis may be acute or subacute and usually follows an acute illness or emotional upsurge. It manifests with general symptoms of hyperthyroidism such as loss of weight with increased appetite, sweating, intolerance to heat, tachycardia and tremors in hands. The patient is irritable, anxious and fatigued. The basal metabolic rate is high. The ocular signs are mild in form of lid retraction, lid lag and mild exophthalmos. Most cases present with frightened and staring look due to upper lid retraction resulting in wide palpebral aperture. Patient attends the clinic due to his frightened look observed by his relatives. Prognosis is very good. The malady responds well to antithyroid drugs orally.

Thyrotropic Orbitopathy

Thyrotropic exophthalmos is a kind of infiltrative ophthalmopathy.

It is characterized by infiltrative ocular signs and symptoms with exophthalmos and external ophthalmoplegia of varying degrees. The malady affects middle-aged persons and runs a self-limiting course with remissions and relapses (Fig. 3.2).

Management needs to control thyrotoxicosis if associated and prevent ocular complications threatening the vision.

Etiology

Thyroid orbitopathy may be a part of Graves' disease—a syndrome of hyperthyroidism, goiter and ocular signs or may be associated with hypothyroidism or even euthyroidism. There is no direct causative association between thyroid dysfunction and ocular involvement. It has an autoimmune basis.

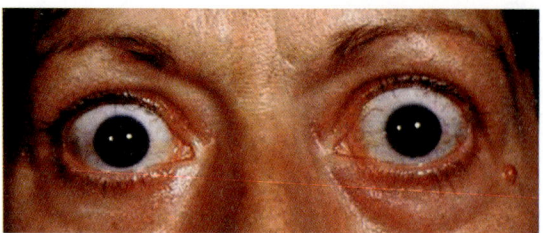

Fig. 3.2: Thyroid orbitopathy—Thyrotoxic exophthalmos

Pathogenesis

The pathogenesis appears to be associated with autoimmune basis. Autoimmune antibodies target extraocular muscles initiating an antigen-antibody reaction. This inflammatory reaction leads in production of mucopolysaccharides by the fibroblasts resulting in swelling followed by production of collagen that results in restriction of ocular movements. Females are more predisposed than males.

Differential Diagnosis

Lid Retraction

- Thyroid myopathy.
- Marcus Gunn syndrome.
- Duane's retraction syndrome.
- Malingering.
- Hysteria.
- Drugs, like phenylephrine, prostigmine, tensilon.
- Physiological, as in surprise and paying attention.

Lid Lag

- Thyroid myopathy.
- Myotonic dystrophia.
- Congenital.
- Mechanical due to scar.
- Physiological.

CLINICAL FEATURES AND MANAGEMENT

Exophthalmos

Exophthalmos is an active proptosis. It is a classical sign of Graves' ophthalmopathy. As a rule both the eyes are involved symmetrically yet it is common to find one eye showing more proptosis than the other eye or even the proptosis may remain unilateral.

Retropulsion

In early stage, the exophthalmos is reducible by firm pressure and at this stage of reducibility, the proptosis disappears with sleep, anesthesia and death.

Lid Signs

Dalrymple's sign—Retraction of Upper Lids

Normally with the eyes in primary position, the upper lid border covers the cornea for about 2 mm. When the upper lid border is resting at the level of the limbus or above the limbus, then it is true retraction of the upper lid. In a case with marked retraction, the sclera is exposed for about 5 mm. Retraction of the upper lid is usually bilateral but may affect only one eye in early stage.

Retraction of lids gives a staring and frightened look to the patient. This look is diagnostic for Graves' ophthalmopathy.

von Graefe's Sign—Lid Lag

There is failure of the upper lid to maintain its relative position with respect to the eyeball. When the patient is asked to look downwards well below the horizontal level then the upper lid lags behind in its descent with the eyeball.

Enroth's Sign—Puffy Lids

The lids appear full puffy and edematous due to infiltration behind the orbital septum. There is no dipping of the lid edema on pressure.

Stellwag's Sign—Infrequent Blinking Reflex

There is decreased frequency and incompleteness of the blinking reflex.

Conjunctival Signs

Conjunctival Hyperemia

There is congestion of the conjunctiva especially on the temporal aspect. It is due to conjunctival venous stasis due to increased tissue pressure within the orbit.

Chemosis

The conjunctiva to begin with appears glossy then waterloged and finally chemosed. In few cases of marked infiltrative ophthalmopathy, the chemosed conjunctiva may protrude between the lids usually overhanging the entire lower lid margin.

Pupillary Signs

Some cases may show inequality of dilation of pupils. Some cases may show ill-sustained or jerky papillary reaction on eliciting consensual light reflex. In late stage due to optic neuropathy the pupil reaction is sluggish or no reaction to light reflex.

Ocular Motility

Moebius's sign

There is weakness in the convergence for near work due to infiltration and fibrosis of medial rectus muscle.

Ballet's Sign

There is partial or complete immobility of the eyes without internal ophthalmoplegia. To begin with there is restriction of ocular movements which soon becomes fixed in position of depression. Usually there is limitation of elevation due to involvement of inferior rectus and inferior oblique muscles, followed by limitation of lateral movement due to involvement of medial rectus muscle, followed by fixation of the eye in position of depression due to involvement of lateral and superior rectus muscles in severe cases of thyrotropic infiltrative ophthalmopathy. The globe is fixed in position of depression mechanically as the eyes cannot be moved passively with forceps in the forced duction test. It is not unusual for ocular myasthenia to be associated with thyrotropic or endocrine exophthalmos.

Superior Limbic Keratoconjunctivitis

Cornea is involved due to upper lid retraction, proptosis, lagophthalmos, inability to move the eye upwards, infrequent and incomplete blinking reflex.

Optic Neuropathy

Optic neuropathy occurs due to direct compression of the nerve or its blood supply due to increased volume of orbital contents with increased intraorbital pressure. It is associated with slowly progressive visual loss with field defects.

Classification

Class 0

No ocular signs and symptoms.

Class 1

Lid signs: These are limited to upper lid retraction with or without lid lag and proptosis that may be minimal, moderate or marked.

Class 2

Soft tissue: There are signs and symptoms such as chemosis, puffy lids, extrusion of orbital fat, palpable lacrimal gland and visible extraocular muscles. These signs and symptoms may be minimal, moderate or marked.

Class 3

Proptosis: It is present in all the class from 2 to 6. Proptosis may be minimal, moderate or marked.

Class 4

Extraocular muscles involvement: There is restriction of ocular movements that may be minimal at extreme gaze, moderate or marked with no ocular movements.

Class 5

Corneal involvement: It may be minimal in form of exposure keratitis, moderate in form of ulcer or marked in form of necrosis.

Class 6

Vision loss: It is due to involvement of optic nerve in form of optic atrophy or papilledema.

Management

It is better to refer the case to consusltant in endocrinology or nuclear medicine to control thyrotoxicosis. Involve neurogeon in the surgery for orbital decompression.

Medical Therapy

a. Antithyroid drugs.
b. Radioactive iodine.
c. *Topical artificial tear drops:* These are effective in protecting the cornea from exposure keratitis in cases of mild proptosis with retraction of the upper lid.
d. *Guanethidine 5% eyedrops:* It may be effective in decreasing the retraction of the upper lid caused by over action of Muller's muscle.
e. *Systemic steroids:* It is indicated in a case with rapid progress of the exophthalmos with chemosis and optic neuropathy. Start with initial high dose of 80–100 mg of prednisolone and taper it off in about three months if there is a favorable response.
f. *Radiotherapy in the cases wherein steroids are contraindicated:* It is indicated in cases which are unresponsive to steroids or steroids are contraindicated.

Surgical Therapy

i. *Lateral tarsorrhaphy:* Tarsorrhaphy is indicated only when there is exposure keratitis due to lid retraction. Exophthalmos and lid retraction may occur independent of each other.
ii. *Surgery on extraocular muscle:* It is indicated when there is diplopia in primary position of gaze and on reading. It is done when there is no evidence of infiltrative ophthalmopathy.
iii. *Blepharoplasty:* The excess of fatty tissue and redundant skin from and around the eyelids is removed.
iv. *Orbital decompression:* Involve neurosurgeon for orbital decompression.

One-orbital Wall Decompression

In one-orbital wall decompression, the surgeon can decide to perform decompression by using either lateral or medial wall of the orbit depending on the case. Decompression of one-orbital wall usually achieves only 2 to 4 mm of retroplacement of the globe. This is not enough to save neither exposure of cornea nor the optic neuropathy.

Two-orbital Wall Decompression (Antral-ethmoidal)

The decompression is performed by removing part of floor of the orbit and the posterior portion of the medial wall of the orbit. It achieves about 3 to 16 mm of retroplacement of the globe that is effective to save cornea and optic nerve.

This two-wall decompression is cosmetically acceptable to the patient and the surgeon.

Three-orbital Wall Decompression

In this the surgeon removes part of the floor of the orbit, posterior portion of the medial wall of the orbit and portion of the lateral wall of the orbit. It provides about 6 to 10 mm of retroplacement of the globe.

Four-orbital Wall Decompression

The surgeon removes part of the floor of the orbit, portion of lateral and medial wall of the orbit with lateral half of the roof of the orbit. It provides about 10 to 16 mm of retroplacement of the globe.

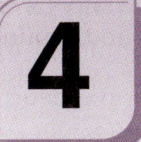

4

A Case with Cyst at Supraorbital Angle

History

Record the history with reference to the following

- Age of onset.
- Duration.
- Any change in the size.
- Any tenderness.
- Any pulsation.
- Any watering of the eye.
- Any associated systemic lesion.
- Any discharge from the eye.
- Any acute or chronic inflammation in past.

CLINICAL EXAMINATION

Inspection

- Look for the situation of the cyst.
  A dermoid is usually situated in the upper supraorbital angle.
  A swelling due to chronic dacryocystitis is below the level of the medial palpebral ligament.
- Look for the surface of the cyst.
  It is smooth in dermoid.
  There is a black spot—a punctum in a sebacious cyst.
- Look for any signs of inflammation.

Palpation

- Feel for any rise of temperature of the skin of the cyst.
- The skin over the cyst is free or firmly attached.

- The cyst is free and mobile or fixed.
- Any tenderness on touch or pressure.
- Feel for the consistency of the cyst whether soft or hard.
- Feel for fluctuation.
- Feel for any indentation in the underlying bone, at the margin of the cyst.

Regurgitation Test

If there is a regurgitation of mucus or muco-pus, then it confirms the diagnosis of chronic dacryocystitis. A negative test does not rule out the sac involvement.

Syringing Test

If the fluid regurgitates from the same or upper punctum then it is diagnostic for chronic dacryocystitis. The fluid will pass down the nose and throat if the passage is patent.

X-ray

X-ray of the paranasal sinuses, specially, ethmoid and frontal is essential to rule out any involvement of sinuses for mucocele.

X-ray orbit to know about any bony deformity at the site of cyst.

Nasal Examination

It is a must in a case with a cyst in the supraorbital angle to rule out any nasal pathology.

Clinical features and management

1. Dermoid cyst.
2. Sebaceous cyst.
3. Inflamed sebaceous cyst.
4. Cold abscess.
5. Mucocele of the anterior ethmoidal sinus and frontal sinus.
6. Tumor of the lacrimal sac.

DERMOID CYST

Dermoid cyst is a smooth, tense, round or hour glass shaped lesion varying in its size from a small pea to an orange. The skin over the cyst is freely mobile. The cyst may be free or adherent to the underlying bone. There is depression of the bone or if the bone is absent then it is in direct contact with the dura matter. The cyst grows very slowly but shows a rapid growth at puberty.

Periorbital Dermoid Cyst

Periorbital cyst is most commonly seen at the outer and upper or inner and upper angle of the orbit (Fig. 4.1). They may occur anywhere in any position along the cranial sutures.

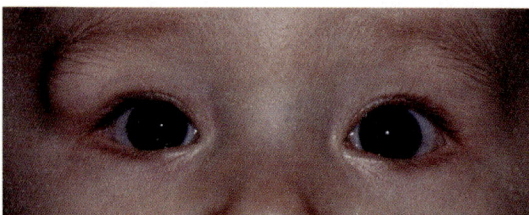

Fig. 4.1: Dermoid cyst at outer angle of orbit

Orbital Dermoid Cyst

These are situated outside the muscle cone. A large cyst behind the eyeball can cause proptosis.

Etiology: The etiology of the dermoid cyst is explained by the theory of dermal inclusion.

Treatment: A complete excision is the only treatment. A periorbital cyst should be removed along with the associated periosteum. An intraorbital cyst can be removed by Kronlein's operation. It is advisable to remove the complete cyst.

SEBACEOUS CYST

- It is due to blockage of the duct of the sebaceous gland which opens mostly into the hair follicle.
- There is always a black spot on the swelling.
- The overlying skin is fixed.
- The swelling is freely movable over deeper structures.
- The sebum can be squeezed out of the cyst through the punctum over the swelling.
- There is no history of watering of the eye.
- The lacrimal syringing shows the patency of the passage.
- Complete excision is the only treatment.

INFLAMED SEBACEOUS CYST

An inflamed sebaceous cyst occurs at the inner side of brow and inner canthus. It is a smooth, globular and subcutaneous mass. The skin at the summit is attached with a waxy black plug at the site of opening of the gland. The inflammatory changes may develop in the cyst due to trauma. When inflamed all the signs and symptoms of acute inflammation such as redness, tenderness and edema are present. Treat by antibiotics and general therapy. After subsidence of symptoms excision is the best choice.

COLD ABSCESS

- It is mostly tubercular.
- The swelling is soft.
- There is no pain or any sign of inflammation.
- There is no history of watering of the eye.
- Syringing shows the patency of the passage.
- Look for a tubercular lesion in the system carefully.

A course of anti-tubercular treatment is the need for therapeutic and diagnostic purpose.

MUCOCELE OF ANTERIOR ETHMOID AND FRONTAL SINUS

- The mucocele of the frontal sinus is in the upper medial angle of the orbit.
- There is no history of epiphora.

- The mucocele of the anterior ethmoid is likely to push the eye outwards.
- X-ray paranasal sinuses shall help.
- Rhinological examination shall be helpful
- The lacrimal passage is patent.

Refer the case to ENT surgeon for advice and treatment.

TUMOR OF THE LACRIMAL SAC

- It is rare.
- There is a long history of epiphora.

- In early stage it simulates as a case of chronic dacryocystitis with regurgitation of mucus or mucopus.
- An appearance of blood on the regurgitation test or on syringing the passage must arouse the suspicion of a tumor most likely a polyp.
- Usually the tumor is detected at the time of surgical removal of the lacrimal sac and later on biopsy report.

Excision is the only treatment.

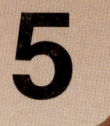
History

Record the history with reference to the following
- Age of onset.
- Family history.
- Ptosis is congenital or acquired.
- Any associated lesions of the system.
- Unilateral or bilateral.
- Ptosis is symmetrical or asymmetrical.
- Any associated diplopia.
- Any generalized weakness of the muscles. Ask about tiredness after a brisk walk, cycling, and mild exercise. Ask about difficulty in mastication.
- Any change in the amount of ptosis in morning and evening or after day's work.
- Any diminution of vision.
- Any change in the expression of face.
- Any associated eye lesion especially of lids.
- Any history of injury to lids or surgery on lids.
- Any change in head-posture.

CLINICAL EXAMINATION

Inspection

- Look for the amount of ptosis.
- Ptosis is unilateral or bilateral.
- Look for facial expression and furrows on the forehead.

An expression less face indicates myasthenia.

- Look for palpebral fissure width.
  In congenital ptosis the palpebral fissure width on down gaze is greater on ptosis side than on normal side while in acquired ptosis the opposite is true.
- Look for associated squint.

Visual Acuity

Assess visual acuity to detect presence of amblyopia.

Lid Crease

Absence of lid crease indicates poor levator action.

Ocular Movements and Cover Test

Test for ocular movements in all the direction to exclude any disturbances of ocular motility. If there is disturbance of ocular motility then assess whether it is symmetrical or asymmetrical and bilateral or unilateral. All the muscles are involved or only few or an isolated muscle is defective. Look for squint.

A horizontal squint does not affect the outcome of ptosis surgery. A patient with a unilateral ptosis and squint involving horizontal muscle can be operated in the same sitting.

If there is hypotropia then it is better to correct the hypotropia. The correction of hypotropia may relieve the ptosis.

Pupillary Reaction

The pupillary reaction shows a light-near dissociation in a case of dystrophia myotonica. It may show abnormal reaction in a case of neurogenic ptosis.

Ophthalmoscopy

Pigmentary changes are seen in a case of dystrophia myotonica and Kearns-Sayre syndrome.

Lens opacities are seen in a case of dystrophia myotonica.

Slit Lamp Examination

It is essential to exclude any pre-senile changes in the lens.

Jaw Winking Phenomenon

This phenomenon is to be elicited to exclude synkinetic ptosis. Ask the patient to open and close the mouth and observe for any movement of the lid with ptosis. Ask the patient to move his jaw from side to side and observe the lid for any associated movement. If it is a case of synkinetic ptosis then the plan for the surgery will change. In this case, levator resection will aggravate the movements of the lids with movement of the jaw. In these cases, the choice is to excise the levator muscle on each eyelid and give a bilateral facialata frontalis sling. This will cure the patient from the social and cosmetic embarrassment of movement of the lid with the movement of the jaw.

Phenylephrine Test for Function of Muller's Muscle

Instill 10 percent phenylephrine eyedrops several times in the conjunctival sac of the affected side with ptosis. The test is positive if the lid assumes a normal position in 10–15 minutes after instillation of the phenylephrine drops. The positive test indicates that the operation to resect Muller's muscle and conjunctiva can relieve the ptosis. The phenylephrine stimulates the sympathetically innervated Muller's muscle and thus gives an idea about what can be achieved by resection of Muller's muscle and the conjunctiva.

Bell's Phenomenon Test

To perform this test, the surgeon separates the lids and at the same time the patient is instructed to close the eyes tightly. The Bell's phenomenon is present, if the eyes move upwards. The eyes may not move at all in the upward direction or move in the opposite direction in a condition of inverse Bell's phenomenon. There is always lagophthalmos following ptosis surgery. A good Bell's phenomenon is in favour of good postoperative results as there shall be no exposure keratitis following ptosis surgery.

Fluorescein Test for Corneal Staining

A patient of residual ptosis following ptosis surgery may show corneal staining in the lower part of the cornea. If there is exposure keratopathy then it is a contraindication for further ptosis surgery. Treat keratopathy.

Measurement of Amount of Ptosis

The central palpebral fissure width in the primary position of gaze gives the amount of ptosis.

- In unilateral ptosis the amount of ptosis is the difference between the palpebral fissures width on each side with fixation of the frontalis muscle.
- In a case of bilateral ptosis the amount of ptosis is the differences between the normal average palpebral fissure width of 10 mm and the width actually measured. To measure the width the surgeon lifts the lid of one eye so that patient can fix in primary position of gaze and the width in the other eye is measured.

Measurement of Levator Muscle Function

With Burke's method, the patient is asked to look to extreme down gaze. The zero mark of the millimeter ruler is placed adjacent to the central upper eyelid margin. The frontalis muscle is fixed with direct pressure on the eyebrow by the surgeon. Keeping the frontalis muscle fixed the patient is asked to look in extreme up gaze. Measure directly on the ruler the excursion (movement) of the lid from down gaze to up gaze position. The normal levator movement ranges from 15 to 18 mm (Fig. 5.1).

Grading of levator function
- Normal   15 mm
- Good   8 mm or more
- Fair   5 mm or more
- Poor   4 mm or less

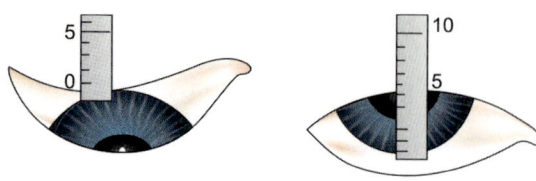

Fig. 5.1: Levator function

Measurement of the Eyelid Crease

To give a better cosmetic result, it is essential to measure the "Margin Crease Distance (MCD)" preoperatively. The margin crease distance is the distance from the center of the upper eyelid margin to the center of the upper eyelid crease when the eye is in down gaze position. If the eyelid crease is not visible then the skin of the upper lid may be slightly elevated to expose the lid crease. At the time of surgery the site of the crease is chosen that corresponds to the measurement.

CLINICAL FEATURES AND MANAGEMENT

Congenital Ptosis (Fig. 5.2)

1. Simple ptosis.
2. Ptosis with congenital deformities of the lids.
3. Ptosis with congenital external ophthalmoplegia.
4. Sympathetic ptosis due to congenital sympathetic lesion.
5. Synkinetic ptosis-paradoxical movement of the lid with the movement of the eye or the jaw, (Jaw winking phenomenon).
6. Periodic ptosis.
7. Intermittent pseudoptosis occurs with retraction syndrome.

Acquired Ptosis

1. Apparent or pseudoptosis.

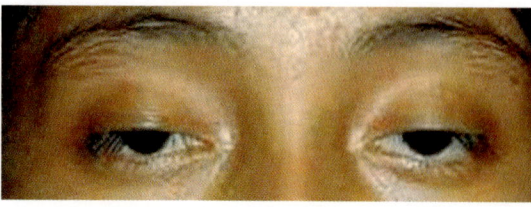

Fig. 5.2: Congenital bilateral ptosis

2. Pseudo-paralytic ptosis.
3. Mechanical ptosis.
4. Neurogenic ptosis.
5. Sympathetic ptosis.
6. Toxic ptosis.
7. Traumatic ptosis.
8. Myogenic ptosis.

CLINICAL FEATURES OF CONGENITAL PTOSIS

Simple Ptosis

It is the most common type of ptosis covering about 77% cases of ptosis. It has a strong hereditary tendency. There is a dropping of the lid since birth. The lid is smooth, unwrinkled, thin, without a tarsal fold, may cover the pupil. If the pupil is covered then to have a vision, the patient adopts a typical posture. The chin is raised, head is tilted backwards, forehead on the affected side shows horizontal furrows, vertical folds at the root of the nose and the eyebrow is arched. The pathogenesis in these cases is lack of peripheral differentiation of the muscles. There may be only affection of the lid or it may be associated with paresis of ipsilateral superior rectus muscle. It is most amenable to surgery of resection of the levator muscle.

Ptosis with Congenital Deformities of Lids

Epicanthus is the most common type of deformity occurring with ptosis. Epicanthus is a semi-lunar fold of skin arising in the upper lid that takes a crescentic shape round the inner canthus and gets lost in the lower lid. It is usually bilateral. In most cases it disappears with age. It is normal in mongoloid race. Epicanthus can be corrected by surgical excision of a vertically elliptical area of skin over the bridge of the nose.

Blepharophimosis is a congenital malady in which the palpebral fissure is narrow. It can be treated by canthoplasty.

Treat ptosis by surgery.

Ptosis with Congenital External Ophthalmoplegia

On testing ocular movements, there may be a varying degree of external ophthalmoplegia.

The most common affection is the palsy of the superior rectus and inferior oblique muscle. A paresis of medial rectus muscle shall cause a divergent squint. There may be involvement of the entire third nerve. Ophthalmoplegia may be complete or partial. A congenital external ophthalmoplegia without ptosis is exceptional.

Sympathetic Ptosis

Sympathetic ptosis is a rare congenital anomaly. A lesion of sympathetic in its course or central manifests as Horner's syndrome-comprised of ptosis, narrow palpebral aperture, relative miosis and enophthalmos.

Synkinetic Ptosis

The paradoxical movement of the affected lid in an association with the movements of the other extraocular muscles of the eye or with the muscles of the mastication is a rare congenital anomaly.

There is ptosis since birth. Mother complains that the affected lid moves while the infant is in the act of sucking the milk. It is typically unilateral and is always associated with ptosis.

While testing the patient for ocular movements and the movements of jaw, observe the movement of the lid. The lid which is covering the upper part of cornea shoots upwards on opening the jaw or on the lateral movements of the jaw or on movement of the eyeball. It is due to abnormal nervous connection in the central nervous system between the nerve supply to levator and the associated muscles.

This phenomenon of movement of the affected lid with the jaw movement is known as 'Jaw winking phenomenon or Marcus Gunn's phenomenon'.

Marcus Gunn's Phenomenon (Jaw Winking)

In typical case, when the jaw is opened, the apparently paretic lid shoots upwards to a level higher than that of the lid in the opposite eye. The lid up-shoots on opening the jaw but the lid cannot maintain the upward position even if the jaw is kept open. All kinds of variations have been reported

- Ptosis increases if the jaw is moved towards the affected eye and there is extreme retraction of the lid if the jaw is moved towards the opposite normal eye.
- The lid shoots upwards if the jaw is opened but not when the jaw is moved laterally.
- The lid shoots upwards on moving the jaw laterally in a grinding movement but not when the jaw is opened.
- The lid shoots upwards on protrusion of the jaw but not on the lateral movement.
- The lid shoots upwards when the jaw is closed and not when the jaw is opened.
- The lid shoots upwards whether the jaw is closed or opened.
- There is no movement of the lid with deglutition.
- The lid may shoot upwards with inspiration.
- There is movement of the lid with lateral movement of the eye.

The lid moves upwards with downward movement of the eye. This kind of synkinetic movement of the lid and the eye is known as "pseudo-Graefe phenomenon" wherein the action of the levator is linked with inferior rectus muscle.

In a case of ptosis with jaw-winking phenomenon excise the levator on both the sides and give a bilateral frontalis sling. This surgery will abolish the synkinetic phenomenon and correct the ptosis also.

Results are gratifying.

Periodic Ptosis

It is seen in cyclic oculomotor spasm. In the mydriatic phase there is a complete oculomotor paralysis with ptosis. In the miotic phase, there is lid retraction, convergence, miosis and spasm of accommodation.

Intermittent Pseudoptosis

It is associated with retraction syndrome wherein the affected eye retracts on attempted adduction resulting in narrow palpebral fissure giving an appearance of pseudoptosis. Under-action of medial and lateral rectus muscle in the same eye without any history of surgery is diagnostic for "Retraction syndrome".

CLINICAL FEATURES OF ACQUIRED PTOSIS

An Apparent or Pseudoptosis

This is due to lack of support to the upper lid seen in the following conditions:
- Phthisis bulbi.
- Enophthalmos.
- In old age due to loss of orbital fat.
- Facial hemiatrophy.
- Microphthalmos.
- Improper and ill-fitting prosthesis.
- Empty socket without prosthesis.
- Blow out fracture of the orbit causing downward displacement of the eyeball.

Pseudo-Paralytic Ptosis

It occurs due to loss of the tone of orbicularis muscle. It is seen in old age after prolong bandage of the eye.

Mechanical Ptosis

In mechanical ptosis, the lid droops down due to increased weight and volume of the lid. It is usually seen in cases of:
- Trachoma—due to involvement of levator and Muller's muscle apart from its thickness due to fibrosis.
- Edema of lids due to inflammation.
- Neoplastic lesions—due to increase in its weight.
- Hypertrophy of the lid.
  Treat the cause.

Neurogenic Ptosis due to Oculomotor Nerve Lesion

A lesion of oculomotor (third) nerve is the most common cause for neurogenic ptosis. It can be affected by any lesion during its long course intracranially, in the cavernous sinus, in the superior orbital fissure and in the orbit. Ptosis due to oculomotor nerve is always associated with palsy of other extraocular muscles supplied by it. It is to be kept in the mind that all the extraocular muscles are supplied by the oculomotor nerve except the lateral rectus and superior oblique muscle. The lateral rectus is supplied by the sixth and the superior oblique by the fourth cranial nerves.

The following facts must be kept in mind while thinking of a neurological lesion for ptosis.
- Levator is the only extraocular muscle which has a separate representation in the central cortex therefore an isolated ptosis can occur in cerebral lesions.
- A unilateral ptosis with a dilated pupil is a characteristic of a temporal lobe lesion.
- A unilateral ptosis with a constricted pupil is a characteristic of a midbrain lesion.
- In supranuclear lesions, the eyes maintain parallelism and there is no diplopia.
- In nuclear lesions, the parallelism of the eyes is lost and patient complains of diplopia.
- In basal lesions there is involvement of other cranial nerves. The syndrome of the apex of the orbit is the most common cause for basal lesion in which the ptosis may be the only presenting symptom.
- Parinaud's syndrome is due to lesion in the posterior commissure of midbrain. There is a bilateral ptosis of sympathetic type with small and inactive pupils. Some cases may show loss of upward movement of the eyes. Treat the causative factor.

Sympathetic Ptosis

It is typically seen in a case of a Horner's syndrome. The clinical features show
- Slight ptosis.
- Narrowing of the palpebral aperture.
- Slight miosis.
- Slight enophthalmos.
- Transitory lowering of intraocular pressure.
- Increased temperature and decreased sweating on the affected side.
- Slight decoloration of iris.

Ptosis due to a sympathetic lesion is slight. The levator is active and can raise the lid. The lid fold is intact. The common causes for sympathetic paresis are pleural effusion, cervical rib, mediastinal tumor, aneurysm of aorta and cervical lymph nodes. Treat the cause.

Toxic Ptosis

Ptosis is seen in all the cases of toxemia. It is seen commonly in toxemia of diabetes and eclampsia.

Traumatic Ptosis

The levator is a weak and slender muscle. It can get involved even in a mild trauma. Trauma to the levator muscle or its tendon or to the nerve to levator can result in a ptosis. History of trauma shall help to diagnose the malady. The scar may help.

Myogenic Ptosis

Chronic Progressive External Ophthalmoplegia

It is a rare disease usually called as ocular myopathy. It is characterized by symmetrical slowly progressive ptosis with ocular immobility. There is no diplopia because of symmetrical involvement of muscles. It can be easily differentiated from myasthenia by symmetrical involvement and no diplopia. It manifests as a primary ocular myopathy without any other feature. It may manifest as oculopharyngeal dystrophy in which there is an association of involvement of pharyngeal muscles and temporalis muscles. It may be associated with Kearns-Sayre syndrome characterized by ocular myopathy, pigmentary retinopathy and heart block which may cause sudden death.

Dystrophia Myotonica

It is an uncommon genetic disorder affecting many parts of the body. It is characterized by excessive contractility and difficulty in relaxation of skeletal muscles, hypogonadism, baldness, cardiac anomalies, and ocular features.

Ocular Features

- Ptosis with weakness of facial muscles giving an expression less face with a mournful appearance.
- Ocular motility disturbances.
- Pigmentary retinopathy involving macula or peripheral retina.

- Pupillary reaction shows light-near dissociation.
- Pre-senile cataract with cortical or sub-capsular opacities.

Myasthenia Gravis

Please refer Chapter 7 (A Case with Myasthenic Ptosis).

MANAGEMENT OF PTOSIS

The aim of the treatment is for cosmetic and visual improvement.

Lid Crutches

It supports the lid. A semilunar wire loop is soldered to the spectacle frame at one end. It helps to support the lid. It does cause irritation but gradually the patient learns to adjust to tolerate.

Contact Lens

A haptic contact lens with a shelf on which the margin of the upper lid rests has been devised. Patients do not tolerate it.

Elevation of Lid by Magnetic Force

A strip of a magnetic metal is implanted in the upper lid.

A magnet is placed behind the upper rim of frame. It shall pull the upper lid.

Two small cobalt platinum magnets are placed one on the lid fixed by an adhesive tape and the other on the frame.

SURGICAL MANAGEMENT

The treatment of congenital ptosis is surgical. The treatment of the acquired ptosis is to treat the cause and surgery only when all other means have failed and the condition has become stabilized.

Each case must be examined and assessed for the type of surgery he will need.

For Congenital Ptosis

The surgery is the only choice for congenital ptosis. In most cases the surgery shall be rewarding and gratifying. Surgery should never be done in cases wherein there are chances to leave the eye open thereby threatening the vision by exposure keratitis. Surgery should never be undertaken if there are chances to unmask the diplopia.

For Acquired Ptosis

The treatment of the acquired ptosis is to treat the cause and surgery only when all other means have failed and the condition has become stabilized.

Each case must be examined and assessed for the type of surgery he will need.

There are four basic surgical procedures to correct the ptosis.

- Resection of the levator muscle.
- Resection of the Muller's muscle and conjunctiva.
- Frontalis sling.
- Re-insertion of a detached and recessed levator aponeurosis.

Resection of Levator Muscle

1. Conjunctival approach (Blaskowic's operation).
2. Skin approach (Everbusch's operation).

The skin approach gives better results.

Skin approach (Everbusch's operation) is preferred for the following reasons:

- Exposure of the levator is easy.
- Extensive exposure can be achieved for large resection of the muscle.
- It is easy to identify all the attachments of the levator muscle.
- It is easy to attach the resected muscle at the site of insertion, the anterior surface of the tarsal plate.

Clinical Points of Importance for Levator Surgery

- In a case with 4 to 7 mm of ptosis the levator muscle can be resected from 15 to 22 mm.
- The resection of levator is indicated in all the cases of congenial ptosis where 4 mm or more of levator function is present.
- Resection of about 3 to 4 mm of levator muscle corrects the ptosis by 1 mm. This

varies with the tone and power of the levator muscle and weight of the upper lid in that patient.

- The effect of resection of levator muscle is less in congenital ptosis than acquired ptosis, in children with congenital bilateral ptosis and ptosis associated with involvement of ipsilateral superior rectus muscle.
- A case of congenital ptosis needs minimum of 10 mm of resection of levator.
- Division of abnormally taut lateral expansions of levator muscle helps to correct further 1 to 2 mm of ptosis. The surgeon can reduce resection of levator muscle accordingly.
- The levator resection should not be more than 22 mm.
- An operation involving advancement and resection of the levator muscle yields better result.
- Resection of levator muscle gives good results functionally and cosmetically if there is a reasonable degree levator muscle action is present. Clinically it has been observed that resection of levator gives good results even in cases with no levator action.
- The levator resection operation is the first choice for surgery rewarding patient and gratifying the surgeon.
- Overcorrection can be avoided by proper preoperative assessment. Some adjustment can be made by the surgeon at the time of insertion of the muscle with mattress sutures. The surgeon can either tighten or loosen the sutures as per requirement. Overcorrection results in cosmetic embarrassment and exposure keratitis in the lower part of the cornea periphery.
- Undercorrection occurs due to improper assessment of the ptosis and levator action.
- It is better to undercorrect than overcorrect the ptosis. It is to be kept in the mind that if the levator action is good then it is advisable to under-correct by 1 mm. and if the levator action is poor then it is advisable to overcorrect by 1 mm.

Resection of Muller's Muscle and Conjunctiva (Fassanella Servat operation (Traso-conjunctivo-Mullerectomy)

It is indicated in congenital or acquired ptosis cases who have a positive phenylephrine test response. Its Indications are congenital ptosis and Horner's syndrome. In this surgery-vertical shorting of the lid is achieved by resecting a strip of upper part of tarsus along with conjunctiva and Muller's muscle. Its main complication is dry eye.

Frontalis Sling

This surgery aims to attach the tarsal plate to frontalis muscle as the levator function is poor.
  It is indicated in the following conditions
  - Congenital ptosis with less than 4 mm of levator function.
  - Marcus Gunn jaw winking phenomenon.
  - Myopathic ptosis.
  - Ptosis with external ophthalmoplegia.
  - Ptosis due to third nerve paralysis.
  - Ptosis due to myasthenia gravis in which a residual ptosis persists after full medical therapy.
  - Ptosis with epicanthus or blepharophimosis.
  - Ptosis due to essential spasm.
  - An autogenous facialata is better tolerated and maintains strength therefore it is the first choice for frontalis sling procedure in cases of the congenital ptosis.
  - Other materials used are strips of sclera, silicon rods or bands and synthetic sutures. Supramid is best suited for cases of ptosis with myasthenia, neurogenic ptosis, ptosis with external ophthalmoplegia. The advantage is that the supramid can be removed if there is severe exposure keratitis.
  - Some surgeons prefer a bilateral frontalis sling with excision of normal levator muscle in a unilateral severe ptosis. It forces the patient to raise both eyebrows simultaneously.

Reinsertion of Detached and Recessed Levator Aponeurosis

  - The common cause of acquired ptosis is disinsertion of the levator aponeurosis from its anterior tarsal attachment and recession of the aponeurosis to the level of the orbital septum, where it remains attached. The cause of disinsertion and recession is not known. It may occur following massage of the globe or local anesthetic.

Complications of Ptosis Surgery

  - Lagophthalmos.
  - Overcorrection.
  - Undercorrection.
  - Entropion/ectropion.
  - Conjunctival prolapsed.
  - Asymmetrical lid fold.
  - Hemorrhage, edema and infection.

  If there is vertical squint, then correct squint before ptosis surgery.

6

A Case with Congenital Simple Ptosis

Congenital ptosis is due to failure in the differentiation of the muscles. The levator palpebrae superioris and the superior rectus muscles are closely associated therefore the congenital anomaly frequently involves both the muscles. It is hereditary with autosomal dominance with a relatively high penetrance. It affects both the sex and transmits the condition equally.

The congenital anomaly may manifest as;
1. Simple uncomplicated ptosis.
2. Ptosis with paresis of the ipsilateral superior rectus muscle.

Simple ptosis is a common congenital anomaly of the lid. It may be unilateral or bilateral. It remains stationary for the whole life (Fig. 6.1).

Simple ptosis is the most common type of ptosis covering about 77% of cases of ptosis. There is dropping of the lid since birth. The lid is smooth, unwrinkled and thin without a tarsal fold and may cover the pupil. If the pupil is partially covered then to have clear vision the patient adopts a typical posture. It is most amenable to surgery of resection of the levator muscle. Results are rewarding.

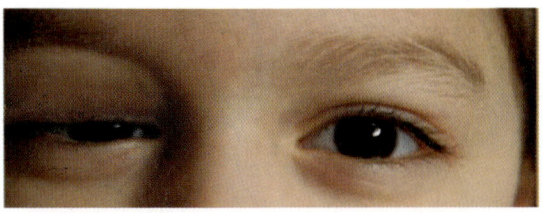

Fig. 6.1: Congenital simple ptosis right eye

CHARACTERISTIC CLINICAL FEATURES

- Occurrence of simple uncomplicated ptosis is common.
- Unilateral ptosis is more common than bilateral ptosis.
- Ptosis is characterized by drooping of the upper lid with inability to raise it.
- The skin of the affected lid is smooth, unwrinkled and thin without a tarsal fold.
- The lid overhangs the cornea with varying degree.
- The pupil may get covered or remains uncovered by the drooping lid.
- If the pupil is covered partially by the drooping lid then the child adopts a characteristic posture to uncover the pupil for better vision.
- The characteristic posture is due to compensatory continued over action of the occipitofrontalis muscle which produces deep horizontal furrows of the forehead and also draws up the eyebrows into a high arch. To further uncover the pupil the child tilts his head backwards.
- The visual acuity, papillary reactions and accommodation are normal.
- If the pupil is covered entirely by the drooping lid then there is no compensatory effort on the part of the patient. It is rare.
- A movement of ptosis lid of 4 mm or more is an indication for surgery with good results.
- Advancement and resection of levator muscle shall correct the malady.

- Surgery by the external route gives better results.

TESTS FOR PLANNING PTOSIS SURGERY

Measurement of Amount of Ptosis

The central palpebral fissure width in the primary position of gaze gives the amount of ptosis.

- In unilateral ptosis the amount of ptosis is the difference between the palpebral fissures width on each side with fixation of the frontalis muscle.
- In a case of bilateral ptosis the amount of ptosis is the differences between the normal average palpebral fissure width of 10 mm and the width actually measured. To measure the width the surgeon lifts the lid of one eye so that patient can fix in primary position of gaze and the width in the other eye is measured.

Measurement of Levator Muscle Function

With Burke's method, the patient is asked to look to extreme down gaze. The zero mark of the millimeter ruler is placed adjacent to the central upper eyelid margin. The frontalis muscle is fixed with direct pressure on the eyebrow by the surgeon. Keeping the frontalis muscle fixed the patient is asked to look in extreme up gaze. Measure directly on the ruler the excursion (movement) of the lid from down gaze to up gaze position. The normal levator movement ranges from 15 to 18 mm. Grading of levator function (Fig. 6.2):

- Normal   15 mm.
- Good   8 mm or more.
- Fair   5 mm or more.
- Poor   4 mm or less.

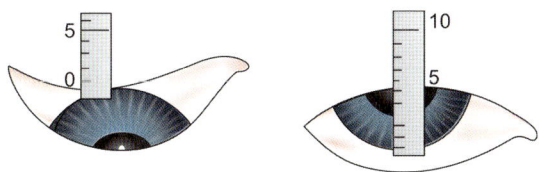

Fig. 6.2: Levator function

In all cases of primary congenial simple ptosis the levator resection operation is indicated if the levator muscle shows movement of 4 mm or more.

Measurement of the Eyelid Crease

To give a better cosmetic result, it is essential to measure the 'Margin Crease Distance' (MCD) preoperatively. The margin crease distance is the distance from the center of the upper eyelid margin to the center of the upper eyelid crease when the eye is in down gaze position. If the eyelid crease is not visible then the skin of the upper lid may be slightly elevated to expose the lid crease. At the time of surgery the site of the crease is chosen that corresponds to the measurement.

Photographic Record

In the present era of mobile photography, it is advisable to maintain a photographic record of the patient ptosis in its primary position as well as in up and down gazes to have a better assessment and plan surgery accordingly.

MANAGEMENT

Resection of the Levator Muscle

1. Conjunctival approach (Blaskowic's operation).
2. Skin approach (Everbusch's operation).

The skin approach gives better results.

Skin approach (Everbusch's operation) is preferred for the following reasons:

- Exposure of the levator is easy.
- Extensive exposure can be achieved for large resection of the muscle.
- It is easy to identify all the attachments of the levator muscle.
- It is easy to attach the resected muscle at the site of insertion, the anterior surface of the tarsal plate.

Clinical Points of Importance for Levator Surgery

- In a case with 4 to 7 mm of ptosis the levator muscle can be resected from 15 to 22 mm.

- The resection of levator is indicated in all the cases of congenial ptosis where 4 mm or more of levator function is present.
- Resection of about 3 to 4 mm of levator muscle corrects the ptosis by 1 mm. This varies with the tone and power of the levator muscle and weight of the upper lid in that patient.
- The effect of resection of levator muscle is less in congenital ptosis than acquired ptosis, in children with congenital bilateral ptosis and ptosis associated with involvement of ipsilateral superior rectus muscle.
- A case of congenital ptosis needs minimum of 10 mm of resection of levator.
- Division of abnormally taut lateral expansions of levator muscle helps to correct further 1 to 2 mm of ptosis. The surgeon can reduce resection of levator muscle accordingly.
- The levator resection should not be more than 22 mm.
- An operation involving advancement and resection of the levator muscle yields better result.
- Resection of levator muscle gives good results functionally and cosmetically if there is a reasonable degree levator muscle action is present. Clinically it has been observed that resection of levator gives good results even in cases with no levator action.
- The levator resection operation is the first choice for surgery rewarding patient and gratifying the surgeon.
- Overcorrection can be avoided by proper preoperative assessment. Some adjustment can be made by the surgeon at the time of insertion of the muscle with mattress sutures. The surgeon can either tighten or loosen the sutures as per requirement. Overcorrection results in cosmetic embarrassment and exposure keratitis in the lower part of the cornea periphery.
- Undercorrection occurs due to improper assessment of the ptosis and levator action.
- It is better to undercorrect than overcorrect the ptosis. It is to be kept in the mind that if the levator action is good then it is advisable to undercorrect by 1 mm and if the levator action is poor then it is advisable to overcorrect by 1 mm.

Syndromes Associated with Ptosis

- Ehlers-Danlos syndrome.
- Erb-Goldman syndrome (myasthenia gravis).
- Homer's syndrome (cervical sympathetic paralysis).
- Marcus Gunn syndrome (jaw winking phenomenon).
- Mobius syndrome (congenital paralysis of sixth and seventh nerve).
- Kearn's Sayre syndrome (ophthalmoplegic retinal degeneration).
- von Recklinghausen's syndrome (neurofibromatosis).
- Tolosa-Hunt syndrome (painful ophthalmoplegia).

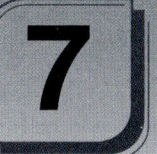

7

A Case with Myasthenic Ptosis

Myasthenia gravis is an autoimmune malady in which auto-antibodies are produced against the acetylcholine receptor, resulting in dysfunctional transmission of nerve impulses at the neuromuscular junction manifesting as generalized weakness.

CLINICAL EXAMINATION

It is characterized by fatigue of striated (skeletal) muscles. The myasthenia gravis may be generalized or ocular. About 50% of patients with generalized myasthenia have ocular symptoms and about 80% of patients with ocular myasthenia will develop symptoms of generalized myasthenia.

It typically affects females between 20 and 40 years of age.

Lids

Ptosis and diplopia are presenting symptoms. Lid may show fatigability and lagophthalmos secondary to poor lid closure.

Pupil

Pupil and papillary reactions are normal.

Test for Myasthenia Gravis

Prostigmine test: Inject intramuscular prostigmine methylsulphate combined with atropine and watch for the response in the improvement of the ptosis, ocular movements and expression on the face. The ptosis due to an organic nervous lesion is unaffected. The ptosis due to myasthenia gravis usually shows a measurable improvement within few minutes of injection. The response to prostigmine is diagnostic of myasthenia and no other condition.

Tensilon test: This test is also to confirm the diagnosis of myasthenia gravis. There is a significant improvement in the ptosis and ocular motility, following an intravenous injection of tensilon (edrophonium) a fast acting anticholinesterase drug.

Inject atropine 0.3 mg intravenously. Fill a tuberculin syringe with tensilon 1 ml (10 mg) and inject 0.2 cc intravenously as a test dose and observe the patient for full one minute. If there are no signs and symptoms of hypersensitivity (e.g. salivation, sweating, lacrimation) then inject remaining 0.8 ml of tensilon. The beneficial effect is visible in 2 to 5 minutes.

- Assess the improvement in ptosis motility by observation and measurement.
- Use maddox rod to assess the change in ocular motility.
- The test is positive in cases of polymyositis and Graves' ophthalmopathy also therefore use clinical judgment.

Cogan test (Lid twitch sign): This test if positive in an early stage of myasthenia when the patient has lid movement or when there is only a partial ptosis.

Ask the patient to fix his gaze on an object in the lower field. Then ask him to fix his gaze on the object in the upper field and keep his gaze fixed in its upper gaze. Observe the movements of the upper lids. On looking upwards, the upper lid elevates quickly upwards with the gaze and then though the gaze is fixed upwards on the object in the upper field, the upper lid slowly drops down to several millimeters with a twitch.

Electromyography

Electromyography may be used to document the improvement with tensilon test or to demonstrate the fatigue of the neuromuscular junction.

Tensilon Tonography

Glaser has suggested that tensilon tonography is helpful in making diagnosis. Tonography is performed while tensilon is injected intravenously. If there is a positive response the acute co-contraction of the ocular muscles will result in a sudden increase in intraocular pressure which is plotted on the graph.

Serum Acetylcholine Receptor Antibodies

Anti-acetylcholine receptor antibodies are present in about 90% of patients with myasthenia gravis. A therapy with plasmapheresis can be given to remove anti-acetylcholine antibodies.

CT Scan

CT scan of chest is mandatory to rule out thymoma, present in 10% cases of myasthenia gravis.

CLINICAL FEATURES AND MANAGEMENT

Ocular Symptoms

Ptosis

Characteristically the ptosis first appears in the evening when the patient is tired from his day's work and disappears by morning after full night rest. This kind of diurnal variation in the ptosis is diagnostic for myasthenia. Later ptosis appears early during working hours also and gradually becomes permanent.

Ptosis is the one most common symptom of myasthenia gravis. Ptosis becomes evident in about 95% of patients. Myasthenia gravis is the most common cause of a bilateral ptosis in an adult. The ptosis though bilateral is asymmetrical and gets fully manifested by evening when patient is tired from day's work (Fig. 7.1).

It is to be kept in mind that ptosis is often fluctuating but the ophthalmoplegia is more constant.

Diplopia

Diplopia is transient to begin with and gradually becomes permanent.

Patient complains of diplopia due to weakness of the extraocular muscles. All or any of the muscle may be affected. Clinically, it presents like that of supranuclear palsy, internuclear ophthalmoplegia, or isolated extraocular muscle palsy. There is associated intermittent phoria or tropia.

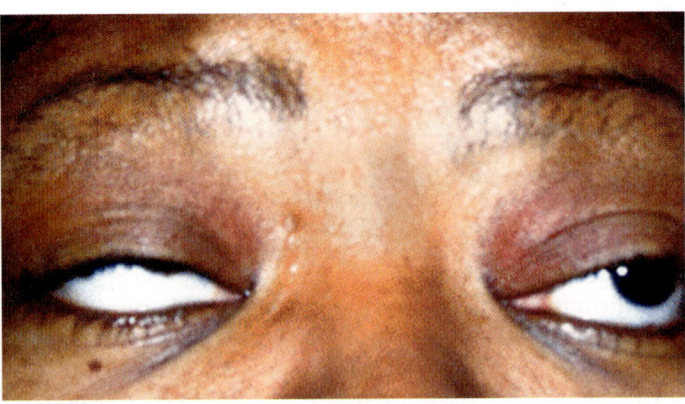

Fig. 7.1: Myasthenic ptosis

Eye Strain for Near Work

Patient complains of eye strain due to myasthenic papillary reaction, paresis of accommodation and insufficiency of convergence. The involvement of the medial rectus muscle leads to insufficiency of convergence.

Management

- The initial treatment is with long-acting anticholinesterase drugs such as pyridostigmine (Mestinon). It shows improvement in the general weakness and ptosis but the ocular motility weakness remains almost unaffected.
- Some cases show marked improvement with addition of systemic steroids. Taper the steroids keeping the side effects in mind for a long-term therapy.
- Surgical treatment by thymectomy has not been beneficial.
- Plasmapheresis to remove anti acetylcholine antibodies have been a recent introduction in therapy.
- A frontalis sling operation for ptosis may help if the frontalis muscle is normal.

8

A Case with Lagophthalmos—Bell's Palsy

History

Record the history with reference to the following
- Ask about any recent exposure to cold.
- Any history of direct cold drafts to the face.
- Any history of recent viral infection.
- It usually affects young and elderly.
- Any history of mild trauma to mandible or temporal bone.
- Any injury at the exit of stylomastoid foramen.
- Any infection of ear such as tympanitis.

CLINICAL EXAMINATION

A simple physical examination is enough to diagnose a case of lagophthalmos due to Bell's palsy.

- There is paralysis of the upper and lower parts of the affected side of the face. It is lower motor neuron type of facial palsy in which both the parts of the face get affected. In the upper motor neuron type of facial palsy the upper part of affected side of the face escapes, i.e. not affected.
- The facial expression is affected.
- Ask the patient to wrinkle the brow. He is unable to wrinkle it.
- Ask the patient to retract the angle of the mouth. He cannot retract the angle of mouth on the affected side.
- Ask the patient to whistle. He cannot whistle as he is unable to use one side of the muscles of face.
- Ask the patient to close the lids. There is lagophthalmos on the affected side. On an attempt to close the eye, the lids cannot be closed and the eye rolls upwards and outwards.

Etiology

The term Bell's palsy is used for cases of isolated facial palsy of unknown origin.

- Bell's palsy occurs due to edema, ischemia and compression of the facial nerve in its canal usually following an exposure to cold weather, wind or mild fever.
- A viral infection has been suggested as an etiological factor since minor epidemics of Bell's palsy occurs occasionally.
- The compression of the facial nerve results in paralysis of the function of the nerve which if not relieved early may sometimes leads to wallerian degeneration of the nerve.
- There may be an associated history of mild trauma to mandible close to exit of the stylomastoid foramen and tympanitis.
- It affects young and elderly people both the sex.

Clinical Features

The patient complains of the following
- Unable to close the eye on the affected side.
- While drinking the fluid escapes from the angle of mouth on the affected side.
- Numbness on the affected side.
- The facial expression is lost on the side affected.

- Patient is unable to wrinkle the brow and forehead.
- Patient is unable to retract the angle of mouth.
- Patient is unable to whistle.
- There is paralysis of the upper and lower parts of the affected side of face (Fig. 8.1).

Differential Diagnosis

Lagophthalmos

- Physiological-many people sleep with slight open eyes, exposing the lower sclera.
- Graves' disease.
- Marked proptosis.
- Seventh nerve paralysis.
- Scar of the lid.

Facial Palsy

- Bell's palsy.
- Otitis media.
- Arteriosclerosis.
- Hypertension.
- Diabetes mellitus.
- Leprosy.
- Secondary syphilis.

- Uveoparotid fever.
- Mikulicz's disease.

Investigations

Electromyography (EMG)

The electromyography of the facial muscles has been used to detect degeneration of the facial nerve. On electromyography if the voltage required to produce contraction of the muscle on the affected side is more than double to that required on the normal side then a Wallerian degeneration has probably set in. The reports obtained are conflicting therefore it cannot be relied on.

CT Scan

An axial and coronal scan can diagnose tumors and fractures in the facial canal.

Magnetic Resonance Imaging (MRI)

The magnetic resonance imaging helps to diagnose lesions in the posterior fossa.

Complications

- Lagophthalmos.
- Ptosis of the eyebrow.

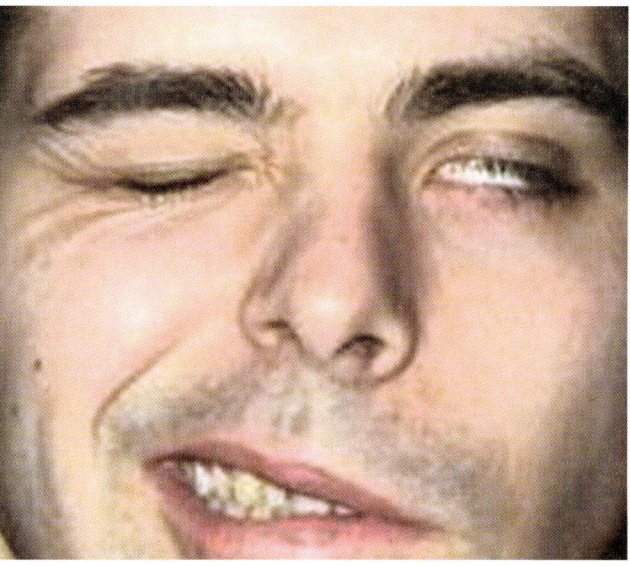

Fig. 8.1: Bell's palsy

- Epiphora.
- Exposure keratitis.
- Cosmetic embarrassment.

Management

The main role of the ophthalmologist is to treat the Bell's palsy and manage ocular complications caused by lagophthalmos as a result of facial palsy.

Treatment of Bell's Palsy

About 75 to 90% of the patients recover spontaneously and completely. The prognosis is good if the patient is young and the palsy is incomplete. The signs of recovery are seen within the first two to three weeks and full recovery occurs within few months. About 10 to 25% patients do not show full recovery. Systemic steroids and supportive treatment are rewarding.

Treatment of Ocular Complications

It is essential to prevent occurrence of exposure keratitis in any case of lagophthalmos especially if there is associated neurotrophic keratopathy. The following measures should be adopted in a case with anticipated early recovery or a case with incomplete palsy of the orbicularis.

- Lubricants such as artificial tears to be used frequently.
- A thin strip of tape can be used to close the palpebral aperture especially during sleep.
- Goggles or spectacles with temporal shields shall help protect the cornea from wind and dust.
- Tarsorrhaphy is the treatment of choice in the cases with anticipated delayed recovery or cases with no recovery.

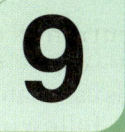

9

A Case with Nodular Lesion of Lid

History

Record the history with reference to the following points
- Nodule is since birth or appeared later in life.
- Is it stationary or growing?
- If growing then its relation with age or trauma?
- Any increase in growth on crying or lowering the head.
- Is there any change in its color?
- Does it ulcerate?
- Any tenderness.
- Any associated conjunctivitis.

CLINICAL EXAMINATION

Inspection

Inspect the nodule with torch light and magnifying loupe or slit lamp.
- Look for its size, shape, color, flat, raised or peduncle.
- Look for its surface, smooth or granular.
- Look for any black head on the surface.
- Look for any crust formation on the surface.
- One or more nodule.
- Symmetrical or asymmetrical.
- Any relation to distribution along the first division of fifth nerve.

Palpation

Palpate the nodule by fingers and note the findings
- The nodule is smooth or uneven.
- Any tenderness to touch or pressure.
- The overlying skin is free or firmly attached to it.
- The nodule is free or attached to underlying structure.
- It is reducible or not.
- Any feeling like hard cords or knobs as if a bag full of worms.

CLINICAL INVESTIGATION

X-ray

It may reveal any bony lesion, bony defect or erosion.

CT Scan

It shall help to rule out the orbital extension or lesion in orbit.

CLINICAL FEATURES AND MANAGEMENT

Non Tumor

1. Chalazion.
2. Xanthelasma.

Benign Tumor

3. Nevus or mole.
4. Molluscum contagiosum.
5. Verruca vulgaris (warts).
6. Simple papilloma.
7. Basal cell papilloma.
8. Capillary hemangioma.
9. Neurofibromatosis.
10. Dermoid cyst.

Malignant Tumor

11. Squamous cell carcinoma.
12. Basal cell carcinoma.
13. Sebaceous gland carcinoma.

Chalazion

Chalazion is the most common type of nodule seen on the eyelids (Fig. 9.1). This is due to chronic lipogranulomatous inflammation of meibomian gland. It presents as a painless, slowly growing, round and firm mass in the tarsal plate. Sometimes it presents as inflamed and tender swelling similar to hordeolum. It seldom subsides spontaneously. A large chalazion may press on the eyeball and cause astigmatism. The majority of the chalazion point towards the conjunctival side. The only treatment is incision and curettage. If there is a recurrence in the same area then biopsy should be performed to rule out malignancy. Quite often a granuloma may grow at the site of the incision of chalazion. Excise it. A meibomian gland carcinoma or a basal cell caracinoma can be mistaken for a chalazion.

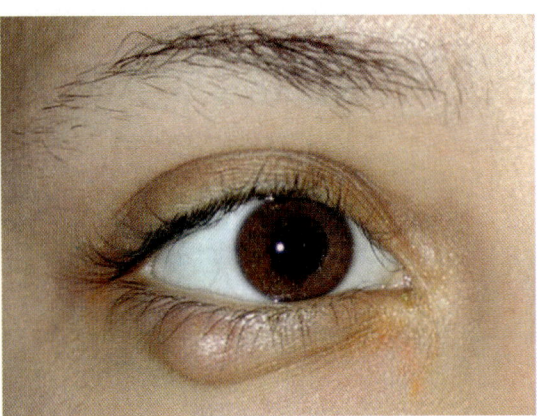

Fig. 9.1: Chalazion

Treatment

Incision and curettage: Infiltrate the eyelid in the region of chalazion by lignocaine. Instill topical anesthetic in the conjunctival sac. Apply the chalazion clamp and evert the lid. Make a vertical incision in the cyst through the conjunctiva and curette the contents. Excise any granulation tissue with scissors. Release the clamp and replace the lid. Apply an antibiotic eye ointment and pad the eye for four hours.

Steroid Intralesional Injection

Inject 0.2 ml of triamcinolone diacetate directly into the cyst through skin or conjunctiva. Second injection can be given after two weeks, Good response in about 80%. Hard lesions are not responsive.

Systemic tetracycline can be given in case with recurrence.

Xanthelasma (Xanthoma)

These are yellow plaques most commonly seen in the upper and lower lids near the inner canthus, symmetrical in two lids on both the sides. These are seen in elderly women and often associated with diabetes. The growth is slow. Treat by excision or cryotherapy. It needs treatment for cosmetic purpose.

Nevus or Mole

A nevus or a mole occurs on the lid margin involving both the skin and the conjunctiva (Fig. 9.2). Two moles may be symmetrically situated on the lids of the same eye indicating their origin at a time when the lids were still united. There is tendency for growth at puberty. It is rare to change in malignancy. Most of these do not require any treatment. Best is to leave these alone. Treat if at all by complete and extensive excision including normal tissue.

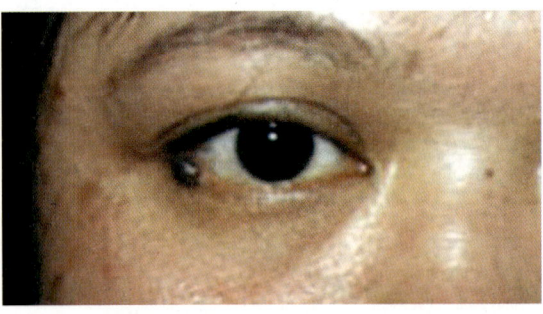

Fig. 9.2: Nevus-right lower lid

Molluscum Contagiosum

This is caused by virus infection which mostly affects children. It presents as a small, pale-white waxy, umbilicated and elevated nodules on both the lids and surrounding area (Fig. 9.3). These may resolve spontaneously in few months. The chronic shedding of cells laden with the viral particle may induce chronic follicular conjunctivitis and superficial keratitis. Treat the case early without waiting for resolution if there is chronic follicular conjunctivitis which do not respond to any therapy. Treat each lesion by incision and expression of sebum like content and follow with cauterization with povidone.

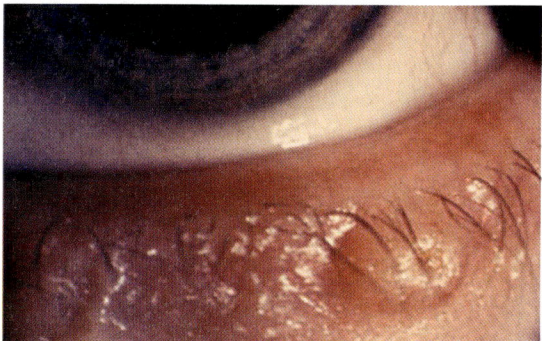

Fig. 9.3: Molluscum contagiosum

Verruca Vulgaris (Warts)

This is caused by a virus infection. It appears as a filiform wart. Occasionally these appear as a crop of lesions simultaneously. Treat by excision and cauterization.

Simple Papilloma

It is one of the most common benign tumor of the lid. It presents as a peduncle lesions on the lid margins. Adults are affected. These are slow growing lesions. Treat by simple excision.

Basal Cell Papilloma

It is common in elderly people. It presents as a slow growing, discrete, greasy, brown or dark, round or oval lesion that appears stuck on the surface like a button. It has a friable surface. Microscopically it is characterized by an outward acanthotic proliferation of basal-like cells (basaloid cells) and may show variations such as hyperkeratosis or even an adenoid or glandular pattern. The basaloid appearance can lead to confusion with basal cell carcinoma. The presence of accumulations of keratin in crypts helps to differentiate it.

Capillary Hemangioma

Capillary hemangioma typically presents at birth or soon after as a periocular swelling in the anterior part of the orbit. It may show increase in size during crying and straining. There is no pulsation or a bruit. A lesion involving surrounding subcutaneous tissue gives a dark red or bluish color to the skin of the lids. Superficial 'strawberry' naevi may also be found on the lids. The tumor grows in the first year of life then stabilizes and eventually shows regression and disappearance by the age of five. Hemangioma often follows the area of distribution of first and second division of fifth nerve. In the Sturge-Weber syndrome, it is associated with the hemangioma of choroid and glaucoma and also hemangioma of leptomeninges. Only retrobulbar hemangiomas need surgical treatment for optic nerve compression and proptosis causing keratopathy. Others may need for cosmetic purpose. It can be treated by systemic steroids, steroid injection in the tumor, radiation and surgical excision using cutting diathermy. Sclerosing agents and cryotherapy should be avoided.

Neurofibromatosis (von Recklingausen's disease)

It involves lid, temporal region and orbit. A neurofibroma represents a proliferation of all the various components of the peripheral nerve, i.e. the axon, its sheath and its supporting connective tissue cells. The swollen lid and temporal region forms a characteristic picture. The hypertrophied nerves can be felt through the skin like hard cords. On palpation, the cord-like masses in the lid feels like a "bag of worms", a feeling once felt cannot be mistaken. Operative measures are not satisfactory.

Dermoid Cyst

Dermoid cysts are congenital in origin, believed to result from an embryonic displacement of epidermis to a subcutaneous location. It remains unnoticed during the early years of life because of its small size. Later it enlarges to form a smooth, painless swelling located in the upper nasal or upper temporal quadrant of the orbit. It also appears as a swelling in the upper nasal or temporal quadrant of superior orbital margin involving the lid. The overlying skin is free. The cyst may be attached to the underlying bones, giving support to the theory that dermoid cysts represent the sequestration of surface ectoderm owing to closure of suture lines of the bony orbit. Sometimes there may be a stalk connecting the cyst to intracranial dura through the opening in the bone. Excision is the only treatment. Deep seated dermoid cyst must be evaluated with X-ray and CT Scan. The cyst contains cheesy material. Remove the cyst in total as the cheesy material in the cyst is irritating to the orbital tissue.

Squamous Cell Carcinoma (Epithelioma)

Squamous cell carcinoma is an invasive epithelial malignancy arising from squamous cell layer of the epidermis. Squamous cell carcinoma occurs commonly at the sites where the character of the epithelium changes, the common site being lid margin and limbus. It appears as a small nodule at the lid margin in elderly people. It grows slowly with involvement of the pre-auricular lymph nodes. Treat by excision biopsy with frozen section or Moh's micrographic soon a nodule is noticed in an elderly person without any reason.

Basal Cell Carcinoma (Rodent Ulcer)

Basal cell carcinoma arises from the basal cells of the epidermis. It shows predilection for the lower lid near inner canthus. It commences as a small pimple which ulcerates. On removing the scab, the ulcer shows raised and indurated margins (Fig. 9.4). The ulcer spreads slowly. The epithelial growth extends under the skin in all the direction like fingers and also deeply destroying the lids, orbit and bones. It is a locally malignant tumor. Lymphatic nodes are not involved. Treat by excision biopsy with frozen section or Moh's micrographic surgery. It should be removed when it is a small nodule or ulcer. Later it is difficult to eradicate it completely and require extensive surgery with radiation.

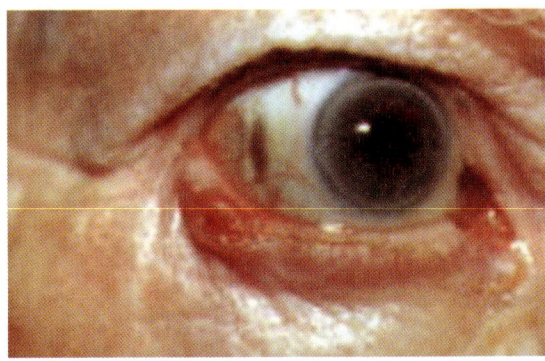

Fig. 9.4: Basal cell carcinoma

Sebaceous Gland Carcinoma

This arises from the meibomian glands. It appears as a discrete, yellow, firm nodule on the lids. It may be isolated or multicentric. There may be an associated chronic blepharitis. These are likely to be mistaken for a chalazion. A nodule in elderly must be seen with suspicion and if there is recurrence then histopathology is a must. Treat by local excision.

MANAGEMENT

Local Surgical Excision

Local surgical excision with at least 3 mm margin outside the extent of tumor is the choice. Excised specimen must be sent for histopathology to confirm the diagnosis and also to ensure that the margin of the specimen is free of tumor cells.

Radiotherapy

It is indicated in the cases that are unsuitable for surgery or for those who refuse surgery.

The complications of radiotherapy include loss of eyelashes, keratinization of the conjunctiva, dry eye and damage to the skin of lids.

Cryotherapy

Cryotherapy is good for a small and superficial basal cell carcinoma. During therapy achieve temperature to minus 30° C to cause tissue death.

Moh's Micrographic Technique (Chemosurgery)

The technique involves excising the tumor in successive layers and microscopically scanning the entire underside of each layer by the systematic use of frozen sections. This is a technique of choice if the tumor is recurrent and diffuse with indistinct margins so that entire tumor can be dissected with no chance of recurrence.

10

A Case with Lid or Lacrimal Gland Lesion

History

Record the history with reference to the following
- Age of onset. It may be a congenital disorder.
- Any associated eye lesion.
- Any history of trauma, burn or surgery of the lid.
- Any history of epilation at home if yes, then since when.
- Any nodule with or without tenderness or pain.
- Any itching, swelling, blisters, vesicles, puffiness, solid edema, patches, erythema, cyst, ulcer, etc.
- Any loss of eyebrow or cilia.
- Any poliosis or vitiligo.
- Any unusual sign in any form.

CLINICAL EXAMINATION

Inspection

Inspect the lesion; Inspection itself shall lead you to diagnosis easily.
- Look for its size, shape, color, flat, raised or peduncle.
- Look for its surface, smooth or granular.
- Look for any black head on the surface.
- Look for any crust formation on the surface.
- One or more nodule.
- Symmetrical or asymmetrical.
- Any relation to distribution along the first division of fifth nerve.

Palpation

Palpate the lesion by fingers and note the findings. Palpation shall further contribute to arrive at diagnosis.

- The lesion is smooth or uneven.
- Any tenderness to touch or pressure.
- The overlying skin is free or firmly attached to it.
- The lesion is free or attached to underlying structure.
- The lesion is reducible or not.
- The lesion is tender or not.

CLINICAL INVESTIGATION

X-ray

It may reveal any bony lesion, bony defect or erosion.

CT Scan

It shall help to rule out the orbital extension or lesion in orbit.

CLINICAL FEATURES AND MANAGEMENT

Lid Lesions

1. Acne vulgaris.
2. Acne of meibomian glands.
3. Furuncle.
4. Carbuncle.
5. Staphylococcal impetigo.
6. Erysipelas.
7. Lupus vulgaris.
8. Leprosy.
9. Herpes simplex.
10. Herpes zoster.
11. Molluscum contagiosum.
12. Myxedema.
13. Xanthelasma.
14. Scleroderma.

15. Blepharochalasis.
16. Vitiligo.
17. Alopecia and madarosis.
18. Sebaceous cyst.
19. Squamous cell carcinoma.
20. Basal cell carcinoma.
21. Ecchymosis of lids.
22. Hyperpigmentation of lid.

Lacrimal Gland Lesions

23. Sjögren's syndrome.
24. Mikulicz's syndrome.
25. Sarcoidosis.
26. Heerfordt's disease.
27. Mixed lacrimal gland tumor.

LID LESIONS

Acne Vulgaris

Acne vulgaris is a condition in which there is a crop of "black heads" due to plugging of sebaceous glands by inspissated secretion. It may become indurated and occasionally it may develop in a superficial cutaneous abscess which heals with a pitted scar. Treat by extraction of black heads and with low fat diet. Vaccination of acne bacillus and staphylococci has been tried.

Acne of Meibomian Glands

Acne of Meibomian gland is the result of retention of meibomian secretion. Inspissation of secretion appears usually in old people as yellow deposits shining through the palpebral conjunctiva, known as "Meibomian Infarcts". Deposition of lime salts in these results in hard mass "Meibomian Lithiasis" which may break through the conjunctiva and abrade the cornea causing marked irritation. These can be removed by a curette. These should be differentiated from conjunctival lithiasis.

Furuncle

A furuncle or boil is an acute infection by a virulent *Staphylococcus aureus*. It is always associated with a hair follicle or skin gland. There is a localized infection. The inflammation commences as a small tender indurated nodule. It may resolve at this stage or usually progresses to suppuration or necrosis and heals with a pitted scar. Its frequent occurrence indicates poor general health and low resistance to staphylococci. Exclude diabetes. Improve general health by good diet rich in proteins. Treat it with respect care to avoid occurrence of orbital cellulitis or even cavernous sinus thrombophlebitis.

Carbuncles

It occurs rarely in aged in the region of eyebrows especially in diabetics and debilitated persons. It is same as a furuncle except that the infection is deeper involving the subcutaneous tissue therefore more widespread. It opens on surface of skin by several openings followed by necrosis, sloughing ulcer and heals with a ragged scar. There is fever with lymphadenopathy. It needs energetic treatment to prevent spread of infection and metastasis.

Staphylococcal Impetigo

It is a superficial and widespread intra-epidermal infection of skin by staphylococci. It is characterized by a crop of yellow blisters which burst to leave thin crusts. The face and lids and scalp are common sites. Treat by local and systemic antibiotics with improvement in general health.

Erysipelas

It is due to streptococcal infection usually due to a wound or abrasion. It is an acute localized inflammation of the skin and subcutaneous tissue manifesting with local signs of redness, edema, induration and constitutional symptoms of fever, malaise and toxemia. The causative organism is virulent and contagious therefore isolation of the patient is essential. The involved area of skin is red, hot and indurated with shining and glazed surface with a sharp spreading margin dotted with minute vesicles—an important diagnostic feature. Local complications include an abscess of lid, orbital cellulitis, cavernous sinus thrombophlebitis, keratitis and even panophthalmitis if not treated properly and energetically.

Lupus Vulgaris

Lupus vulgaris is a chronic and slowly progressive tuberculous infection of the skin. It is characterized by "soft apple-jelly like tubercles". It starts as a small nodule under the epithelium that pushes to surface and appears as a translucent mass varying in size from a pin head to pea. It spreads slowly eventually forming a lupus patch in which the periphery shows active changes while center shows retrogressive changes. It leaves a permanent scar.

Leprosy

Leprosy involves the eyebrows and lids with great frequency affecting about two-thirds of all cases. The lesions include the following
- Loss of cilia or eyebrows.
- Skin nodules.
- Paralysis of orbicularis.
- Paralysis of orbicularis with facial paralysis.
- Diffuse infiltration of lids.
- Anesthetic patches on lids.

The lid involvement is very frequent and thus the malady is diagnosed easily by the physician and even by common man.

Herpes Simplex

Herpes simplex may attack the lids particularly the lower lid within the distribution of the infraorbital branch of the trigeminal nerve. Clinically, there is slight edema and erythema of the lid skin with a patch of vesicles, usually of pin-head size. The vesicles are filled with clear fluid. On drying up there is formation of crust.

Herpes Zoster

In herpes zoster ophthalmicus, the attack is confined to the first division of the fifth nerve the most common being the frontal nerve, the lacrimal and nasociliary nerve. There is edema, redness, with vesiculation. It is a very painful condition. It heals leaving pitted scars.

Molluscum Contagiosum

It is a mildly contagious disease of skin characterized by the appearance of small globular and umbilicated nodules on the skin of lids, face and lid margins. Its importance lies in the incidence of ocular complications the commonest being the follicular conjunctivitis. Treat the molluscum contagiosum nodules by incision and squeezing out the contents and swabbing the cavity with povidone.

Myxedema

Myxedema causes solid edema of the lids. The characteristic picture is puffiness of the lids associated with the expressionless face. The lower lids are baggy with dry and rough skin and no pitting on pressure. The hairs of the lateral third of the eyebrows fall out. Treat myxedema.

Xanthelasma

There are symmetrical and bilateral yellow patches in the skin of the lids usually at the inner angle. It is due to deposition of lipoid materials. It is symptomless and permanent. The patches can be removed surgically to give cosmetic improvement.

Scleroderma

The scleroderma is a condition of skin in which the skin is hard and stiff. The affected area looks ivory like. The skin is bound to underlying tissue. The face becomes immobile, mask like and expressionless. The lids show no movement with difficulty in closure and there is entropion with keratitis. It is of unknown etiology. It is a serious disease and untreatable. Steroids have been found to be useful.

Blepharochalasis

It is the looseness of the skin of the upper or lower lid associated with chronic or recurrent edema of the lid and defect in the orbital septum allowing the fat to herniate in the lids. The skin of the lid is so loose that it hangs down in loose folds over the lid margin. Treat by excision of the loose skin and also remove prolapsed orbital fat at the same time.

Vitiligo

It is an acquired depigmentation characterized by presence of white patches in the skin surrounded by a hyperpigmented areola. The hairs (eyebrows and eyelashes) in the patch are also white. It is seen in Vogt-Koyanagi syndrome characterized with uveitis, alopecia, poliosis and deafness. It is seen after local skin disease in syphilis, psoriasis, leprosy, neurodermatitis or lupus erythematosus. Pathologically there is absence of melanin and melanoblast. No treatment.

Alopecia and Madarosis

Alopecia is a condition of falling out of the hairs, from scalp, brows, lashes and other hairy regions. Acquired alopecia can be due to the following causes:

Alopecia Areata

It is characterized by sudden appearance of bald patches on the scalp in a normal person without any obvious factor. Anxiety, worry and nervous shock may be playing some part.

Alopecia of Brows and Lashes

It is seen after furuncle, sycosis, rosacea, mycoses and erysipelas. Any acute or chronic infection which can cause destruction of hair follicles can cause alopecia of brows and lashes.

Idiopathic alopecia: It occurs in young people as a premature senile alopecia.

Symptomatic alopecia: It occurs in the following conditions:

- Vogt-Koyanagi syndrome.
- Idiopathic.
- Myxedema.
- Thyrotoxicosis.
- Squamous blepharitis.
- Trachoma.
- Burns.
- Syphilis.
- Leprosy.
- Acute infective fevers.
- Use of arsenic and thallium.
- Irradiation.

Madarosis: Madarosis is a condition of falling out of eyelashes due to destructive process. It is seen following ulcerative blepharitis, trachoma and burns.

Sebaceous Cyst

Sebaceous cyst occurs in the lids as elsewhere usually in the region of brows and inner canthus. Clinically, it is a smooth, globular mass which is subcutaneous with skin attached at the summit and at the site of orifice which is plugged with the inspissated sebum. The presence of a black plug at the summit of the cyst which is smooth and globular is a diagnostic feature. Treat by complete excision along with a small elliptical piece of skin containing the orifice of the gland.

Squamous Cell Carcinoma

It commences as a small hard nodule which grows slowly and painlessly. After few months it shows erosions and fissures which tends to crust and eventually develops in an ulcer. The base of ulcer is sharply defined, indurated and hyperemic. The edges of the ulcer are hard and undermined. It extends locally destroying skin, connective tissue, cartilage, bone, periostium, lids, conjunctiva and anything coming in its way. Any indurated nodule after the age of forty without any obvious reason must be suspected. It is better to excise it and send it for biopsy.

Basal Cell Carcinoma

It begins as a shiny small translucent nodule or a scaly patch. It grows very slowly. After few weeks or months, an ulcer develops in the center with small pearly satellite nodules in the periphery at the edges. A typical rodent ulcer appears with raised nodular border and indurated base (Fig. 10.1). Treat soon by excision.

Ecchymosis of Lids

Etiology

Direct trauma over the eye, such as a blow over the eye, trauma by ball, stone, etc.

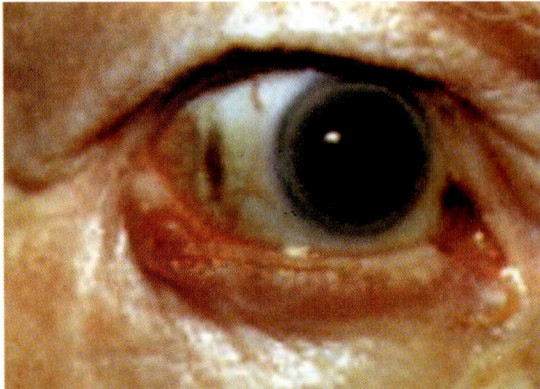

Fig. 10.1: Basal cell carcinoma

Fracture of the orbital wall, nose, nasal sinuses and base of skull.

Violent coughing, vomiting, or pressure on thorax.

Clinical Features

In Ecchymosis of the lids, the blood tends to diffuse through the loose connective tissue of the lids. The blood is checked from further spread to cheek, upper lip and forehead, by the firm adhesion of the fascia at the eyebrows, and at the naso-jugal and malar folds. The lids become swollen and the eye is closed, even the uppet lid overhanging the lower lid. The blood has an easy way to cross over the nasal bridge and spread into the tissue of the opposite eyelid. The skin over the bridge of the nose is thick, so that the skin over it appears normal. The presence of the blood in the opposite lid makes the patient alarmed. The passage of the blood to the opposite lid helps to diffuse the blood and reduce the swelling of the affected eyelid. Assure the patient that it is a normal natural phenomenon to diffuse the blood.

Hyperpigmentation of Skin of Lids

Dark rings round the eyes: It is very common and patient is alarmed. This may be due to hyperpigmentation but some times, it is an appearance due to dilation of deep venules of the skin in a ring shape along the lower orbital margin. It is common in females in the state of fatigue, menstruation, and after debilitating illness. It seems to be due to lack of facial support, allowing vasodilation. This must disappear with increase in weight. If the dark rings do not disappear then it is due to hyper-pigmentation.

Hyperpigmentation
- Melanotic hyperpigmentation.
- Utero-overian disturbances.
- Menstruation.
- Pregnancy.
- Addison's disease.
- Diabetes.
- Secondary syphilis.
- Tuberculosis.
- Graves' disease.
- Myxedema.
- Cirrhosis of liver.
- Rheumatoid arthritis.
- Dermatomyositis.
- Lichen planus.
- Xeroderma pigmentosa.

LACRIMAL GLAND LESIONS

Sjögren's Syndrome

Sjögren's syndrome is an autoimmune disease. In a primary Sjögren's syndrome, there is involvement of salivary glands with involvement of mucous membrane of bronchial tree and vagina. The involvement of salivary glands results in dry mouth (Xerostomia), therefore, there is a difficulty in mastication and thus patient requires liquid for mastication and swallowing. In a secondary Sjögren's syndrome, there is an association of connective tissue disorder the most common being the sero-positive rheumatoid arthritis. Other systemic diseases associated include: systemic lupus erythematosus, systemic sclerosis, psoriatic arthritis, juvenile chronic arthritis, and polymyositis.

Mikulicz's Syndrome

It is characterized by symmetrical enlargement of the lacrimal and salivary glands. It is of varied etiology but the swelling is of lymphomatous nature. In uveoparotitis (Heerfordt's disease), there is an enlargement of salivary (parotid) glands along with uveitis.

Sarcoidosis

Sarcoidosis is a chronic granulomatous disease of unknown etiology characterized by multiple cutaneous and subcutaneous nodules with similar nodules in the viscera and bones. There are periodic exacerbations and remissions. There is no caseation. A positive biopsy of the cutaneous nodule is diagnostic. Most cases develop chronic bilateral uveitis-anterior and posterior. The anterior uveitis is nodular. The posterior uveitis is characterized by retinal exudates and perivasculitis.

With the involvement of the parotid glands the disease is known as uveoparotid fever (Heerfordt's syndrome). With the involvement of the lacrimal glands it is called Mikulicz's syndrome.

Heerfordt's Syndrome
(Uveoparotitis, uveoparotid fever)

It is characterized by bilateral simultaneous affection of uvea (uveitis), parotid gland enlargement and cranial nerves. It affects young persons with onset of malaise and fever followed by either uveitis or painful swelling of the parotid glands or both. Patient may complain of diplopia due to palsy of oculomotor nerve or there is facial paralysis.

Mixed Lacrimal Gland Tumor

All the conditions which cause swelling of the lacrimal gland lead to restriction of the movement of the eyeball. The eyeball is pushed downwards and inwards. There is a limitation of the movement of the eyeball in the outward or outward and upward. There is slight proptosis. A benign mixed lacrimal gland tumor grows slowly without any pain and no involvement of the bone. A malignant lacrimal gland tumor grows fast, with pain and destruction of bone. Early surgical removal is the best treatment available for both.

A Case with Epiphora

History

Record the history with reference to the following:
- Age of onset.
- Duration watering.
- Unilateral or bilateral.
- Any recent history of conjunctival inflammation.
- Any recent history of instillation of topical idoxuridine which may cause punctum stenosis.
- Any past history of Bell's palsy.
- Any change in the epiphora with change in weather.
- Any history of trauma involving the medial canthus of the affected eye.
- Any surgery near the medial canthus.

CLINICAL EXAMINATION

Inspection

Punctum

Normally when the eye looks upward then the lower punctum should not be visible without slightly everting the lower lid. If it is visible then there is eversion of the lower puncta which may be cause of epiphora. Inspect the punctum for misplacement, stenosis, foreign body (eyelash) in the punctum and pouting of the punctum. A pouting of the punctum indicates infection of canaliculi.

Canaliculi

Apply pressure over the canaliculi and look for any reflux from it. Presence of reflux indicates canaliculitis which may be bacterial or fungal. Collect the material for culture and sensitivity.

Marginal Tear Strip

In a case of epiphora the marginal tear strip is higher than normal. It can be appreciated better with fluorescein staining of the tear fluid.

Punctum on Lid Closure

On gentle lid closure the two puncta are in opposition. In a patient with laxity of the lid the puncta are not in opposition. The lower lid may be slightly everted which may be the cause epiphora in elderly.

Regurgitation Test

Reflux of a mucopurulent material indicates chronic dacryocystitis. A negative test does not rule out involvement of the lacrimal sac as a cause for epiphora.

Syringing of the Lacrimal Passage

Instill topical anesthetic in the conjunctival sac. Make the patient lie down on the operation table. Syringing is done from the lower punctum with saline. The passage is patent if the fluid passes down the throat. In case of obstruction the fluid regurgitates from the same punctum or through the upper punctum. If there is regurgitation of fluid from the same lower punctum then perform syringing from the upper punctum. A regurgitation of fluid from the upper punctum also indicates a block at the canaliculi-sac junction. A patent passage on syringing through the upper punctum indicates block of the lower canaliculi.

Examination of Nose

Examine the nose for any nasal pathology like, atrophic rhinitis, chronic rhinitis, hypertrophied turbinate, inflammation, deviated septum, etc.

LACRIMAL APPARATUS

The lacrimal apparatus consists of two parts:
1. The lacrimal gland and the accessory glands which secrete the lacrimal fluid.
2. The lacrimal drainage system which comprises of the punctum, canaliculi, sac and nasolacrimal duct. It drains the lacrimal fluid from the conjunctival sac to the nose.

The disorders of the lacrimal apparatus give rise to annoying and social embarrassing symptoms of lacrimation, epiphora and dry eye.

Lacrimation

Lacrimal Hypersecretion

Lacrimation is an active process of excessive secretion of lacrimal fluid—the tear fluid due to irritation or inflammation of conjunctiva, cornea, uvea, nose, sinuses and emotional factors.

Though the lacrimal drainage system is functioning normally yet it fails to cope with drainage of excessive secretion of lacrimal fluid resulting in the annoying and embarrassing symptom of overflow of the lacrimal fluid—commonly referred as watering of the eye or flowing of tears.

- Reflex trigeminaal irritation, due to any painful disease or injury of the eye, e.g. keratitis, iritis, eyelids, glaucoma, etc.
- Reflex visual irritation. The lacrimation is bilateral.
- In association with tabes and thyrotoxicosis.
- Due to lacrimal gland disease, like cysts, tumors and Mikulicz's syndrome.

Lacrimal Hyposecretion

- Keratoconjunctivitis, sicca.
- Sjögren's syndrome.
- Obstruction of lacrimal ductules due to trachoma, burns and xerosis.

Bloody Tears

- It is invariably due to conjunctival bleeding.
- Conjunctival angioma.
- Granuloma.
- Vicarious menstruation.
- Trauma to conjunctiva.
- Epistaxis.
- Pannus or any other corneal vascular lesion.

Epiphora

- Punctum-atresia, misplacement, eversion and spastic occlusion of the punctum.
- Canaliculi—atresia, inflammation or stenosis of the canaliculi.
- Sac—the sac may be atrophic.
- Duct—obstruction of the duct.
- Nose—atrophic rhinitis, chronic rhinitis, hypertrophied inferior turbinate.

EPIPHORA

Epiphora is a passive process in which though the secretion of the lacrimal fluid is normal yet the lacrimal drainage system fails to drain the fluid due to obstruction in its passage resulting in accumulation and overflow of the tear fluid—manifesting as watering of the eye-an annoying and embarrassing symptom.

Etiological Factors

Punctum: There may be atresia, misplacement, eversion or spastic occlusion of the punctum.

Canaliculi: There may be atresia, inflammation or stenosis of the canaliculi.

Lacrimal sac: The lacrimal sac may be stenosed or atrophic. There may be functional block. There may be chronic inflammation.

Nasolacrimal duct: The congenital obstruction of the nasolacrimal duct is the most common cause for epiphora in newborn and infants.

Nose: A nasal pathology in the form of atrophic rhinitis, chronic rhinitis, hypertrophied inferior turbinate, deviated septum can produce the symptom of epiphora.

Clinical features and management

1. Congenital absence of punctum.
2. Spastic occlusion of punctum.
3. Congenital absence of lower canaliculi.
4. Occlusion of lower canaliculi.
5. Total occlusion of both canaliculi.
6. Chronic dacryocystitis.
7. Congenital obstruction of nasolacrimal duct.
8. Probing of nasolacrimal duct.

Congenital Absence of Punctum

Locate the appropriate site of the lower punctum under an operating microscope. Give a verticle incision of 2 mm through this site on the conjunctival side to open the ampulla of the lower canaliculi.

If the above procedure fails then open the lacrimal sac and perform a retrograde probing of the lower canaliculi through the sac and incise the conjunctiva at the tip of the probe to 3 mm medially to open the canaliculus.

Spastic Occlusion of Punctum

In a case of spastic occlusion of the punctum one to three snip operation is an ideal surgery with very good response.

One snip surgery: Some patients may need only one snip from the punctum to the junction of the ampulla to relieve epiphora. This one snip surgery keeps the capillary attraction and the pump of ampulla intact.

Two snip surgery: Some patients who do not respond to one snip then perform a two snip operation. Repeat the first vartical incision. Make a horizontal incision from the lower end of this first verticle incision along the canaliculi for 2 mm.

Three snip surgery: A three snip operation is indicated in all the cases who show a stenosed punctum soon after repeated dilation of the punctum. In this operation repeat the two incisions. The third incision joins the end of

second incision to begining of first incision. Thus a triangular piece of tissue is removed with its base between the punctum and ampulla and apex in the lower canaliculi.

Congenital Absence of Lower Canaliculi

In this case transplant the upper canaliculi.

Occlusion of Lower Canaliculi

Canthocystostomy: An incision in the lateral wall of the lacrimal sac from the entrance of the upper canaliculi to sac-duct junction is indicated.

Total Occlusion of Both Canaliculi

Conjunctivodacryocystostomy: The fundus of the lacrimal sac is mobilised in the lacus lacrimalis where it is stitched to the conjunctival incision through which the sac is brought in. The fundus of the sac is excised and the cut end of the sac is sutured with cut end of the conjunctiva to create a passage from the conjunctiva to the sac.

Conjunctivodacryocystorhinostomy: In this the conjunctiva is sutured to the sac with usual procedure for dacryocystorhinostomy.

Chronic Dacryocystitis

Dacryocystorhinostomy is the ideal operation for all the cases having chronic dacryocystitis. It relieves the symptom of epiphora for which the patient seeks the advice of surgeon. It relieves the surgeon from threatening source of infection to the eye.

Congenital Obstruction of Nasolacrimal Duct

About 30% of the newborn infants are born with closure of the nasolacrimal duct due to membranous occlusion of the lower or upper end of the canal, presence of epithelial debris in the canal or due to failure in the canalization of the nasolacrimal duct. The symptom of watering of the eye appears in the majority of the cases within the first three days of the life. It may be unilateral or bilateral. The diagnosis is obvious in most cases with the history of constant watering since birth or one to three weeks after. Most of the cases resolve within 4–6 weeks after birth. Parents need proper counseling and to follow conservative treatment.

Conservative Management

Regular check up: Every week until epiphora resolves.

Crigler's lacrimal sac massage: Massage the lacrimal sac area by sliding finger tip with gentle pressure in an inferior direction using the antibiotic ointment as a lubricant.

Topical antibiotic drops: If there is discharge from the eye.

Surgical Management

Probing of Nasolacrimal Duct

Probing is an ideal surgery in infants. It should not be delayed more than the age of three months if the infant shows epiphora with block of the passage by syringing. It is a simple and rewarding procedure.

Steps of operation
- Irrigate the lacrimal sac by syringing with saline and antibiotic drops.
- Evert the upper lid and dilate the upper punctum with the punctum dilator.
- Irrigate the lacrimal sac again through the upper punctum and canaliculi, to assess the passage before passing the probe. The lacrimal cannula must pass easily and smoothly without any obstruction.
- Take a probe of No 3 or 4 (0.6 to 0.8 mm) and pass it into the upper punctum and canaliculus so as to enter the sac and touch the medial wall of the lacrimal fossa. The surgeon is able to feel the touch of the probe to the bony wall of the lacrimal fossa. Keeping the probe in light contact with the lacrimal bone, the probe is gradually swing into the vertical position, through an angle of about 90° to the approximate anatomical direction of the nasolacrimal canal (a line upon face running from the middle of the medial palpebral ligament above to the base of ala

nasi below) so as to reach the upper end of the canal. A light push downwards shall engage it in the canal and with further push it will enter into the canal. If the probe is engaged into the duct then it will not move when it is released by the operator. Further if the probe is lightly moved from side to side the head of the infant also moves with it confirming about it proper entry into the duct. Do not insert the probe more than twelve millimeters. At this stage it is a good practice to withdraw the probe few mm and push it back four to six times and then leave it in situ for ten minutes. This procedure of leaving the probe in situ helps in hemostasis preventing hemorrhage from the rich capillary plexus of the canal and in dilating the fibrous stricture in the duct.
- Withdraw the probe as the child comes out of anesthesia.
- Irrigate the eye and apply eye ointment.
- Hand over the child to the waiting mother with instruction to keep the head end raised and neck slightly extended for free breathing and no feed for two hours.
- Surgeon must keep watch on the baby making her sit under his direct observation.

Postoperative Care

- Instill antibiotic eye drops 4 to 6 times a day for 10 days. Syringe the lacrimal sac next day. If the passage is patent then advice instillation of eyedrops for 10 days more. If the passage is not patent then call the patient for syringing daily for 3 weeks. Most of the cases will show patency in this period. Repeat the nasolacrimal duct probing if the passage is not patent even after 4 weeks of first probing.
- In some cases there may be reflux of mucus from the lacrimal sac even though there is patency of the passage on the lacrimal syringing. This reflux is due to atony of the sac. Usually the sac regains its tone in course of time. It is advisable to continue to use antibiotic eyedrops in such cases for few weeks.

- Advise mother to consult eye surgeon whenever there is nasal catarrh, as it may cause partial block of the duct. Use of antibiotic and decongestant eyedrops shall be helpful.

Complications

Rupture of canaliculi: The punctum may not dilate and forceful entry of the probe may cause rupture of the canaliculi. This can be avoided by proper dilation of the punctum or to slit open the upper canaliculus.

False Passage

The eversion of the upper lid to expose the upper punctum may give rise to a kink in the canaliculus and therefore difficulty in passing the probe or may become a cause for false passage of the probe. The kink in the canaliculus can be avoided by pulling the upper lid outwards and passing a cannula before attempting to pass a probe to assess the passage. The cannula or the probe must pass freely and smoothly without any obstruction. On swinging the probe and pushing it downwards to get engaged in the opening of the duct, it may miss the opening. It can be tested by releasing the probe. If it is engaged then the probe retains its position. If not engaged then withdraw it back to its horizontal position and try to swing it in position again.

Failure of Procedure

With all the care and precaution, by the surgeon there may be a tear in the canaliculi, creation of false passage and the probe may not get engaged in the opening of the duct.

Non-engagement of the probe indicates thick membranous block at the upper end of the duct. Such cases needs two or three probing to activate absorption of epithelial debris of the upper end. The child needs syringing every alternate day in between.

Results: Results are rewarding and gratifying.

A Case with Dacryocystitis

History

Record the history with reference to the following:
- Age of onset.
- Duration of watering from the eye.
- Watering is unilateral or bilateral.
- Any recurrent conjunctivitis.
- Any history of emptying the contents of the sac by pressure on it in the nose.
- Any history of previous acute inflammation.
- Any previous surgery minor or major.
- Any nasal pathology.

CLINICAL EXAMINATION

Inspection

- There is a swelling in the sac region near the medial canthus.
- There is watering of the eye. The eye appears wet with the fluid collecting at the medial canthus. The tears may be rolling out of the eye at the medial canthus.
- There may be some discharge at the medial canthus.
- The conjunctiva may be slightly congested indicating chronic conjunctivitis.
- Look for any mark of scar or fistula.

Palpation

- The swelling feels soft.
- Presence of tenderness to touch indicates inflammation.
- Some cases may give a feeling of a hard nodule as in a case of encysted chronic dacryocystitis.

Clinical Investigation

- Fluorescein dye disappearance test.
- Regurgitation test.
- Syringing of the lacrimal passage.
- Radio-active tracer.
- Dacryocystography.
- X-ray paranasal sinuses and orbit.
- Nasal examination.

Fluorescein Dye Disappearance Test

Instill two drops of dye in the conjunctival sac of both the eyes and observe after two minutes. In a patient with normal drainage system no dye is seen in the conjunctival sac. The presence of the dye in the conjunctival sac indicates inadequate lacrimal drainage that could be due to atonic sac or obstruction in the passage. Such a case needs further investigation.

Regurgitation Test

Make the patient sit comfortably on a chair facing the surgeon and at a slightly lower level. Hold the face of the patient by both the hands on the side with fingers spread out to get a good hold. Retract the lower lid of left eye with the thumb of the right hand. Apply the pressure at the lacrimal sac region by the thumb of the left hand keeping the hold on the face all the time. It prevents the patient to pull his head backwards when the surgeon is applying pressure at the sac region for the test.

Interpretation of Regurgitation Test

- In chronic dacryocystitis, the contents of the sac shall regurgitate through the lower or lower and upper punctum.
- In chronic dacryocystitis with functional block the contents of the sac shall empty in the nose.
- In chronic dacryocystitis with encysted lacrimal sac there is no regurgitation of the contents. The nodule like swelling is there but it does not discharge its contents neither in the conjunctival sac nor it empties in the nose.
- In chronic dacryocystitis with atrophic sac there is no regurgitation. There is no swelling also. Patient just complains of epiphora.

Syringing of the Lacrimal Passage

Make the patient lie on the operation table. Instill one drop of 2 percent lignocaine in the conjunctival sac of the eye to be tested for patency. Wait for five minutes for the effect of local anesthetic. A 2 ml syringe with lacrimal canula is filled with an antibiotic eye drops. Expose the lower punctum by supporting and slightly everting the lower lid by the thumb of one hand. Dilate the punctum with a punctum dilator. Pick up the syringe and insert the lacrimal cannula in the punctum and then push it in the canaliculi to reach the lacrimal sac and push the plunger of the syringe slowly and observe the result.

Interpretation of Syringing Test

- The fluid passes down the throat freely. It indicates the patency of the passage.
- There is regurgitation of the fluid from the upper punctum. It indicates a block at the sac and nasolacrimal duct junction.
- There is regurgitation of the fluid from the same punctum. It indicates a block at the sac and canaliculus junction. In such cases try syringing from the upper punctum. If the fluid regurgitates from the upper canaliculi also, it further confirms the block at the sac and canaliculi junction.
- Syringing is not possible if there is block of the punctum or punctum is absent.

Radio-active Tracer

A radio-active tracer (sulphur colloid or technetium) is instilled in the conjunctival sac and drainage of this radio-active fluid through the lacrimal passage is visualized by using an Anger gamma camera. No extra advantage over other methods for testing the patency is noted.

Dacryocystography

It is a non-invasive technique to evaluate the lacrimal drainage system (Fig. 12.1) in its totality. In this method a radiopaque material; lipiodol, pentopaque or dianosil is pushed in the lacrimal sac and X-rayed.

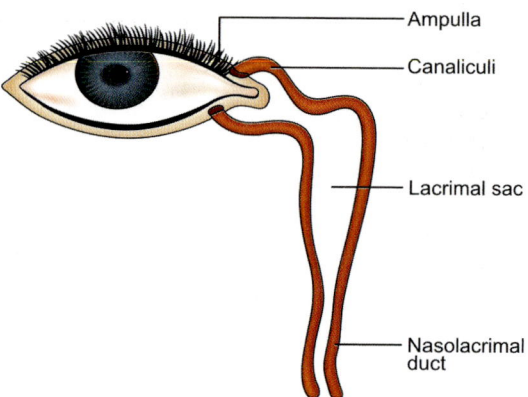

Fig. 12.1: Lacrimal drainage system

Technique

Empty the sac by regurgitation test. It is advisable to syringe the lacrimal passage to clear it of its mucopus. Suck the contents in the sac by syringe. An empty sac allows proper filling of the sac with the radiopaque dye. Inject about 1 ml of the dye in the sac with lacrimal cannula until the dye outflows from the upper punctum. Wipe off the dye from the face and lids. Paint the eyelashes and the lid margin with the dye to have proper orientation of the X-ray film. Take X-ray in the upright-forehead-nose position. Take two exposures-anteroposterior and lateral within two minutes after injecting the dye in the sac. After X-ray, regurgitate the dye.

The film may show the canaliculi, the sac, the duct and frequently some dye on the floor of the nose or in nasopharynx if there is patency of the passage. A dacryocystogram is to be interpreted to have a correct clinical assessment of a case and planning the surgery accordingly.

Interpretation of a Dacryocystogram

- Small shrunken stenosed sac is suggestive of a long-standing chronic catarrhal dacryocystitis of the lacrimal sac. The case is suitable for Dacryocystorhinostomy.
- Dilated sac with smooth regular outline is suggestive of a chronic suppurative dacryocystitis. It is suitable for Dacryocystorhinostomy.
- Dilated sac with irregular outline indicates adhesions of the sac wall due to pericystitis or acute exacerbations of chronic dacryocystitis. Plan for dacryocystorhinostomy and can terminate in dacryocystectomy if there is surgical problem to fashion out the sac flaps due to its friability.
- Pear-shaped dilated sac with regular outline with dye just entering the upper end of the nasolacrimal duct is suggestive of chronic dacryocystitis with functional block. Presence of the dye in the duct or the nasal fossa is confirmatory. It is most suitable for dacryocystorhinostomy.
- Presence of dye in the ethmoidal sinus indicates internal fistula.

Clinical Application of Dacryocystogram

Dacryocystogram gives an idea about the size and shape of the lacrimal sac, any adhesions of the sac wall, any pouches or diverticula, the site of obstruction and whether the block is absolute or functional.

Dacryocystorhinostomy does not depend on the size of the sac but it definitely depends on the condition of the sac wall. Dacryocystogram fails to provide the information about the condition of the sac wall whether it is thin or thick, friable or separable from the surrounding tissue for conditioning the flaps for suturing with nasal mucosa. Therefore, the surgeon must plan for dacryocystorhinostomy in all the cases except the cases presenting with absolute contraindications for anastomotic operation. If the surgeon finds any problem in fashioning the sac flaps due to its friability then he can always terminate the case in dacryocystectomy.

Dacryocystectomy only helps in eliminating the constant source of infection that endangers the cornea and vision but does not provide relief to the patient for his annoying and embarrassing symptom of watering for which he came to the hospital.

Dacryocystorhinostomy provides relief from the embarrassing and annoying symptom of constant epiphora as well as eliminating the source of infection by providing proper drainage of lacrimal fluid.

Dacryocystorhinostomy is rewarding and gratifying surgery both for the patient and the surgeon.

Dacryocystogram helps the surgeon to plan and perform anastomosing operation in most of the cases.

Plain X-ray of Orbit and Paranasal Sinuses

The X-ray of orbit and paranasal sinuses shall give information about any bony lesion and inflammation of sinuses which might have direct or indirect relation with the etiology of dacryocystitis.

Nasal Examination

A nasal examination is a must in any case having a swelling in lacrimal sac region or near the nose. Look for deviated nasal septum, polyp, granuloma, neoplasm, condition of the nasal mucosa, infection, abnormal air cells and hypertrophied turbinate. Transillumination of the maxillary sinus shall be helpful.

The nasal pathology in the form of deviated septum, hypertrophied turbinate and hypertrophied nasal mucosa is no contraindication for dacryocystorhinostomy.

The nasal pathology in the form of atrophic rhinitis, granuloma or papilloma are contraindication for anastomotic operation as these affect the nasal mucosa required to fashion out the flaps.

Investigations

Culture of ocular and nasal region: It may prove useful to determine appropriate antibiotic therapy.

CT Scan

It is useful to rule out malignanacy or a mass as a cause for dacryocystitis.

DACRYOCYSTITIS

Symptom

Epiphora

Epiphora is the one universal symptom of dacryocystitis. The tears are seen rolling over the cheek. It can lead to eczema of the lid and surrounding skin. Constant wiping may result in manifestation of ectropion of the lower lid in the affected side. Epiphora is an annoying symptom with social embarrassment.

Recurrent Unilateral Conjunctivitis

Any patient with a history of recurrent unilateral conjunctivitis must be investigated for the patency of the lacrimal drainage system. Chronic dacryocystitis is a constant source of infection. Rarely it can endanger the cornea with ulcer and thereby loss of vision.

Clinical Features and Management

1. Dacryocystitis neonatorum (congenital dacryocystitis).
2. Acute dacryocystitis.
3. Chronic dacryocystitis.
4. Chronic dacryocystitis with fistula.
5. Chronic dacryocystitis with functional block.
6. Chronic dacryocystitis with encysted sac.
7. Chronic dacryocystitis with atrophic sac.
8. Chronic dacryocystitis with pseudo sac.

Dacryocystitis Neonatorum
(congenital dacryocystitis)

About 30% of the newborn infants are born with closure of the nasolacrimal duct due to membranous occlusion of the lower or upper end of the canal, presence of epithelial debris in the canal or due to failure in the canalization of the nasolacrimal duct. The symptom of watering of the eye appears in the majority of the cases within the first three days of the life. It runs a chronic course.

Treatment

Massage and antibiotic: The only treatment in early stage is to massage over the lacrimal sac area and topical antibiotic eyedrops four times a day and regular check up. Massage increases hydrostatic pressure in the lacrimal sac and it helps to open up the membranous block at the upper or lower end of the duct.

Syringing with antibiotic eye drops: Syringing once or twice a week helps to open up the membranous block by exerting hydraulic pressure.

Massage, antibiotic drops and syringing prevents infection of the lacrimal drainage system. Most of the cases respond to it as there is tendency for the passage to get canalized in due course of time.

Probing of the nasolacrimal duct: If the watering persists even after the age of three months and the syringing shows non-patency of the lacrimal passage then probing of the nasolacrimal duct should be undertaken without further delay to avoid setting up of a chronic inflammation of the sac.

Probing is a safe procedure with gratifying results:

See Chapter 11 "A Case with Epiphora" for details.

Acute Dacryocystitis

It can occur spontaneously without any history of epiphora. It can occur as a sudden exacerbation in a case of chronic dacryocystitis or as an acute peridacryocystitis. All the signs and symptoms of acute inflammation appear such as swelling with redness, edema, pain, local tenderness and heat (Fig. 12.2). If the patient seeks the treatment early then it usually resolves. A course of an antibiotic having a wider spectrum and analgesic is needed in all the cases. If the pus has already formed then it needs an incision and drainage. If not treated then it forms an external fistula. On resolution perform surgery either

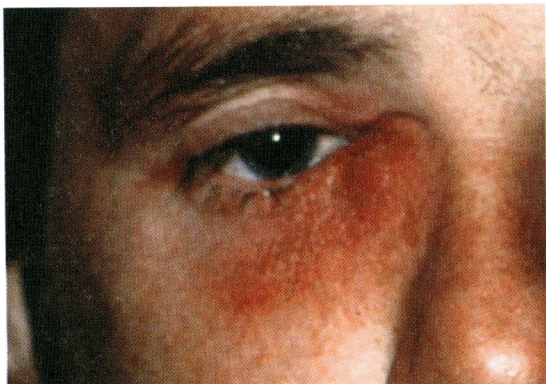

Fig. 12.2: Acute dacryocystitis

dacryocystectomy or dacryocystorhinostomy depending on the clinical signs, dacryocystogram and nasal pathology. Dacryocystorhinostomy provides relief to the patient from annoying symptom of epiphora and infection.

Chronic Dacryocystitis

It is a chronic inflammation of the lacrimal sac. The patient presents with history and symptom of watering of the eye and mild congestion of the conjunctiva. There is a nodule in the lacrimal sac region below the level of the inner canthus. The nodular swelling is not mobile (Fig. 12.3). The skin over the swelling is free and normal. There is no tenderness. The regurgitation test is positive. The syringing shows non-patency of the lacrimal passage. It is most suitable case for dacryocystorhinostomy.

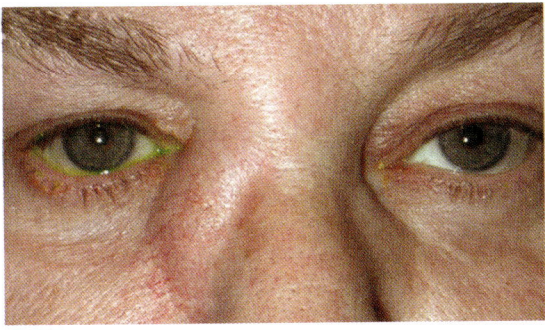

Fig. 12.3: Chronic dacryocystitis

Incidence

- *Age:* Usually it affects people in the fifth decade of life. It does affect the newborn infants as a congenital anomaly.
- *Sex:* There is a significant sex incidence; females to males ratio is 80% to 20% attributed to narrow canal and high nasal index in females.
- *Race:* It is rare among Negros due to shorter, wider and less sinuous canal with large ostium.
- *Heredity:* It is transmitted as a dominant characteristic.
- *Social infrastructure:* It is seen more commonly in persons in the low social, economic and hygienic infrastructural setting.

Pathogenesis

The vicious circle of stasis and mild infection of long duration is a well established causative factor.

The common source of infection is from the neighboring structures like nose, sinuses and conjunctiva. Mild and low grade infection leads to congestion and edema of the mucosa of the nasolacrimal duct resulting in partial blockage favoring stasis. Stasis further favors inflammation. Thus a vicious circle is set up that ultimately leads to complete blockage manifesting as chronic dacryocystitis.

Etiological Factors for Stasis and Infection

Anatomical factors: The narrow nasolacrimal duct, folds and valves in the duct mucosa favor stasis. Hypertrophy of the inferior turbinate, deviated septum, atrophic rhinitis and polyps in the nose also favor stasis.

Infection from neighboring structures: Mild infection from conjunctiva, nose and sinuses leads to chronic congestion and edema of the mucosa lining the duct resulting in partial stasis. Recurrent episodes of inflammation lead to complete blockage of the duct.

General infections: An attack of influenza, mumps, malaria, chickenpox and any malaise or fever causes generalized congestion. The congestion of the mucosa of the nasolacrimal duct results in stasis. Repeated attacks may lead to complete blockage of the duct.

Lacrimation: Lacrimation denotes excessive secretion of lacrimal fluid. The excessive lacrimal fluid rolls out of the eyes as tears and a part of it is retained by the fibroelastic lacrimal sac as a compensatory phenomenon. Repeated episodes may lead to the atony of the sac favoring stasis and blockage.

Treatment

The ideal treatment is Dacryocystorhinostomy to provide relief to the patient from his embarrassing symptom of epiphora and threatening source of infection.

Chronic Dacryocystitis with Fistula

In some cases of chronic dacryocystitis the contents of the sac may discharge into the ethmoid sinus resulting in an internal fistula. In these cases the contents drain into the nose which may lead to marked diminution of the symptom of the watering of the eye. An acute exacerbation in a case of chronic dacryocystitis results in formation of the pus which results in formation of an external fistula. These cases require surgical therapy either a dacryocystectomy or a dacryocystorhinostomy again depending on the clinical signs, dacryocystogram and the nasal condition of the case.

Chronic Dacryocystitis with Functional Block

The clinical features are like any case of a chronic dacryocystitis except that on the regurgitation test the sac empties its contents in the nose as well as in the conjunctival sac. Most of the patients are able to demonstrate this phenomenon as they have learned themselves to empty the contents of the sac to get relief from the symptom of watering for few hours. The pathogenesis of the functional block lies in the fibro-elastic nature of the lacrimal sac and the rich venous plexus around the nasolacrimal duct. The engorgement of the venous plexus around the duct results in the partial block. The lacrimal sac dilates to accommodate the tear fluid. In due course of time the sac losses its power to

pump the fluid. The sac becomes atonic. In these cases due to pressure in the regurgitation test, most of the sac contents empty in the nose. These cases are ideal cases for dacryocystorhinostomy.

Chronic Dacryocystitis with Encysted Sac

In few cases of chronic dacryocystitis both the exits the canaliculi and the nasolacrimal duct becomes blocked leaving a cyst of a sac with mucus or muco-pus. There is a swelling at the lacrimal sac region with watering of the eye. The regurgitation test is negative. On syringing the fluid regurgitates from the same punctum indicating block at the canaliculus-sac junction. It is a fit case for a dacryocystectomy.

Chronic Dacryocystitis with Atrophic Sac

The patient complains of watering. There is no swelling at the lacrimal sac region on inspection. There is no swelling felt even on palpation. The regurgitation test is negative. There is no history of recurrent unilateral conjunctivitis. Syringing shows regurgitation of clear fluid from the upper punctum. A dacryocystogram shows only the canaliculi and a very small sac. During surgery the sac wall appears hypertrophied with a small lumen. A dacryocystorhinostomy can be performed as a hypertrophied sac gives thick sac flaps for suturing.

Chronic Dacryocystitis with Pseudo Sac

The recurrence of dacryocystitis though not common yet occurs following dacryocystectomy. The recurrence occurs due to regeneration of the epithelium lining the sac wall or the nasolacrimal duct. In dacryocystectomy there is always a chance that inadvertently a small piece of the sac specially the fundus of the sac or the sac at the cupola may have been left. The serous discharge from the surrounding tissue may excite a fribroblastic reaction which results in the fibrous lining of the cavity left after extirpation of the sac. The sac fascia itself may collect the fluid and evolves as pseudo sac. The clinical features are like any other case of a chronic dacryocystitis but with a history of an operation and a scar may be visible. The case needs dacryocystorhinostomy as surgical therapy.

MANAGEMENT

Management is only surgical.
- Dacryocystorhinostomy, Endoscopic DCR or Laser DCR.
- Dacryocystectomy.

Dacryocystorhinostomy

Indications

Dacryocystorhinostomy is the first choice for all the clinical types of chronic dacryocystitis. On operation table, if the condition of the sac wall does not allow the proper formation of even one superior flap then the case can always be terminated in dacryocystectomy. Energetic effort should be made to perform Dacryocystorhinostomy operation to relieve the patient of his social and cosmetic embarrassment of watering and annoying symptom of recurrent conjunctivitis with discharge.

Contraindications

- Neoplasm of the sac.
- Tuberculosis of the sac.
- Osteomyelitis of the bone.

Operation Steps

- Irrigate thoroughly the lacrimal sac and the conjunctival sac with normal saline.
- Pass suture in both the lids and close the lids with the first tie of a surgical knot.
- Incision in the skin, 3 mm away from the canthus starting 5 mm above the inner canthus to 25 mm downwards and slightly curved at the lower end.
- Incise the orbicularis fascia and the orbicularis muscle in the line of skin incision.
- Undermine the skin and muscle to expose the medial palpebral ligament and apply the retractor to expose the field of operation.
- Expose the medial palpebral ligament up to its attachment at the lacrimal crest.

- With the sharp dissector make an incision in the periostium just above the attachment of the medial palpebral ligament and extend it below and upwards along the anterior lacrimal crest.
- Seperate the periostium from the crest and lacrimal fossa reflecting the sac along with periostium laterally, thereby exposing the lacrimal fossa up to canal.
- Make an ostium 10 mm in the bone.
- Prepare nasal flaps from the nasal mucosa exposed.
- Prepare lacrimal sac flaps.
- Suture the lower nasal and lower sac flaps.
- Suture the upper nasal and upper sac flaps.
- Apply subcutaneous suture to skin.
- Clean the area of operation and apply an eye ointment in the eye.
- Apply dressing to the wound and shift the patient.

Postoperative Care

- Make the patient mobile.
- Patient can have light meals.
- Advise patient not to strain or blow the nose.
- Change the dressing the next day.
- Syringe the passage with an antibiotic eye drops.
- Remove sutures on fifth day.
- Advice to use antibiotic eyedrops 4 times a day for 10 days.

Complications

Hemorrhage: Hemorrhage from the angular vein, bone and nasal flaps. Legate the angular vein. Use bone wax for bleeding from the bone. Pack the nose for 10 minutes if the nasal flaps show bleeding.

The Angular Vein

The angular vein is the most important vessel to be taken care of during surgery on the lacrimal sac. It is a subcutaneous vessel visible through the skin about 8 mm from the inner canthus.

It is formed by the union of the supraorbital and frontal veins and runs down at the side of nose lateral to angular artery passing across the nasal edge of the medial palpebral ligament piercing the orbicularis below the ligament. It has communication with the superior ophthalmic vein and facial vein. The facial vein runs obliquely downwards and backwards across the face. It crosses the mandible and joins the posterior facial vein to form a common facial vein which opens into the internal jugular vein. The facial vein communicates with the nasal veins and pterygoid plexus of veins, and inferior ophthalmic vein. This explains that any septic lesion on the face can result in cavernous sinus thrombosis. Tributaries of angular vein are:

- Supraorbital vein.
- Frontal vein.
- Superficial nasal veins.
- Facial vein.

Abnormal Air Cells

In some cases there may be abnormal air cells and one finds a problem in locating the nasal mucosa. Pass a probe from the nostril. If the probe is not felt then clear the air cell and you reach the mucosa.

Thin and Friable Sac Wall and Nasal Mucosa

The nasal mucosa may be thin and friable. It may get torn or damaged during triphining a hole in the bone. If the nasal flap is not available, then suture the upper sac flap to the periostium on the bone in the fossa. The lower flaps have no part in keeping the anastomosis open. It is the upper flaps that play an important role in keeping the communication. Therefore suture the upper flap to anything available on the opposite side the connective tissue, muscle or the periostium. Similarly, if the sac wall is friable then suture upper nasal flap to any tissue on the opposite side.

Block of Anastomosis

Usually the passage is patent on the next day on syringing. If there is regurgitation of the fluid from the upper punctum and no fluid passes down then examine the nose and try to remove the clots from the nose if any. In spite of block, the surgeon must continue to syringe the passage daily. In most case the patient develops patency. If the block occurs after few days then probably the block is due to formation of granulation tissue or the sac flaps have given way. In such cases the case must be taken for surgery again and explore the area and clean the field with all the tissue there and close the wound. Somehow in these cases the tear fluid finds way to flow down by capillary action and the patient does not complain of epiphora.

Results

The results of dacryocystorhinostomy have been 95 to 98% by almost all the surgeon performing anastomotic operation. Thus an eye surgeon must plan for a dacryocystorhinostomy operation in each suitable case. If there is a complication which cannot be overcome on the operation table the surgeon can terminate the case in dacryocystectomy without any harm to the patient.

Dacryocystectomy

Indications

- Elderly, debilitated, malnourished people with long-standing chronic dacryocystitis.
- Tuberculosis of the lacrimal sac.
- Primary neoplasm of the lacrimal sac.
- Severe atrophic rhinitis.
- Chronic dacyocystitis with encysted lacrimal sac.
- Chronic dacryocystitis with pseudo lacrimal sac.

Contraindications

- Young healthy people with long standing chronic dacryocystitis with dilated sac.

Operation Steps

- Irrigate thoroughly the lacrimal sac and the conjunctival sac with normal saline.
- Pass a suture in both the lids and close the lids with the first tie of a surgical knot.
- Give a 20 to 25 mm long incision from 5 mm above the inner canthus and about 3 mm away from the inner canthus in the skin.

- Incise the orbicularis fascia and the orbicularis muscle in the line of skin incision.
- Undermine the skin and muscle and apply the retractor to expose the field of operation.
- Expose the medial palpebral ligament up to its attachment to the bone. The medial palpebral ligament is attached to the anterior lacrimal crest.
- With the sharp dissector make an incision in the periostium just above the attachment of the ligament and extend it below and upwards along the anterior lacrimal crest.
- Seperate the periostium from the lacrimal fossa and reflect it laterally exposing the lacrimal fossa upto the canal. Thus the sac along with its fascia and periostium lining the fossa is reflected.
- Incise the medial palpebral ligament at its lateral attachment.
- Hold the ligament and snip the sac along with its fascia from all sides and cut at its lower end. Thus the sac along with its fascia and the periostium has been excised.
- Curettage the nasolacrimal duct and pass a probe to confirm free passage. It helps to drain the lacrimal fluid.
- Apply subcutaneous suture to close the wound.
- Clean the area of the operation and the conjunctival sac.
- Apply an eye ointment in the eye.
- Apply dressing over the incision and shift the patient.

Postoperative Care

- Change the dressing next day.
- Remove dressing from the third day.
- Remove sutures on fifth day.
- Advice to use antibiotic eyedrops four to six times a day for 15 days.

Complications

- Injury to angular vein. It can be ligated.
- Opening of the orbital septum and herniation of fat. It occurs only if the anatomical plane is not kept in mind. There is no harm but operator may miss the sac completely.
- Recurrence of chronic dacryocystitis with formation of pseudo-sac. With the above technique, wherein the sac along with its fascia, tissue around and periostium has been removed, there is no chance for recurrence.
- Allergic reaction to local anesthetic agent due to entry in vein.
- Abrasion of cornea
- Fracture of lacrimal bone and connection between ethmoid and orbit.
- Tear of the sac wall.
- Part of the fundus of the sac may be left undissected.
- Improper suturing.

Results

Results are gratifying as patient is relieved of its source of infection that threatens the eye every moment of life. Anyhow, most of the patients are also relieved of epiphora also.

13

A Case with Dry Eye Syndrome

History

Record the history with reference to the following:

- An intelligent patient may straight complain of feeling of dryness in the eyes, discomfort in the movement of lids, collection of stingy mucus and less formation of tears.
- Any complain of itching and burning sensation.
- Excessive mucus collection at the canthus or eyelid margin.
- Foreign body sensation.
- Difficulty in mastication or swallowing.
- Needs water or any liquid to help masticate and swallow.

CLINICAL EXAMINATION

Inspection

Examine the eye with the help of torch light and loupe.

- The eye appears normal except mild redness.
- Bulbar conjunctiva is lusterless and hyperemic.
- Lid margin may show blepharitis.

Slit Lamp Biomicroscopy

- The marginal tear strip at the lower lid margin is reduced or absent.
- Mucus strands in the lower fornix.
- Bulbar conjunctiva appears lusterless. It may be thick, hyperemic and may show edema.
- Mucus strands in the precorneal tear film. The mucus strands in the precorneal tear film tends to move with each blink. In a normal eye the mucus is washed out with blinking.
- Fluorescein staining may show minute epithelial erosions in the lower part of the cornea.
- Filaments are seen on the cornea with unattached end moving with each blink.

Test for Tear Film

1. Tear film break-up time (BUT).
2. Schirmer I and II test.
3. Rose Bengal staining.
4. Giemsa staining of scraping of conjunctiva.
5. Levels of lysozyme and lactoferrin in tear fluid.
6. Tear osmolarity.
7. Conjunctival impression cytology.

Tear Film Break-up Time Test

The tear film break-up time is the time interval between the last blink and the appearance of the first dry spot on the cornea.

This test assesses the stability of the precorneal tear film. Deficiency of the mucin content of tear fluid affects the stability of the tear film resulting in an early break-up time.

Technique

Adjust the patient on the slit lamp with a cobalt blue filter and broad beam of light. Now apply a moist fluorescein strip to the bulbar conjunctiva or lower fornix and ask him to blink few times. Scan the tear film while refraining the patient from blinking. After few seconds black spots or lines appear in the tear film on the cornea indicating formation of dry spots. The tear film break-up time is the time interval between the last blink and the appearance of the first dry spot. It is advisable to have the average of three measurements of tear film break-up time.

Interpretation

- Appearance of dry spot in the same location should be ignored as it could be due to local defect in the corneal epithelium.
- The normal tear film break-up time varies from 15 to 34 seconds.
- The tear film break-up time is always shorter than normal in eyes with mucin deficiency.
- The normal break-up time is more than 10 seconds.
- A break-up time of less than 10 seconds is taken as abnormal.

Schirmer Test

This test assesses the total tear secretion. This test is performed by measuring the amount of wetting of the Whatman-41 filter paper 5 × 35 mm strip.

Schirmer I

It is done without prior instillation of a topical anesthetic in the conjunctival sac. This test measures the total secretion, i.e. basic and reflex tear secretion. The filter paper folded at 5 mm from one end is inserted in the lower fornix at the junction of lateral one-third and medial two-thirds. Patient is asked to look up and keep the eyes open and not to blink. After five minutes of insertion the filter paper is removed and the wetting of the filter paper is measured from the fold. A normal eye wets the filter paper more than 15 mm. A measurement between 5 and 10 mm is considered as borderline. A measurement of less than 5 mm is indicative of deficiency of tear secretion if same reading is obtained on repeated test.

Schirmer II

This test measures reflex tear secretion. It is performed after using topical anesthetic in the conjunctival sac. After placing the strip in the lower fornix, irritate the ipsilateral nasal mucosa with a cotton swab. Measure the wetting of the strip after two minutes. A wetting of less than 15 mm is indicative of decreased reflex secretion. It is seldom used as the reflex secretion is usually intact.

Rose Bengal Staining

Do not anesthetize the conjunctiva to avoid false positive results.

Instill a small drop of rose bengal 1% solution in the conjunctival sac and scan the conjunctiva and cornea by slit lamp. Rose bengal has an affinity for devitalized epithelial cells and mucosa thus it is very useful in detecting even mild cases of dry eye-keratoconjunctivitis sicca. Three staining patterns have been described:

In the pattern 'A', the scan shows confluent staining of the conjunctiva and cornea-indication for severe keratoconjunctivitis sicca (dry eye).

In the pattern 'B', the scan shows extensive staining of the cornea-indication of moderate keratoconjunctivitis sicca (dry eye).

In the pattern 'C', the scan shows fine punctuate staining of the cornea in the inter-palpebral area-indication of mild kerato-conjunctivitis sicca (dry eye).

Giemsa Staining of Scraping of Conjunctiva

A smear examination of scraping from the conjunctiva will show increased number of goblet cells.

Lysozyme Assay

This test is based on the fact that there may be reduction in the concentration of lysozyme in tears in a case of keratoconjunctivitis sicca (dry eye).

Tear Osmometry for Tear Hyperosmolarity

Osmolarity increases in keratoconjunctivitis sicca (dry eye).

Conjunctival Cytology

In mucin deficiency the number of goblet cells will be reduced.

Clinical features and management
1. Tears-tear film and break-up time (BUT).
2. Dry eye syndrome (keratoconjunctivitis sicca: KCS).
3. Sjögren's syndrome.

TEARS-TEAR FILM AND BREAK-UP TIME (BUT)

Tears

The lacrimal glands—the orbital and the palpebral portion secretes about 95% of the aqueous component of the tears. The remaining 5% of the tears are produced by the accessory lacrimal glands of Krause and wolfring lodged in the fornices.

Basic and Reflex Secretion of Tears

Basic secretion of tears is the resting secretion occurring normally. The reflex secretion of tears is much more and occurs due to stimulus derived from parasympathetic reflex. Reflex secretion occurs in both the eyes following superficial stimulus of one eye. The main and accessory lacrimal glands both respond to reflex stimulus as one unit.

Tear film and Tear film Break-up Time

The pre-corneal tear film has three layers which from posterior to anterior are mucin layer, aqueous layer and lipid or oily layer (Fig. 13.1).

The Inner Mucin Layer

It is innermost and thinnest layer of the precorneal teal film. The mucin is secreted by the globlet cells in the conjunctiva and also by the crypts of Henle and glands of Manz. Its function is to convert the corneal epithelium from a hydrophobic to a hydrophillic surface. Mucin is a glycoprotien which becomes adsorbed onto the cell membrane of the epithelial cells making them hydrophillic.

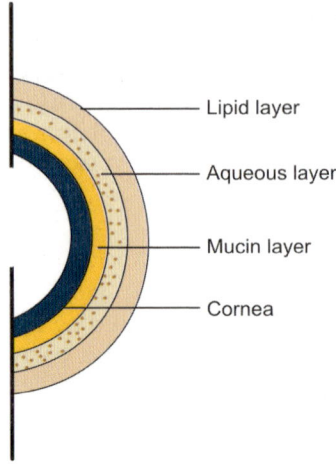

Fig. 13.1: Tear film

The Middle Aqueous Layer

The aqueous component is secreted by main and accessory lacrimal glands. Its functions are:

- Supply atmospheric oxygen to corneal epithelium.
- It has antibacterial enzymes; lysozyme, lactoferin and betalysin.
- Provides a smooth optical surface of cornea.
- Keeps the eye clean by washing action.

The Outer Lipid Layer

The lipid layer is secreted by the Meibomian glands.
   Its functions are:
- Retard the evaporation of aqueous layer.
- Increase surface tension so the film is stable.
- Lubricate the eyelids.

Pathogenesis of Tear Film Break-up

Tear film cannot remain stable for a long time. The formation of tear film is a complex process which requires a normal blinking reflex, a normal lid condition and normal corneal epithelium. With each blink the mucin is distributed over the corneal epithelium making it hydrophilic and allows the aqueous and lipid layer to spread forming three layers of tear film. Evaporation beings immediately and the tear film starts to thin. Some of the superficial lipids will migrate to the tear-epithelial interface usually within a minute creating an area of high interfacial tension over which the tear film becomes unstable, breaks up and forms so called **'dry spots'**. With each new blink, the surface is recoated and the cycle repeats itself.

Tear Film Break-up Time

The time interval between the blink and appearance of a dry spot in a normal eye is called "Tear film break-up time". This time is usually greater than the time between the two blinks. The normal break-up time varies from 15 to 34 seconds. A break-up time of less than 10 seconds is taken as abnormal. There is a wide variation of values obtained in same individual. A break-up time of less than 10 seconds obtained on repeat test can be considered positive along with other positive signs of dry eye.

DRY EYE SYNDROME KERATO-CONJUNCTIVITIS SICCA: KCS

Deficiency in any of the components of the pre-corneal tear film results in dryness of the eye due to the appearance of dry spots on the corneal and conjunctival epithelium. So, dry eye syndrome is a symptom complex that occurs as sequelae to deficiency in any component of pre-corneal tear film.

Dry eye syndrome is a disease of the ocular surface exposed to different disturbances of the natural function and protective mechanism of the external ocular surface leading to an unstable tear film during open eye. It is important to realize that the external ocular surface has to maintain the integrity during; force of blinking, air currents, humidity, minute foreign bodies and micro-organisms.

Etiology

Aqueous Deficiency Dry Eye

It occurs in Sjögren's syndrome, Sarcoidosis, Lymphoma, Leukemia and Amyloidosis.

Aqueous deficiency can occur in idiopathic hyposecretion and affection of the lacrimal glands.

Mucin Deficiency Dry Eye

It occurs when goblet cells are damaged as in xerophthalmia and conjunctival scarring which may be due to trachoma, Stevens-Johnson syndrome, ocular pemphigoid, chemical burns, chronic bacterial or viral conjunctivitis and irradiation.

Lipid Deficiency Dry Eye

Lipid deficiency is rare. Lipid abnormality is seen in patient with chronic Blepharitis and Meibomitis.

Miscellaneous

- Effect of drugs like atropine and diuretics.
- Mumps.
- Deficient blinking.
- Lid surgery not allowing proper polishing.
- Impaired eyelid function as in cases of Bell's palsy, symblepharon, pterygium, lagophthalmos and ectropion.
- Exposure keratitis.

Symptoms

- Scratchy or a sandy feeling in the eye.
- Foreign body sensation in the eye.
- Excessive secretion of mucus.
- Burning sensation especially under the fan, air-conditioning, watching television, study and on exposure to heat.
- Difficulty in opening the eyelids as if they are stuck up.
- Itching, photophobia, mild pain and redness.
- Less flow of tears even when exposed to irritant odors and fumes and emotional situations.

Signs

- Lusterless ocular surface.
- Conjunctival xerosis.
- Mild redness of the conjunctiva with mucus in fornix.
- Mild blepharitis

- Punctate epithelial erosions on the lower part of cornea taking fluorescein stain.
- Filaments on the cornea moving with each blink and takes rose bengal stain.
- Deficient or absent lower lid marginal tear strip.

Test

- Tear film break-up time reduced or even less than 10 seconds.
- Rose bengal staining shows devitalized epithelium of conjunctiva in the inter-palpebral area and mucus plaques on the cornea.
- Schirmer's test-I is positive.
- Giemsa staining of the conjunctival scraping may show increased number of goblet cells as in a case of a Sjögren's syndrome.

Differential Diagnosis

- Hypofunction of lacrimal gland.
- Sjögren's syndrome.
- Sarcoidosis.
- Lymphoma.
- Leukemia.
- Amyloidosis.
- Mucin deficiency.
- Vitamin A deficiency.
- Conjunctival scarring due to the following.
- Trachoma.
- Stevens-Johnson syndrome.
- Pemphigoid.
- Chemical burns.
- Chronic bacterial or viral conjunctivitis.
- Irradiation.
- Miscellaneous.
- Effect of drug like atropine, diuretics.
- Mumps.
- Deficient blinking.
- Lid surgery not allowing proper polishing.
- Exposure keratitis.

SJÖGREN'S SYNDROME

Sjögren's sydrome is an autoimmune chronic inflammatory disease with multi system involvement.

Siögren's syndrome is characterized by triad of the following:
- Keratoconjunctivitis sicca-dry eye due to aqueous deficiency.
- Xerostomia (dry mouth) with or without enlargement of salivary gland.
- Rhemumatiod arthritis or other connective tissue diseases like systemic lupus erythematous, periarteritis nodosa, polymyositis, progressive systemic sclerosis, psoriatic arthritis, juvenile chronic arthritis, Hashimoto's thyroiditis, and primary biliary cirrhosis. Sjögren's syndrome affects more females. Ocular symptoms appear in 4th to 6th decade. The histopathologic changes of the lacrimal gland consist of lymphocytic infiltration and occasional plasma cells leading to atrophy and destruction of the glandular tissue. This results in dryness of mouth, eyes and mucus membranes. A labial salivary gland biopsy helps in a suspected case. The tear lysozyme is reduced or absent in over 90% of cases. Treatment is aimed to provide relief to symptoms. Steroids are helpful in cases with rheumatoid factor.

MANAGEMENT

Conventional management of dry eye is palliative either by tear substitutes or tear fluid conserving therapy.

Counseling—Assurance and Advice

- There is no cure for dry eye syndrome but there are options to relieve the symptoms.
- Assurance that nothing serious will happen.
- Advice the patient to avoid heat, wind, and strong light to avoid evaporation of tear fluid.
- Protective spectacles shall help to preserve tear fluid.
- Dry eye syndrome is a progressive disease. Aim is to treat the malady early by all the means available to prevent its progress to a severe level.
  1. *Topical cyclosporine A (0.05% to*

long period of 6 to 12 months has been found to be very effective.

2. *Unpreserved tear substitutes:* Artificial tears in form of eye drops, ointment are the main therapy to provide relief to the patient from his annoying and depressive signs and symptoms. Most of the available artificial tear drops contain either cellulose derivatives or polyvinyl alcohol.

3. *Mucolytics:* Acetylcysteine 5% as drops instilled four times a day in the eyes with excessive mucus as in Sjögren's syndrome. Mucolytics helps to decrease the tear viscosity.

4. *Topical steroids:* Helpful in controlling symptoms.

5. *Topical antibiotics:* A patient of dry eye has an increased susceptibility to infection. Take care of the associated blepharitis, corneal and conjunctival infection.

6. *Topical retinoids:* It helps in reversing the cellular changes.

7. *Autologous serum*

8. *Occlusion of punctum:* It can be done to save tears from drainage. It can be a temporary occlusion or a permanent occlusion, depending on the individual case. It can be carried out by collagen implants, adhesive tissue, electro-cauterization, argon laser and surgical occlusion.

9. *Tarsorrhaphy*

10. *Systemic therapy:* Steroids and antibiotics may be needed in associated systemic diseases or to control associated chronic inflammation.

11. *Supportive therapy:* Nourishing diet with vitamins, minerals and antioxidants with change in the lifestyle.

14

A Case with Chlamydial Follicular Conjunctivitis

History

Record the history with reference to the following

- Duration and onset whether acute or chronic.
- Any instillation of drugs like neomycin, atropine or epinephrine.
- Any history of exposure to an individual with conjunctivitis.
- Addiction to alcohol.
- Socioeconomic and literary status.
- Household pets.
- Recent vaccination.
- Trauma by vegetative material.

CLINICAL EXAMINATION

Inspection

- Look at the eye for swelling of lids, discharge and scales.
- Expose the lower fornix and examine for follicles.
- Evert the upper lid and examine for follicles.

Palpation

Palpate for preauricular lymph node.

LABORATORY INVESTIGATION

Scrapings

Conjunctival scraping should be taken during active stage. The material is placed on the glass slides for gram and Giemsa staining.

Gram Staining

It helps to identify and differentiate gram-positive from gram-negative bacteria.

Giemsa Staining

It is used to identify the type of inflammatory and epithelial cells.

CHLAMYDIAL FOLLICULAR CONJUNCTIVITIS

Chlamydia trachomatis belongs to PLT: Psittacosis-Lymphogranuloma-Trachoma group. *Chlamydia trachomatis* produces intracytoplasmic inclusion bodies known as H.P. bodies (*Halberstaedter Prowazeke* bodies). Eleven serotypes of Chlamydia—A, B, Ba, C, D, E, F, G, H, J and K have been identified by the microimmunofluorescence (micro-IF) technique. Serotypes A, B, Ba, and C are associated with trachoma while serotypes D, E, F, G, H, J and K are associated with paratrachoma-oculogenital chlamydial follicular conjunctivitis popularly known as adult inclusion conjunctivitis.

Clinical Features and Management

1. Trachoma.
2. Adult inclusion conjunctivitis.

TRACHOMA

Trachoma is a chronic keratoconjunctivitis, primarily involving the superficial epithelium of conjunctiva and cornea simultaneously. It is characterized by papillary and follicular conjunctival response. It is common among poor and malnourished population living in an unhygienic conditions. It is contagious in acute stage being spread by transfer of the conjunctival secretions directly by fingers and common linen used by family members. The common fly acts as a major vector in the infection-re-infection cycle. Trachoma is common cause of preventable blindness in the world.

Etiology

Trachoma is caused by serotypes A, B, Ba, and C of "*Chlamydia trachomatis*".

Symptoms and Signs

- Mild irritation and foreign body sensation in the eyes.
- Very frequent blinking.
- Mild lacrimation.
- Lid appears thick and swollen.
- Conjunctival congestion.
- Follicles and scarring in the tarsal conjunctiva.
- Epithelial keratitis in upper part of cornea.
- Progressive or regressive pannus.
- Superior limbal follicles.
- Herbert's pits.

Conjunctival Signs

The essential lesion is follicles. Clinically these appear as multiple, discrete, elevated nodules. Each follicle is encircled by a tiny blood vessel. The size of follicles may vary from 0.5 mm to 5 mm (Fig. 14.1). The follicles heal by cicatrization which appears as a minute star shaped scars visible by slit lamp.

Corneal Signs

Superficial Keratitis

There are numerous epithelial erosions in the upper part of cornea. These stain with fluorescein and can be seen by slit lamp.

Pannus

The pannus develops as a lymphoid infiltration with vascularization of cornea

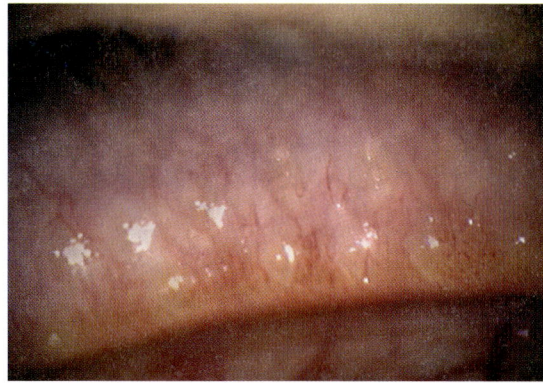

Fig. 14.1: Follicular conjunctivitis

which is usually limited to the upper limbus but later may involve the entire cornea from all sides. In early stage of pannus the vessels are superficial and lie between Bowman's membrane and epithelium carrying with them a small amount of granulation tissue. Later the Bowman's membrane disappears and superficial layers of substantia propria get involved which on healing leaves opacity of cornea.

Progressive Pannus

The vessels are parallel with little or no anastomosis. The vessels are directed vertically downwards and extend to a level to form a horizontal line and beyond this line there is a narrow strip of infiltration and haze of cornea.

Regressive Pannus

In this, the line of infiltration and haze of cornea recedes therefore the vessels appear to extend beyond the line of infiltration and haze.

Resolution of Pannus

The pannus resolves completely leaving cornea clear apart from the fine obliterated vessels if the case has received treatment before the disappearance of the Bowman's membrane.

The cases in which the Bowman's membrane has been destroyed with involvement of the substantia propria ends up with permanent opacity of the cornea.

Superior Limbal Follicles and Herberts Pits

The follicles at the limbus on healing leaves the pitted scars called as Herbert's pits. The follicles at the limbus appear as gelatinous, semi-opaque, dome-shaped elevations surrounded by pannus. Herbert's pits appear as small depressions (pits) in the connective tissue of limbo-corneal junction. There is no depression as they are filled with epithelium and look like small lucid circles or semicircles in the semi-opaque limbus.

Corneal Ulcers

Ulcers are usually at the advancing edge of the pannus.

THE WORLD HEALTH ORGANIZATION (WHO) CLASSIFICATION (FISTO)

Trachomatous Follicles (F)

There are five or more follicles of at least 0.5 mm diameter on the upper tarsal plate with visible palpebral conjunctival blood vessels. Few papillae may be visible. Treatment at this stage leaves no scarring or minimal scarring.

Trachomatous Intense Follicles (I)

More than 50% of the palpebral conjunctival blood vessels are not visible due to numerous follicles and papillae. This stage indicates high risk of serious complications.

Trachomatous Scarring (S)

There is scarring of the tarsal conjunctiva with white fibrous bands.

Trachomatous Trichiasis (T)

It shows presence of at least one trichiatic eyelash.

Trachomatous Opacities (O)

Presence of corneal opacity covering part of pupillary region resulting in blurred vision.

Complications and Sequelae

- Herbert's pits.
- Trachomatus ptosis.
- Entropion.
- Trichiasis.
- Trachomatous xerosis.
- Trachomatous tylosis (thickening of lid margin).
- Trachomatous madarosis.
- Pannus.
- Corneal opacity.

Clinical Diagnosis

The presence of any two of the following sings is diagnostic.
- Follicles.
- Pannus.
- Epithelial keratitis.
- Scarring in the conjunctiva.

Laboratory Diagnosis

- *Conjunctival cytology:* Giemsa stained conjunctival smear shows predominantly polymorphonuclear reaction with presence of plasma and leber cells.
- *Detection of inclusion bodies* in conjunctival smear.
- *Micro-immuno-fluorescence (micro-IF)* method to detect the specific antibodies by serotyping of TRIC agents.
- *Direct monoclonal fluorescent antibody microscopy* of conjunctival smear.
- *McCoy cell culture.*
- *Polymerase chain reaction (PCR)* is also useful.
- *ELISA:* Enzyme-linked immune-sorbent assay for Chlamydial antigens.

MANAGEMENT

Topical Therapy

Tetracycline or Erythromycin 1% eye ointment four times a day for six weeks or Sulfacetamide 20% eyedrops three times a day with tetracycline 1% eye ointment at bed time for six weeks.

Intermittent Regime

This continuous topical treatment should be followed by intermittent regime in endemic areas by applying 1% Tetracycline eye ointment twice a day for 7 days in a month for at least six months.

Systemic Therapy

Tetracycline or erythromycin 250 mg four times a day for 3–4 weeks or doxycycline 100 mg twice a day for 3–4 weeks.

Combined Therapy

Trachomatous intense follicular inflammation needs combined topical and systemic therapy with intermittent regime.

Supportive Therapy with Counseling

- Early and energetic treatment is the key to save the eye from severe complications.
- Improve general health and environment.
- Regular treatment is essential to get rid of this blinding malady.
- Explain to the patient that it will take at least 3–6 months to get cured from this blinding malady.

ADULT INCLUSION CONJUNCTIVITIS

It is a type of acute follicular conjunctivitis. It affects young adults during their sexually active period.

Etiology

It is caused by the serotype D, E, F, G, H, J and K of *"Chlamydia trachomatis"*.

The conjunctivitis manifests after a week of sexual exposure and may be associated with nonspecific urethritis in males and cervicitis in females. The infection may be transferred from the genitals by the fingers. Another common mode of infection is through the water of the swimming pools, which may cause local epidemics known as **"swimming bath conjunctivitis"**.

Clinical Features (Fig. 14.2)

- It is an acute bilateral mucopurulent conjunctivitis.
- Follicles are seen in the lower fornix. Later these appear on upper fornix and upper tarsal plate.
- Pre-auricular lymph node is enlarged and tender.

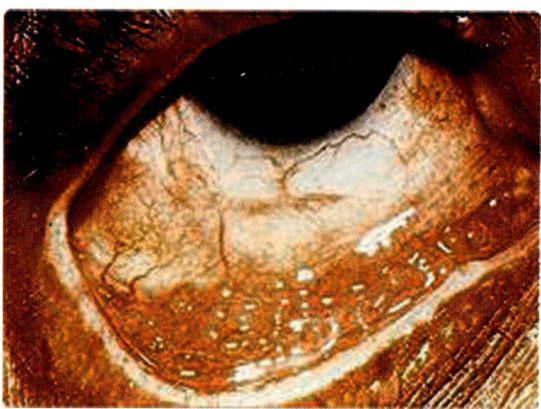

Fig. 14.2: Inclusion conjunctivitis

- Epithelial keratitis is seen in the upper part of cornea.
- Micropannus may be there.
- It runs a benign course and often evolves in chronic follicular conjunctivitis.

SPECIAL INVESTIGATION

- **Giemsa staining** of conjunctival scrapings.
- **FTA-ABS test** (Fluorescent treponemal antibody absorption).

This is a specific test to detect anti-treponemal antibodies. Once positive, the test remains positive for the rest of life. This test should be done seeing the venereal nature of the disease.

- **VDRL** (Venereal Disease Research Laboratory): This is nonspecific test useful for screening.
- **Gram staining:** Gram staining of the smear of the pus discharge from urethra will show the organism.
- **Urine examination with culture and sensitivity:** It is required to diagnose or exclude gonorrhea.

Differential Diagnosis

Adult inclusion conjunctivitis is to be differentiated from viral follicular conjunctivitis (Table 14.1).

Table 14.1: Differential diagnosis of inclusion conjunctivitis and viral follicular conjunctivitis

	Inclusion	*Viral*
Incubation	2–3 weeks	3–7 days
Age	Young adult	Any age
Systemic disease	Genitourinary	Upper respiratory
Discharge	Mucopurulent	Watery
Preauricular lymphadenopathy	Present	Present
Follicles	Fornices	Fornices
Keratitis	Present	Present
Cytology	Inclusion bodies	No inclusion bodies
	Polymorphs	Mononuclear cells
Response to tetracycline	Good	No response

MANAGEMENT

Topical Therapy

Tetracycline 1% eye ointment in the eyes, four times a day for six weeks (Fig. 14.1).

Systemic Therapy

Any broad spectrum antibiotics such as:
- Tetracycline 250 mg four times a day for 3–4 weeks.
- Doxycycline 100 mg twice a day for 1–2 weeks.
- Erythromycin 250 mg four times a day for 3–4 weeks only in pregnant and lactating females.
- Ofloxacin 200 mg twice a day for 7 days.

Supportive Therapy with Counseling

Carefully modifying the life and lifestyle with firm determination

15

A Case with Viral Follicular Conjunctivitis

History

Record the history with reference to the following:
- Duration and onset whether acute or chronic.
- Any instillation of drugs like neomycin, atropine or epinephrine.
- Any history of exposure to an individual with conjunctivitis.
- Addiction to alcohol.
- Socioeconomic and literary status.
- Household pets.
- Recent vaccination.
- Trauma by vegetative material.

CLINICAL EXAMINATION

Inspection

- Look at the eye for swelling of lids, discharge and scales.
- Expose the lower fornix and examine for follicles.
- Evert the upper lid and examine for follicles.

Palpation

Palpate for preauricular lymph node.

Clinical Features (Fig. 15.1)

- It is an acute catarrhal conjunctivitis.
- It shows marked follicular hyperplasia in the lower fornix and lower palpebral conjunctiva.
- Feeling of discomfort and foreign body sensation.

- Mild hyperemia of the conjunctiva with mucoid discharge.
- Lacrimation and photophobia.

LABORATORY INVESTIGATION

Scrapings

Conjunctival scraping should be taken during active stage. The material is placed on the glass slides for gram and Giemsa staining.

Gram Staining

It helps to identify and differentiate gram-positive from gram-negative bacteria.

Giemsa Staining

It is used to identify the type of inflammatory and epithelial cells.

Clinical Features and Management

1. Pharyngoconjunctival fever.
2. Epidemic-keratoconjunctivitis.
3. Herpes simplex conjunctivitis.
4. Newcastle conjunctivitis.
5. Acute hemorrhagic conjunctivitis.
6. Molluscum contagiosum conjunctivitis.

PHARYNGOCONJUNCTIVAL FEVER (PCF)

It is an adenoviral affection commonly associated with subtypes 3 and 7.

It is characterized by acute follicular conjunctivitis associated with pharyngitis, fever and preauricular lymphadenopathy. It affects

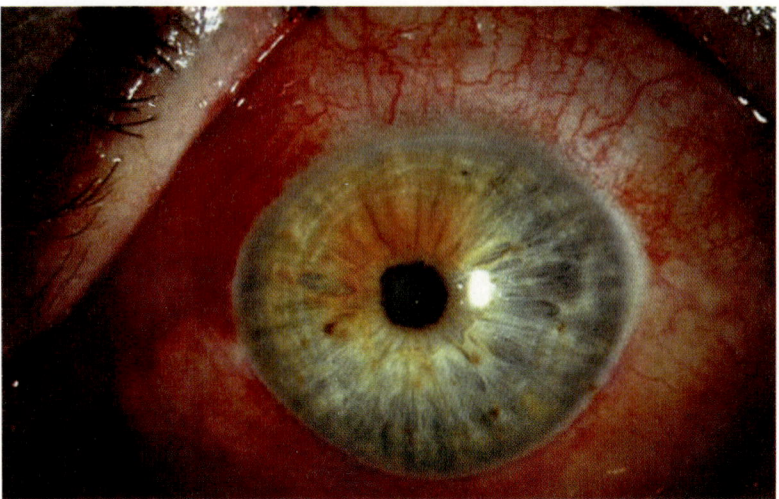

Fig. 15.1: Viral follicular conjunctivitis

primarily children in endemic form. Epithelial punctuate keratitis manifests in about 30% of cases. It needs supportive treatment. Topical instillation of tetracycline 1% eye ointment shall help to ward of corneal affection. Treatment is usually supportive to provide relief from pharyngitis and fever.

EPIDEMIC KERATOCONJUNCTIVITIS (EKC)

It is an adenoviral affection commonly associated with serotype 8 and 19.

It is contagious and spreads through contact with contaminated fingers, solutions and linen. Its incubation period is about eight days and remains contagious for 2–3 weeks.

In the early stage, there is conjunctival congestion with mild lacrimation and chemosis. Soon it is followed by formation of follicles mostly marked in the lower fornix. Some cases may show pseudo membranous conjunctivitis. Involvement of the cornea in form of superficial punctuate keratitis is a distinctive feature that becomes apparent after one week of the onset of the malady.

Preauricular lymphadenopathy is always associated.

Treatment is usually supportive.

Adenine arabinoside (Ara-A) has given good results (Fig. 15.1).

HERPES SIMPLEX CONJUNCTIVITIS

It occurs as one of the clinical manifestation of herpes simplex virus type 1 and spreads by close contact.

In its typical form, it is associated with usual vesicular lesions of face. There is preauricular adenopthy, dedritic figure on cornea, large follicles in the conjunctiva, and reduced sensation of cornea. There are tiny ulcers on the intermarginal portion of the eyelid which takes fluorescein stain. There are minute microdendritic lesions on the cornea which look like punctate keratitis. Reduced corneal sensation and formation of a pannus is strongly suggestive of herpes infection.

In its atypical form, the follicular conjunctivitis occurs without lesions of face, eyelids or cornea, resembling epidemic keratoconjunctivitis.

Treatment

Topical application of Acyclovir eye ointment 3% for 2–3 weeks is effective in controlling the malady.

NEWCASTLE CONJUNCTIVITIS

It is caused by the Newcastle virus. It affects people coming in contact with diseased fowls in a poultry farm. The clinical picture is like that of phyaryngoconjunctival fever.

ACUTE HEMORRHAGIC CONJUNCTIVITIS

It is caused by enterovirus type 70. It affects people from low socioeconomic status living in unhygienic surroundings with poor personal habit of cleanliness. It is highly contagious but self limiting. The conjunctivitis is characterized by multiple conjunctival hemorrhages, conjunctival hyperemia, lacrimation, lid edema and follicular hyperplasia. Some cases may show superficial punctuate keratitis and pre-auricular lymphadenopathy. No effective treatment. It resolves within seven days without sequelae.

MOLLUSCUM CONTAGIOSUM CONJUNCTIVITIS

Molluscum contagiosum is caused by virus which affects childern. The nodular lesions appear as a small, pale-waxy, umbilicated elevated multiple nodules on both the lids and around. Histologically large intracystoplasmic inclusion bodies occur within acanthotic epidermis. The chronic shedding of cells laden with the virus particles may induce chronic follicular conjunctivitis and superficial keratitis. Treat the case early without waiting for resolution. Treat by incision and expression of sebum from each lesion followed by cauterization with povidone. Instill an antibiotic eye ointment in the eyes to prevent secondary infection.

16

A Case with Allergic Conjunctivitis

History

Record the history with reference to the following:
- Working in agriculture field.
- Contact with pets.
- Playing in fields with wild growth of grass.
- Instillation of eyedrops for a prolonged period.
- Any history of hay fever, asthma, and eczema.
- Any relation to season, especially spring season.
- Any use of contact lens.
- Using an artificial eye.
- Systemic use of antibiotics and sulphonamides.
- Exposure to chemical fumes, polluted air, smog and dusty wind.
- Exposure to vegetation, particularly to cactus.
- Any use of hair dye.
- Any change in the brand of cosmetics used especially eyebrow and eyelid pencils and coloring agents.

CLINICAL EXAMINATION

Inspection

- Inspect the eye and surrounding area for any eczema, allergic dermatitis and excoriation of skin.
- Inspect the type of discharge, whether watery, mucus, stingy or filamentous.
- Inspect the lids about swelling.
- Inspect the lower fornix for follicles and mucus strands.
- Evert the upper lid and inspect the conjunctiva for papillae or follicles and their shape, size, color and hue.
- Look for any gelatinous thickening of the conjunctiva around the limbus.

- Palpate for preauricular and sub-maxillary lymph nodes.
- Palpate the lids with finger tip for any signs of roughness or dry skin over the lids.

Slit Lamp Biomicroscopy

- Examine the cornea for epithelial keratitis.
- Examine the follicles at the limbus and in upper tarsus for their configuration.
- Examine for micro-pannus.

Systemic Examination

- Look for any allergic lesion of skin anywhere on the body.
- Examine the nose, mouth, pharynx for any vesicles and bullae.
- A gynecological check up shall be helpful.

Laboratory Investigations

Grams and Giemsa Staining of Conjunctival Scraping

Take a scraping from the lower fornix and place it on the glass slide for grams and Giemsa staining. Presence of eosinophils and eosinophilic granules are suggestive of allergic conjunctivitis.

Total and Differential Count of WBC

Eosinophilia indicates an allergic factor.

Serum IgE Level

It is raised in vernal conjunctivitis.

ACUTE ALLERGIC CONJUNCTIVITIS

Allergic conjunctivitis is a type I hypersensitivity response to external allergens, affecting predominantly males during the first two decades of life.

It occurs due to severe reaction to the allergen entering the conjunctival sac. It is often seen following the lodging of a tiny insect in the conjunctival sac with the flow of wind, exposure to wild grass in a field, stroking the pet animal or exposure to any kind of noxious fumes. Exposure to pollens, grass pollens, animal dandruff, house dust, mites and cockroaches, etc. acts as trigger.

Clinical Features (Fig. 16.1)

- Sudden irritation of eyes with burning sensation.
- Sudden itching in the eyes.
- Sudden lacrimation.
- Intense redness of the eye.
- Chemosis and edema of lids may be seen.

Treatment

- Immediately wash the eyes with clean drinking water or saline.

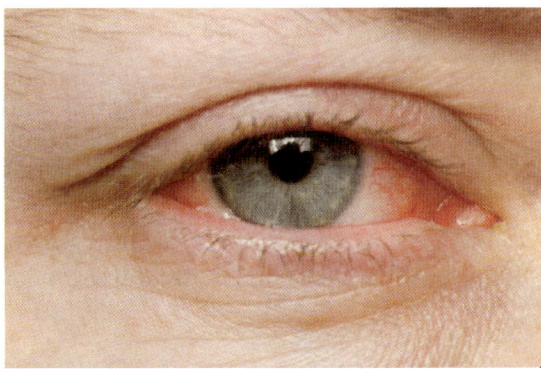

Fig. 16.1: Allergic conjunctivitis

- Topical instillation of steroid eyedrops every half an hour for 4–6 times shall abort the reaction.
- Systemic steroids in severe cases.
- Advise the patient to use goggles to avoid recurrence and exposure to allergens.

CHRONIC ALLERGIC CONJUNCTIVITIS

It is a manifestation of a hypersensitivity or toxic reaction to variety of drugs used for topical instillation in the eyes. The following drugs are known to cause an allergic reaction, idoxuridine, neomycin, pilocarpine, physostigmine, atropine and preservatives like thiomersol.

Clinical Features (Fig. 16.2)

- Mild irritation, itching and redness.
- Fine papillary or follicular response.
- Mild punctate epithelial keratitis.
- Skin of the lids and surrounding area may show signs of allergic dermatitis due to use of atropine or in contact lens wearers.

Treatment

- Withdraw the drug.
- Topical steroids for two weeks shall provide relief.
- Disodium cromoglycate 2% eyedrops for a month or until the symptoms are relieved.
- Systemic antihistamines and steroids in long duration cases.

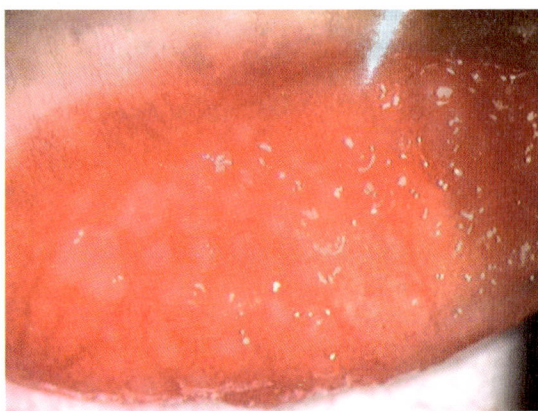

Fig. 16.2: Papillary conjunctivitis

VERNAL KERATOCONJUNCTIVITIS
(Spring Catarrh)

It affects children usually males and show exacerbation during spring season. It is a recurrent, bilateral allergic disorder in which IgE mediated mechanisms play an important role.

Clinical Features (Fig. 16.3)

Palpebral Type

- Marked burning and itching sensation accentuates in warm humid environment.
- Conjunctival hyperemia and chemosis with milky hue.
- Papillary hypertrophy. The papillae may be diffuse or flat with "cobble-stone" or "pavement stone" appearance or giant papillae.
- The lids are swollen and heavy.
- White ropy or sticky conjunctival discharge.
- Micro-pannus is visible.

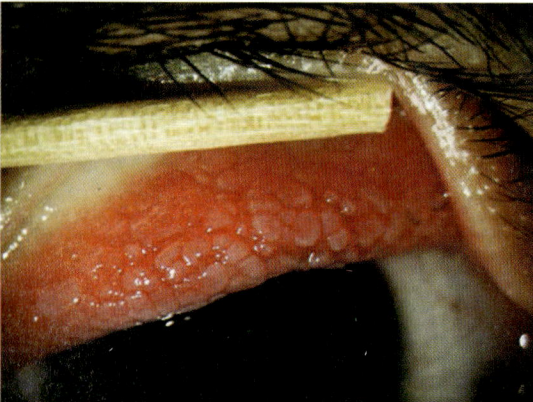

Fig. 16.3: Vernal conjunctivitis

Bulbar Type

- Triangular congestion of bulbar conjunctiva in palpebral area.
- The conjunctiva around the limbus is hyperemic gelatinous thick and assumes appearance of mucoid nodules.
- Presence of white superficial dots (Horner-Trantas' dots) consisting of eosinophils and epithelial debris at the limbus are characteristic features.
- Micro-pannus is visible.

Mixed Type

Some case may show features of both the types.

Vernal keratopathy includes five types of lesions

1. *Punctate epithelial keratitis:* It is seen in the upper cornea sparing the narrow strip adjacent to the limbus.
2. *Epithelial macro-erosions:* The loss of epithelium results in ulceration.
3. *Plaque:* The epithelial macro-erosions are covered by layer of altered exudates which cannot be wetted by tears and resists re-epithelialization.
4. *Sub-epithelial scarring:* It is seen in the form of a ring scar.
5. *Pseudo-gerontoxon:* It resembles arcus senilis and is seen in the previously inflamed upper limbus and shows a classical "cupid's bow" out line.

Clinical Course

It is self limiting and burns out in 5–10 years. Papillaes heal without scarring.

Treatment

Topical therapy
- *Topical steroid* is the main therapy. Start with frequent instillation and taper in few instillations soon to avoid steroid induced complications.
- *Mast cell stabilizer* Disodium cromoglycate 2% eyedrops four times a day for prolonged period. No side effects. It can be used safely. The action of disodium cromoglycate is to prevent the release of vasoactive-amines.
- *Topical antihistamines* are also effective.
- *Acetylcysteine* 0.5% helps to reduce mucus secretion due its mucolytic property and useful in preventing early plaque formation.
- *Topical cyclosporine* 1% eyedrops are effective in severe non-responsive cases.

Systemic therapy

Oral steroids and antihistamines may be needed in some severe cases.

Treatment of large papillae
- Inject steroid in upper tarsal.
- Cryo application.
- Surgical excision.

General treatment
- Cold compresses and ice packs do provide some relief.
- Dark goggles help to provide relief from photophobia.
- Keep the patient in cool area.

PHLYCTENULAR KERATOCONJUNCTIVITIS

It is a delayed hypersensitivity (type IV-cell mediated) response to endogenous microbial proteins of the tubercle bacillus and staphylococcus and also other bacterial antigens. Low resistance due to undernourishment and unhygienic living environment plays an important role.

Its incidence increases markedly in spring and summer seasons. It may follow or precede by mucopurulent conjunctivitis.

Clinical Features

- There is marked photophobia, lacrimation and blepharospasm.
- There may be eczematous lesions on the lids and nose.
- Phlycten may be conjunctival or at the limbus astriding the cornea.
- Conjunctival phlycten appears as a small red elevated nodule with localized congestion around it or general congestion of the conjunctiva.
- A corneal phlycten appears grey white and may progress towards the center of cornea. It may develop in a fascicular ulcer.
- A phlycten may be precede or follow conjunctivitis with mucopurulent discharge due to secondary infection.
- A healed phlycten leaves a triangular scar with its base at limbus. A conjunctival phlycten heals without scar.

- The presenting symptoms of photophobia and lacrimation, with blepharospasm are severe when the disease is tuberculo-protein induced and mild when the disease is staphylococci protein induced.

Phlyctenular conjunctivitis can manifests as:

Simple phlyctenular conjunctivitis is the most common form. It is characterized by the presence of a typical solitary pinkish white nodule with localized congestion on the bulbar conjunctiva usually near the limbus.

Necrotizing phlyctenular conjunctivitis is characterized by the presence of large nodule astriding the limbus. It shows necrosis and may lead to fascicular ulcer if not treated.

Fascicular ulcer is superficial and progressive ulcer towards the pupil followed by prominent parallel leash of vascularization. It heals with band shaped superficial opacity.

Miliary phlyctenular conjunctivitis is characterized by the presence of multiple phlyctens in the form of a ring around the limbus and may even lead to ring ulcer.

Treatment

It needs early and energetic treatment to prevent its evolvement in necrotizing fascicular or ring ulcer.

Topical Therapy

- A short course of topical steroid in form of eyedrops and ointment is very effective. Patient with tuberculo-protein induced phlycten responds well to steroid in comparison to patients with staphylococcal-protein induced phlycten.
- Antibiotic eyedrops and ointment to take care of secondary conjunctival infection.

Systemic Therapy

- Systemic antibiotic may be necessary in some cases to control secondary infection of conjunctiva and any associated blepharitis.
- Treat any septic focus especially in throat (tonsils and adenoids).

- Look for and treat if there is any tubercular focus in the system.
- Look for parasitic infestation by repeated stool examination and treat if positive.
- A high protein diet with vitamins, minerals and hygienic living surrounding is necessary for early cure and to prevent recurrences.

ATOPIC KERATOCONJUNCTIVITIS

It affects young atopic males. The classic atopic skin areas are the lateral neck fold and the antecubital and antepopliteal fossae.

Clinical Features

- Patient complains of itching, soreness, dryness, lacrimation, mucoid discharge, photophobia and blurred vision.
- The lids show fissures, crusts, cracks and roughness.
- The lids appear dry and dark at the places of affection.
- Signs of blepharitis are usually seen.
- Congestion of tarsal conjunctiva with papillae, hyperemia and scarring.
- Cornea may show punctuate epithelial keratitis.
- Cornea may show neovascularization and scars.

Treatment

- Topical steroid as drops and ointment.
- Systemic and topical antibiotics to control blepharitis.
- Antihistamines to treat associated skin lesions.
- Refer the case to skin specialist to look after the atopic dermatitis.

GIANT PAPILLARY CONJUNCTIVITIS

It is a rare disease. It is seen in cases who wear contact lens and artificial eye. It has been postulated that the giant papillary conjunctivitis has an immunological basis in which the protein deposits on the contact lens acts as allergens. The preservative thiomersol used in cleaning solutions for contacts lens has been implicated in altering lens proteins and predisposing patients to this malady of Giant papillary conjunctivitis.

Patient presents after months or years of use of contact lens.

Clinical Features

- There is irritation, itching and photophobia after wearing the contact lens.
- There is increased mucus discharge.
- The upper lid shows papillae which may be small or giant in size depending on the tissue response.
- Some case may show a limbal response like that of a bulbar type of vernal keratoconjunctivitis.
- Patient is unable to tolerate the lens anymore.

Treatment

- Discontinue the use of contact lens for at least three months.
- Topical use of weak steroids and or sodium cromoglycate 2% eye drops for three months.
- With subsidence of symptoms and signs the patient may try again to wear the lens of different polymer.
- Eliminate the cleaning solutions with preservative.

17

A Case with Nodule at Limbus

History

Record the history with reference to the following:
- Duration.
- Slow or fast growing nodule.
- Vascular or non vascular.
- Any history of trauma or surgery.
- Any change in its color.
- Any associated symptom like itching, watering, congestion and discharge.
- Stationary or growing in its size.

CLINICAL EXAMINATION

Inspection

Inspect the nodule for its shape, size, color, surface and location.

Palpation

Anesthetize the conjunctiva and feel the mass with a blunt spatula for its consistency, bleeding, feeling for a foreign body. Ask the patient to close the lids and thereafter palpate the nodule with slight pressure to evaluate consistency and tenderness.

Slit Lamp Biomicroscopy

It helps to evaluate the nodule in magnified view.

Clinical Features and Management

1. Pinguecula
2. Pterygium
3. Phlycten
4. Vernal limbal lesions
5. Episclerits
6. Scleritis
7. Ciliary or intercalary staphyloma
8. Papilloma
9. Naevi
10. Granuloma
11. Dermoid
12. Lipodermoid
13. Intraepithelial epithelioma
14. Squamous cell carcinoma
15. Primary melanoma
16. Retention cyst.

PINGUECULA

Pinguecula appears as a yellowish triangular nodule in the palpebral bulbar conjunctiva on either side of the cornea at the limbus.

Clinical Features

- It appears first on the nasal side thereafter on the temporal side.
- It appears on either side of the limbus in a triangular form the base towards the limbus.
- Usually it is of a moderate size and stationary.
- It is either yellow in color or there are many yellow spots at the edges.
- Occasionally it can become inflamed. Due to inflammation the epithelium becomes thick.
- According to Wilson (1949) both the pinguecula and pterygium, fluoresce in ultraviolet light. This phenomenon is used

to differentiate these from malignant epitheliomata.

Pathology: The pinguecula is of a degenerative nature. There is elastotic degeneration of collagen together with the deposition of amorphous hyaline material.

Treatment: The patient usually comes for cosmetic purpose. It can be excised or cauterized. As such it does not require any treatment.

PTERYGIUM

Pterygium is a diffuse triangular nodular encroachment of the bulbar conjunctiva on the cornea (Fig. 17.1).

Clinical Features

- Its etiological factors include the following:
- Environmental factors like heat, dust and wind.
- Chemical irritants like fumes, gases and smoke.
- Decrease of lacrimal secretion.
- Exposure to ultraviolet rays in solar radiation.
- All the factors do not explain its occurrence on the nasal side of the eye and no progress beyond the middle of cornea.
- It occurs first on the nasal side and later on the temporal side. Both the eyes are usually affected.

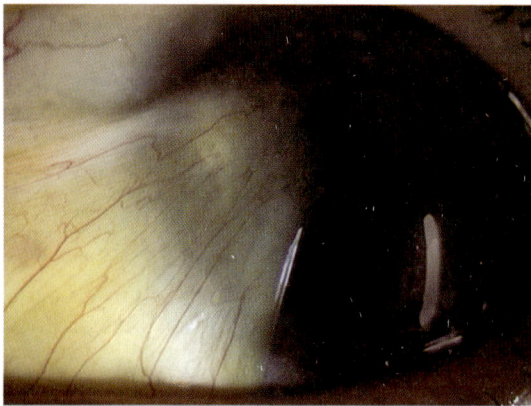

Fig. 17.1: Pterygium

- The early change is the appearance of grey opacities in the cornea near the limbus with shrinkage of the conjunctiva.
- As it grows there is a triangular apex which is blunt. In front of the apex there are small irregular opacities at the level of Bowman's membrane as seen by the slit lamp. Some cases may show a pigmented line just ahead of the superficial opacity.
- The rest of the pterygium appears as a triangular fold of the conjunctiva with overhanging upper and lower borders and the base merging into the bulbar conjunctiva.
- The progressive pterygium is fleshy, thick and vascular.
- The pterygium which ceases to grow appears thin, pale, atrophic but does not disappear.

Symptoms

- The patient consults for cosmetic purpose.
- It can cause astigmatism.
- Dim vision when it reaches the pupil.
- Diplopia due to limitation of abduction.

True Pterygium

It is firmly fixed with the corneal tissue throughout its extent. It occurs only on the nasal or temporal side of the cornea and in the palpebral aperture.

Pseudopterygium

It is adherent to the cornea only at the apex forming a bridge over the limbus under which a probe can be passed. It can occur anywhere around the cornea. It follows an occurrence of a corneal ulcer. A fold of the chemosed conjunctiva gets adherent to the progressive ulcer near the corneal margin and then this is being dragged across the cornea to some extent. Because of this there is a gap at the limbus and a probe can be passed.

Treatment

- Medical treatment is of no value. Surgical treatment is the only answer for a progressive pterygium.

- Simple excision.
- Bare sclera method.
- Excision with plastic repair.
- Transplantation.

PHLYCTEN

It is a pinkish white nodule near the limbus with localized hyperemia (Fig. 17.2). It may astride the limbus. If the overlying epithelium is destroyed then it presents with symptoms of photophobia, lacrimation, blepharospasm and pain. It can resolve spontaneously or progress resulting in a fascicular ulcer and may perforate. It is believed to be a delayed hypersensitivity (Type IV-cell mediated) response to endogenous microbial proteins especially to tubercular, staphylococcal or other bacterial antigens. It responds well to a short course of local steroids. Add antibiotic eye drops if there is an associated conjunctivitis. Improve the general health of the patient who are usually undernourished children living in unhygienic conditions. A healed Phlycten leaves a triangular scar with its base at the limbus.

VERNAL LIMBAL LESIONS

These appear as mucoid nodules. There may be one or more white superficial spots around the limbus. The limbus is surrounded by hyperemic edematous, thick gelatinous looking conjunctiva. Patient presents with

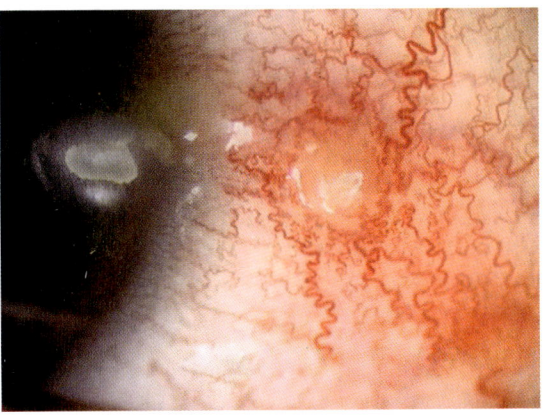

Fig. 17.2: Phlycten at limbus

intense itching, lacrimation, photophobia, foreign body sensation and burning of the eyes. It affects children and show exacerbations during spring season. Recently it has been suggested that it is an allergic disorder in which IgE mediated mechanisms play a role. Topical steroids control the symptoms. Sodium chromoglycate 2% drops are effective with no side effects. Steroids should be tapered to avoid the complication of steroid glaucoma and cataract.

SCLERITIS

- It affects elderly females more commonly than males.
- It is commonly associated with connective tissue disease like rheumatoid arthritis.
- Tuberculosis and sarcoidosis may be associated.
- It manifests as a nodular or diffuse form involving a segment or entire anterior sclera.
- The nodule is fixed and cannot be moved over sclera.
- It is characterized by pain and associated uveitis.
- Treat the cause. Topical steroids are helpful. Systemic indomethacin 50 to 100 mg daily for a long time provides relief. Aspirin is effective.

EPISCLERITIS

- It affects young people. It is benign, self limiting and recurrent disorder.
- It manifests as a nodular or diffuse form.
- It may be asymptomatic or accompanied by pain, tenderness, localized congestion and watering.

Treat by topical steroids. Systemic indomethacin 50 mg twice daily is helpful. Aspirin is effective.

CILIARY AND INTERCALARY STAPHYLOMA

i. *Ciliary staphyloma:* It occurs in the region of the ciliary body where the anterior ciliary arteries penetrate.
ii. *Intercalary staphyloma:* It occurs between the anterior extremity of the

ciliary body and the limbus where the sclera is weak due to presence of the anterior ciliary veins and the canal of Schlemm.

These are usually heavily pigmented. Due to uneven thinning of the sclera the staphyloma appears as lobulated and dark blue protrusions. It is difficult to distinguish the ciliary staphyloma from the intercalary staphyloma yet the location of the anterior ciliary arteries helps. In the ciliary staphyloma the anterior ciliary arteries emerge at the anterior border of the bulge and dark striae of the ciliary processes can be seen on transillumination. In the intercalary staphyloma the anterior ciliary arteries emerge posteriorly.

PAPILLOMA

The papilloma at the limbus can be sessile or peduncle. It is a benign polypoid tumor. It has a tendency to undergo malignant changes. A complete and careful surgical excision is the only treatment.

NAEVI

A naevi usually presents as grey or gelatinous, brown or black or flat or raised nodule near the limbus (Fig. 17.3). Slit lamp examination shows cystic spaces within the substance. It has a tendency to increase during puberty and pregnancy. As it does not undergo malignant change therefore it does not require an excision. Excision is only indicated for cosmetic reasons. Excision should be carried to include the entire lesion with bare sclera technique.

GRANULOMA

A granuloma can occur at the limbus. It grows after a surgical wound or at the site of a foreign body. It consists of granulation tissue. Treat by surgical excision of the tissue with cautery or cryo.

DERMOID

The dermoid appears as yellow whitish tumor mass usually astride the limbus on the temporal side. It consists of epidermoid epithelium with sebaceous glands and hair. The projecting hairs are diagnostic (Fig. 17.4). Treat by surgical excision.

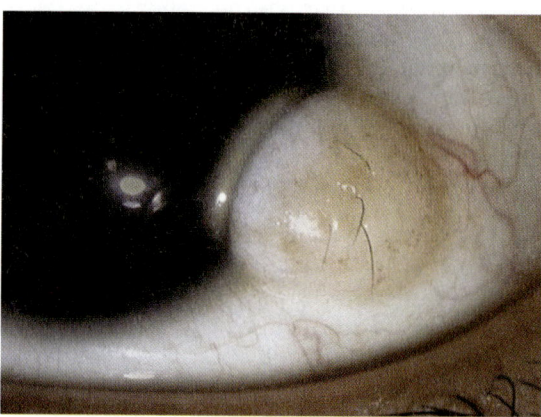

Fig. 17.4: Dermoid at limbus

DERMOLIPOMA

It is a congenital tumor seen at the limbus and may be associated with accessory auricles and other congenital defects. It consists of adipose tissue with surrounding dermis like connective tissue. These are soft, yellow and movable sub-conjunctival mass (Fig. 17.5). Treat by surgical excision.

INTRAEPITHELIAL EPITHELIOMA

It begins at the limbus and spreads to involve the cornea and fornices. It is a premalignant

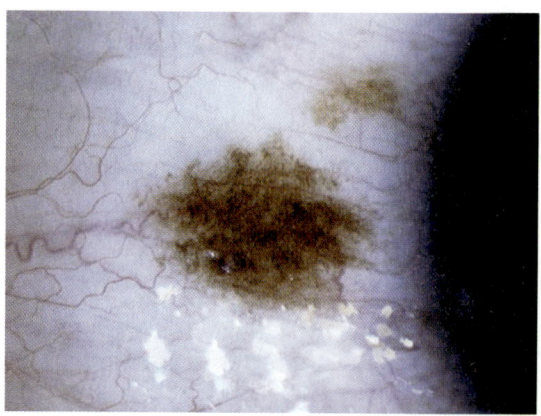

Fig. 17.3: Nevus at limbus

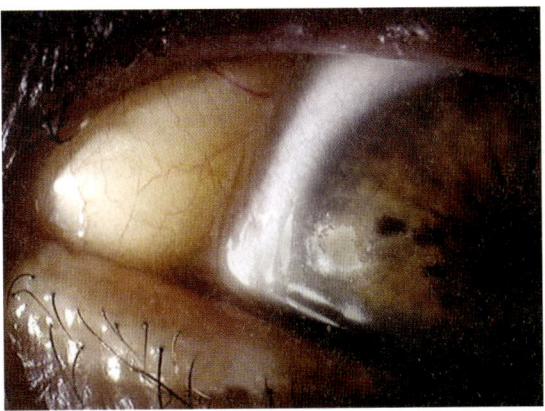

Fig. 17.5: Dermolipoma

tumor of the conjunctival epithelium. It appears as a raised fleshy mass or a gelatinous avascular tumor. Treat by surgical excision, cryo-therapy or both.

SQUAMOUS CELL CARCINOMA

It occurs where one kind of epithelium passes into other. It is common at the limbus. To begin with it appears as a flat granular growth. It is characterized by deep invasion of the stroma with fixation to the underlying tissue. It requires early, complete and careful surgical excision.

PRIMARY MELANOMA

A primary nodular form of malignant conjunctiva melanoma commonly arises at limbus. It may be pigmented or non-pigmented. Treat by complete and careful excision.

RETENTION CYST

It appears as a thin walled cyst with clear fluid and almost symptomless (Fig. 17.6). Treat by surgical excision.

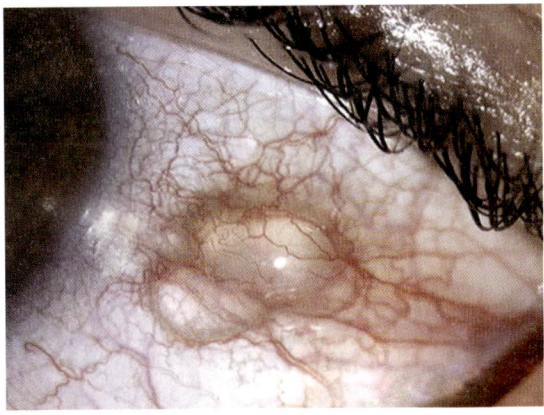

Fig. 17.6: Conjunctival cyst at limbus

18

A Case with Corneal Lesions

History

Record the history. Ask specially about the following symptoms related to corneal lesions.

- *Pain:* The cornea is supplied by the sensory nerve ending of first division of trigeminal (fifth) nerve. Any lesion of cornea wherein the epithelium is disturbed shall cause pain.
- *Photophobia:* Photophobia is an undue sensitivity of cornea even to a normal luminosity. It is due to light induced miosis of inflamed iris.
- *Lacrimation:* Lacrimation is an excessive production of tears. It is due to reflex irritation of corneal nerve endings of first division of fifth nerve.
- Halos: Halos are due to diffraction of light due to edema of the corneal tissue.
- Dim vision: Any lesion in the center of cornea shall result in dim vision. A lesion at periphery does not disturb the vision.
- Lid Edema and blepharospasm: There is swelling of the lid and patient keeps the eye closed to avoid photophobia and pain which occurs even in blinking.
- Systemic disease: Ask for any systemic disease, especially diabetes and use of steroids for any reason.

CLINICAL EXAMINATION OF CORNEA

The cornea is the most accessible structure of the eye for complete clinical examination. Look for the following

- Luster of the cornea.
- Opacity of cornea.
- Circumciliary congestion.
- Edema of cornea.
- Punctate epithelial erosions.
- Filaments.
- Superficial punctate keratitis.
- Neovascularization.
- Deposits on the anterior surface of the cornea.
- Pigmentation of the cornea.
- Keratic precipitates.
- Synechia.
- Abrasions of cornea.
- Ulcer of cornea.
- Hypopyon.
- Mark of injury, scar or adhesion of iris.
- Nodule at the limbus of cornea.
- Any growth of a membrane or vessels on the cornea.
- Dendritic figure on the cornea.
- Scars, pustules, eczema around the eye on the skin.

CLINICAL INVESTIGATION OF CORNEA

Inspection

An examination by a torch and loupe provides basic information about the condition of cornea. In infants and small children torch and loupe is the only method which can be used. Examine the cornea from all sides, throwing the light from all the direction. This helps even to locate a minute lesion or foreign body.

Slit Lamp Biomicroscopy

The slit lamp is the most useful instrument for the examination of cornea. The light beam can be adjusted to vary the width, height and angle of incidence. The microscope and the light beam can be aligned or redirected to view the lesion from different angle (Fig. 18.1).

There are six methods of biomicroscopy by the slit lamp (Fig. 18.2)

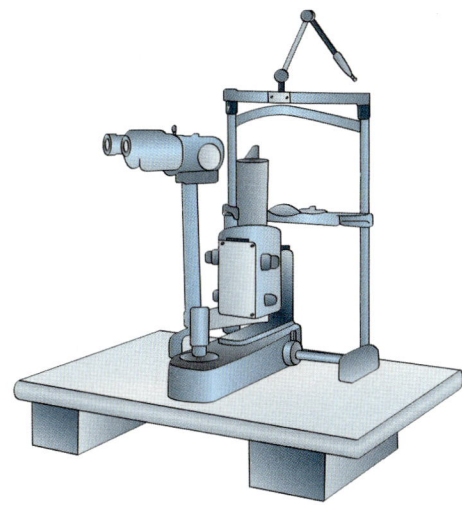

Fig. 18.1: Slit lamp

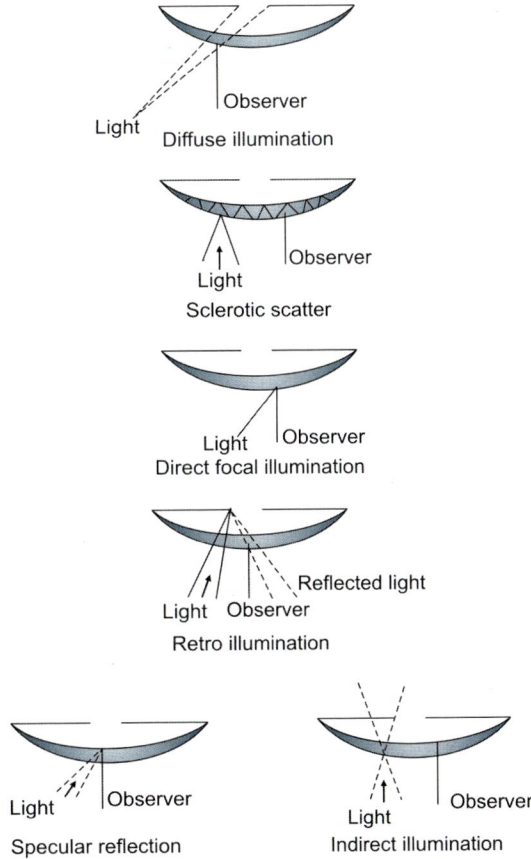

Fig. 18.2: Methods of slit lamp biomicroscopy

Diffuse Illumination

Use a wide beam and keep it slightly out of focus and view the whole cornea from one side to the other. It is like an examination with a torch.

Sclerotic Scatter

Direct a narrow beam at the temporal limbus and focus the microscope centrally on the cornea. In this method, the light from the temporal limbus is transmitted within the cornea by the total internal reflection and exit at the opposite (nasal) limbus. In a normal cornea no light is seen. Any stromal or epithelial opacities gets illuminated. Thus it is useful to diagnose any lesion of stroma or epithelium.

Direct Focal Illumination

In this test focus the slit beam and microscope at coincident points. This technique provides direct view of the structure under observation.

By altering the direction of beam and making it narrow it helps to locate the position of opacity and the depth of the lesion. This is the most common method of examination of cornea by the slit lamp.

Retro-illumination

In this method, the cornea is illuminated by the light reflected from the iris and fundus. Focus the light beam behind the cornea and the microscope on the cornea. By this method any changes in the epithelium, stroma, endothelium and keratic precipitates can be observed with magnification.

Specular Reflection

In this method, the cornea is observed adjacent to the beam. By altering the angle of beam a point is reached at which the reflection of the posterior corneal surface will allow visualization of the endothelial cell mosaic pattern, endothelial changes and folds in the Descemet's membrane. Similarly by altering the angle of beam the reflection of the anterior corneal surface will allow visualization of the pre-corneal tear film.

Indirect Illumination

Direct the beam of the light at the corneal opacity and observe with the microscope. Neovascularization stands out prominently in the scattered light.

Keratoscope

The keratoscope consists of circular disc with concentric circles white in color with gap in between each circle. The observer projects these circles on the cornea of the patient. If cornea is spherical the reflected image of the circles will be uniform. If there is a change in the curvature of the cornea then the image of the circles can be elliptical, irregular or wavy. This test is good for a quick screening of cases. If it shows change in the curvature then the patient can be further examined by keratometer. One can keep a record by photographic keratoscope (Fig. 18.3).

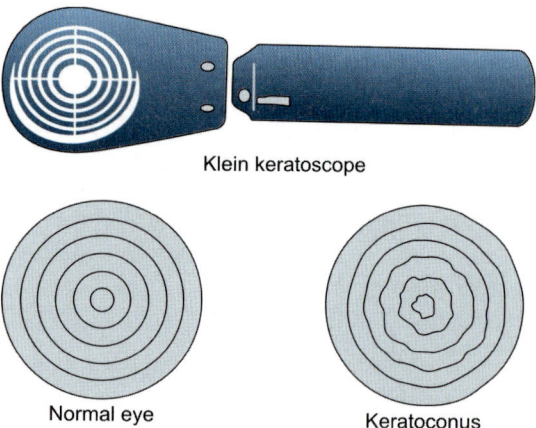

Klein keratoscope

Normal eye   Keratoconus

Fig 18.3: Keratoscope

Keratometry (Ophthalmometry)

It helps to determine the corneal curvature accurately and easily. The mires of the keratometer are seen by the observer when the instrument is in focus. The instrument is rotated to bring the mires in alignment to get the axis of the cylinder. The plus signs are superimposed to determine the radius in the horizontal meridian and the minus signs are superimposed to determine the curvature in the vertical meridian. Rotate the keratometer 90° and remeasure in the vertical meridian by aligning the plus targets. It has a range and it is not possible to measure the highly irregular cornea.

Pachometry

The instrument to measure the corneal thickness is known as a pachometer. The measurement of the thickness of the cornea is helpful to evaluate the cases of corneal decompensation, thickness in the keratoconus and corneal ulcers, cases for corneal transplant and radial keratotomy.

The central corneal thickness ranges between 0.49 and 0.56 mm. A reading of above 0.6 mm is suggestive of endothelial disease.
* Optical pachometry.
  It uses the image splitting device in the Haag-Streit slit lamp.
* Ultrasonic pachometry.
  It is a portable instrument. It is useful in cases for radial keratotomy.

Specular Microscopy

It helps in the study of endothelial cell density. The method helps to find out the various cellular characteristics like size, shape, density and distribution. It gives a photographic record. It is helpful in the surgical techniques of phacoemulsification and intraocular lens implant.

Tear Film Break-up Time

The tear film is composed of three layers
* External lipid layer
* Middle aqueous layer
* Internal mucus layer.

The lipid layer is formed by the lipids from the meibomian glands. The aqueous layer is formed by the tear fluid from the lacrimal glands. The mucus layer is formed from the secretion of the conjunctival goblet cells. The distribution of the tear film depends upon the normal blinking action of the lids which helps to spread the tear film over the pre-corneal surface with every blink. The corneal epithelial surface is hydrophobic. In the eye, the mucin is a natural wetting agent and plays an important role in the formation of a stable tear film. The tear film does not remain stable for a prolonged length of time. The formation of tear film is complex process. With each blink the mucin is distributed over the pre-corneal surface and in addition spreads the aqueous and lipids to form a three-layered tear film. Evaporation begins and tear film begins to thin. Some of the superficial lipids migrate within a minute creating an area over which the tear film becomes unstable, the tear film breaks up and forms the so-called dry spots on the cornea. With each blink the surface is polished and cycle repeats itself. The time taken between each blink and appearance of first dry spot is known as the "tear film break-up time." This is usually greater than the time between each blink. The normal break-up time is between 15 and 34 seconds. A breakup time of less than 10 seconds is taken as abnormal. There are wide variations of values in the same individual so this test is not clinically reliable. A premature rupture of tear film results in the dry state of the eye causing severe damage to the corneal epithelium.

Fluorescein Staining of Cornea

Fluorescein does not stain mucus. The dye remains extracellular. It stains the tear film therefore shows up epithelial corneal defects. It is lipophobic and so will not enter cells. If the lateral attachments between the epithelial cells are disturbed the tear film and dye will pass into the intercellular spaces and appear as staining. If there is epithelial defect then the dye will pass into the hydrophilic stroma and eventually into the aqueous humour. The staining appears as yellow-green hue in cobalt filter.

It is advisable to use fluorescein-impregnated sterile fiter paper strip for corneal staining.

Corneal Sensation

Ask the patient to keep the eye open and explain to him what you are going to do and what cooperation you expect from him. Touch the cornea of one eye with a wisp of moist cotton wool and compare it with the opposite normal eye. Repeat the test few times before coming to a conclusion. The sensitivity of the cornea decreases with age, after wearing a contact lens and after an attack of herpes simplex. The zone of greatest sensitivity is a small area of 5 mm in the center of cornea.

Tonometry

Tonometry is essential in cases of corneal diseases especially in cases with corneal edema, corneal scars, irregular cornea and in corneal transplant cases.

Laboratory Investigations

- Complete blood picture.
- Blood sugar.
- Complete urine examination.
- Stool examination.

Microbiological Investigations

It is required to identify causative organism, confirm the diagnosis and proper management of the corneal ulcer cases.

Instill a drop of local anesthetic (Xylocaine 2%) in the conjunctival sac. Under magnification collect the material by a Kimura spatula or by the bent tip of a 21-gauge hypodermic needle from the base and margin of the corneal ulcer. Transfer the material on to glass slides for staining and in culture media.

- Gram and Giemsa stain for possible identification of causative organism.
- KOH 10% wet preparation for identification of fungal infection.
- Calcofluor white (CFW) stained smears under fluorescence microscope for fungal filaments.

- Culture on blood agar medium for aerobic organisms.
- Culture on Sabouraud's dextrose agar medium for fungi.

Clinical Features and Management

1. Bacterial keratitis.
2. Mycotic keratitis.
3. Herpes simplex keratitis.
4. Herpes zoster ophthalmicus.
5. Mooren's ulcer.
6. Exposure keratitis.
7. Interstitial keratitis.
8. Disciform keratitis.
9. Cogan's syndrome.
10. Keratoconus.
11. Band-shaped keratopathy.
12. Salzmann nodular degeneration.
13. Anterior dystrophy of cornea.
14. Stromal dystrophy of cornea.
15. Posterior dystrophy of cornea.
16. Corneal vascularization.
17. Keratic precipitates.
18. Corneal staphyloma.
19. Cystoid cicatrix and fistula.
20. Krukenberg's pigment spindle.
21. Blood staining of cornea.
22. Vogt's white limbal girdle.
23. Wilson's disease.
24. Posterior keratoconus.
25. Keratoglobus.
26. Rosacea keratitis.
27. Corneal deposits.

BACTERIAL KERATITIS

Clinical Features

- Bacterial keratitis occurs due to pyogenic bacteria such as *Pseudomonas, Staphylococcus aureus and albus, Pneumococcus, Neisseria gonorrhoeae, Escherichia coli which usually invade the cornea by exogenous route.* The organisms which can penetrate an intact epithelium are *Neisseria gonorrhoeae* and *Corynebacterium diphtheriae.*
- Most common predisposing factor is chronic infection of ocular adenexa or trauma or use of steroids.
- A bacterial ulcer due to *Staphylococcus* tends to be oval yellow white with opaque stromal suppuration. The cornea surrounding the ulcer is relatively clear.
- A bacterial ulcer due to *Pseudomonas* tends to be an irregular ulcer with sharp margin, necrosis and the surrounding stroma appear opaque. There is thick mucopurulent exudate. It tends to progress rapidly and cause perforation.
- All the signs and symptoms of corneal involvement are present such as pain, lacrimation, photophobia, circumciliary congestion, swelling of the lid, blepharospasm and blurred vision.
- Fluorescein staining is always positive.
- There may be associated signs of iritis like aqueous flare, hypopyon and posterior synechia.

Management

Bacterial corneal ulcer is a vision threatening or even blinding condition. It demands urgent and energetic treatment. Patient should be hospitalized to provide consistent and intensive therapy under observation.

Topical Antibiotics

Collect the material by scrapping for Gram stain, culture and sensitivity.

Debridement of the ulcer bed and margins to remove the necrosed material by spatula under local anesthesia is essential.

Start initial intense antibiotic therapy to cover both gram-negative and gram-positive organisms. Do not wait for results of culture and sensitivity. Later change the antibiotic according to sensitivity.

- Sub-conjunctival injection and or systemic antibiotics should be given in severe cases.
- Cauterization of the ulcer may be considered in un-responsive cases.
- Keep the intra-ocular pressure low by systemic therapy with acetazolamide 250 mg twice a day for 3–5 days to enhance the healing.
- Use atropine eye drops in every case to treat iritis and prevent posterior synechia and to provide relief from pain due to ciliary spasm.

- Treat any associated systemic disease especially diabetes or causative factor.
- Be careful to differentiate between persistent infection and delay or failure of re-epithelialization due to drug toxicity. Do not over treat the case.
- Supportive therapy in form of analgesics, vitamins, bed rest, nourishing diet, no strain on the eyes and protection by goggles.

MYCOTIC KERATITIS

Clinical Features

- Mycotic keratitis is rare.
- It is common in the persons engaged in agriculture area and during harvesting season.
- It is usually preceded by trauma to cornea with vegetable matter like leaf, straw, hay, thorn, branch of a bush or sapling, any decaying vegetable matter, animal tail, etc.
- It is common among patients who are immune-suppressed systemically or locally such as cases suffering from dry eye or herpetic keratitis.
- Excessive intake of antibiotics and steroids for a long time predisposes the patient to mycotic infection.
- The common causative fungi are *Aspergillus*, *Fusarium* and *Candida albicans*.
- Ulcer presents as a dry-looking, grey white, elevated and rolled out margins with multiple small satellite foci around the ulcer and feathery finger like projection in the adjacent stroma under the intact epithelium.
- The eye shows less reaction in comparison to a bacterial ulcer even with the presence of hypopyon in a small ulcer.
- Corneal vascularization is conspicuously absent.
- Corneal perforation is rare.
- Material for culture should be sent.

Management

- Examination of the wet KOH scrapping under microscope is helpful.

- Gram, Giemsa and Calcofluor white-stained films for fungal hyphae shall be useful.
- Scrapping for culture should be sent.
- **Systemic antifungal drug**—ketoconazole and Fluconazoletosine.
- **Systemic and local antibiotic**—if there is a suspicion of superadded bacterial infection.
- **Topical antifungal eye drops and ointment**—Nystatin 3.5% eye ointment, Natamycin 5% eye drops and or Fluconazol 0.2% eye drops for 6–8 weeks.
- Use atropine eye drops to provide relief from pain and prevent uveitis.
- Do not use corticosteroids.
- Some cases may need a therapeutic corneal graft.
- Most cases with a central ulcer require corneal graft to improve vision as the ulcer leaves a thick leucomatous opacity of cornea on healing.
- Advise prophylaxis to the people working in agriculture field especially by use of plain glasses to avoid injury to cornea.

HERPES SIMPLEX KERATITIS

Keratitis due to herpes simplex virus is quite common. HSV-1 causes infection above the waist involving skin, lips and eyes. HSV-1 infection is acquired by kissing and usually occurs in early years of life from parents or relatives due to expression of love for the child.

HSV-2 causes infection below the waist affecting genitals (genital herpes). HSV-2 infection is acquired by sexual contact and usually occurs in teenage or adult life.

Clinical Features

- Ophthalmologist is primarily concerned with HSV-1 type of infection.
- There is always a stress stimulus for recurrence. It can be: low resistance, following fever, flu, malaria, exposure to extreme heat, cold, and wind, emotional stress, use of steroid-topically or systemically and use of immune-suppressive drugs.

- Skin lesions involving lids, periorbital region and lid margin show vesicles which rapidly forms crusts and heals without scar.
- Preauricular lymphadenopathy.
- Follicular conjunctivitis with mild lacrimation.
- Fine epithelial punctate keratitis.
- Dendritic figure in the cornea (Fig. 18.4).
- Patient may show a geographical ulcer one or more.
- In course of time sub-epithelial infiltration occurs.
- Lesion may progress to disciform keratitis.
- Diminished corneal sensitivity.
- Fluorescein staining is present.
- Anterior uveitis and keratic precipitates occur late.
- It heals leaving scar which is usually thin nebular type.

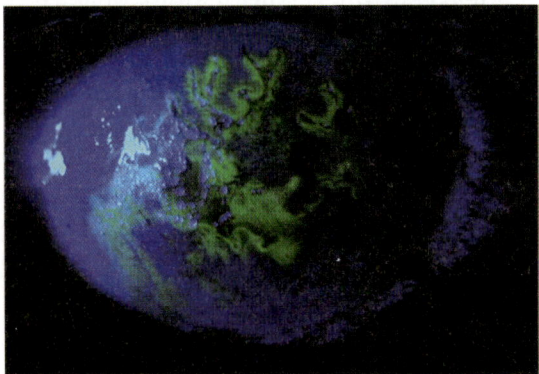

Fig. 18.4: Herpes simplex keratitis

Management

- Antiviral eye drops and eye ointment topically is the first line of treatment. If there is no response in 7 days then change the antiviral drug. If there is good response then taper the instillation and discontinue by 14th day.

Antiviral Drugs in Use

- *Acycloguanosine:* Acyclovir, zovirax 3% ointment-apply five times a day. It is least toxic and most commonly used drug. It gives good response. It gets in viral infected cells. It can penetrate intact corneal epithelium and stroma. It can be used for both the epithelial lesions and stromal lesions. If no response in 7 days then change the drug.
- Trifluorothymidine 1% drops
  It is given two hourly during the day. Ulcer heals in about two weeks. It is more toxic than acyclovir.
- Adenine arabinoside 3% ointment five times a day.
- Ganciclovir (0.15% gel) five times a day. It is more toxic than acyclovir.
- **Cauterization** is needed in few cases.

Debridement

It is an effective way for dendritic ulcers. With advent of effective antiviral drugs it has been abandoned.

Steroids

Steroids in low strength with antiviral drugs cover is indicated for stromal herpes-disciform keratitis. Try to taper and discontinue periodically. Some patients may require one drop daily for several weeks.

- **Supportive treatment** to encounter the stress stimulus that leads to recurrence of the malady.

HERPES ZOSTER OPHTHALMICUS

Herpes zoster ophthalmicus is an acute infection of the ophthalmic division of the trigeminal—the fifth cranial nerve by the *varicella-zoster* virus. This virus produces acidophilic intranuclear inclusion bodies. It is neurotropic in nature.

Clinical Features

- Onset occurs with fever, malaise and pain only in half side of face.
- A severe pain strictly limited to half side of the face must arouse suspicion. Even the air of fan induces neuralgia. Combing of the hair also induces neuralgia. It occurs before the appearance of the vesicles. It is diagnostic. Treatment at this stage shall abort the malady.

- The frontal nerve is more frequently affected than the lacrimal and nasociliary nerves.
- About 10% of all cases of herpes zoster affect the ophthalmic division of fifth nerve.
- Ocular complications occur in 50% of cases. Ocular examination may show follicular conjunctivitis with petechial hemorrhages with preauricular lymphadenopathy.
- Hutchinson's rule—implies that the cornea is mostly involved if the nasociliary branch of the first divisions has been involved showing pox like lesions at the side and or tip of the nose.
- It is soon followed by vesicular rash. It becomes pastular which breaks to form crusting ulcers. There is edema of the lids and edema around the orbit. The active eruptive phase lasts for 3 weeks. The skin lesions heal leaving pitted scars.
- *Keratitis:* Mild cases in which only epithelium is involved show a mild punctate keratitis followed by sub-epithelial infiltrates and heals with thin nebular scar.

  In severe cases there is stromal keratitis which heals leaving a thick scar. It is usually associated with anterior uveitis and keratic precipitates.
- The intraocular pressure is raised.

Sequelae

- Cranial nerve palsies usually affecting the third, fourth, sixth nerve and seventh. The palsy recovers within six months.
- Optic neuritis occurs in about 1% cases. So keep watch on vision.
- Post herpetic neuralgia known as anesthesia dolorosa. It is associated with mild anesthesia of the affected area.
- The scars appear as punched out or pitted scars.
- Iris shows sector atrophy and a moth-eaten appearance.
- Hair loss.

Management

It needs early and energetic treatment to prevent ocular complications, to promote healing of skin lesions and post herpetic neuralgia.

Systemic Therapy

Antiviral antibiotic: Acyclovir (zovirax) 400 mg tablet 5 times a day for 10 days. Start the drug as soon as rash appears. It helps to curtail vesicles and enhances healing. It also helps in reducing the pain during eruptive phase.

Analgesic: It is needed to provide relief from neuralgia.

Steroids: These should be given if there are neurological complications.

Local Therapy

Antibiotic and steroid skin ointment three times a day till skin lesions heal.

Xylocaine skin ointment should be applied over skin lesion to provide relief from pain.

Topical Therapy for Corneal Lesions

Acyclovir (3%) eye ointment five times a day for two weeks.

Atropine 1% drops once a day to prevent uveitis.

Steroid eye drops four times a day-for 2 weeks or so.

Antibiotic eye drops to prevent or cure secondary infection.

With advent of good antiviral drugs and use of steroids the patients usually respond well leaving no complication.

MOOREN'S ULCER
(Chronic Serpiginous Ulcer, Ulcus Rodens)

Mooren's ulcer is a chronic superficial ulcer of unknown etiology.

Clinical Features

- In early stage the ulcer looks like a marginal ulcer with grey infiltration near the margin of the cornea.
- It spreads slowly with undermining the corneal epithelium at its advancing edge

which can be lifted up—a characteristic feature.
- This ulcer can spread round the periphery of the cornea, or in towards the center of cornea or occasionally into the sclera.
- There is a tendency to involve the entire cornea.
- There is no tendency to perforation.
- Healing takes place from the periphery with neovascularization. The healed areas with no superficial layers and heavily vascularized remain permanently cloudy with very low vision.
- Patient complains of severe pain and progress of the ulcer continues.
- Prognosis is bad.

Management

- The classical treatment is the excision of the overhanging edge and free cauterization.
- Conjunctival graft has been tried.
  Lamellar graft has been found to be useful. Treatment is unsatisfactory. Try all the possible means to help the patient to alleviate his pain.

EXPOSURE KERATITIS

Exposure keratitis occurs due to improper wetting of the corneal surface though there is normal secretion of tear fluid. This is due to inability of the lids to polish the cornea with each blink due to lagophthalmos. The common causes are lack of normal Bell's phenomenon, exposure of cornea during sleep or coma, cicatricial entropion or ectropion, seventh nerve palsy, exophthalmos, proptosis and Parkinson's disease.

Pathogenesis

The epithelium of the exposed cornea dries up followed by desiccation. The epithelium is cast off and thereby falls prey to infective organisms. The initial desiccation occurs in the inter palpebral area or lower peripheral part of the cornea resulting in fine punctate epithelial keratitis. It is followed by necrosis then ulcer with vascularization.

Clinical Features

- Diagnosis can be made easily by asking the patient to close the lids normally. Within a minute or two one can observe a small opening between the lids exposing the conjunctiva and lower part of the cornea.
- The exposed conjunctiva and cornea looses the normal luster.
- Superficial vascularization of the cornea.
- Superficial erosions of cornea or even ulcer may be seen in the inferior part of cornea.
- Fluorescein staining may show punctate erosions or ulcer.

Management

- Tarsorrhaphy—If the process is likely to be permanent then tarsorrhaphy is the ideal choice. This will save the eye and relieve the patient of his discomfort.
- If the process is likely to be of temporary nature then use.
- Artificial tear eyedrops.
- Soft bandage contact lens.
- Airtight goggles.
- At night keep lids closed by a piece of tape from lid to cheek.

INTERSTITIAL KERATITIS

It is an inflammation of the stroma of the cornea without primary involvement of the epithelium or endothelium. It is associated with congenital syphilis, tuberculosis and Cogan's syndrome.

Congenital Syphilis

Interstitial keratitis is a late manifestation of congenital syphilis. It is characterized by:
- Bilateral diffuse mid-stromal clouding of cornea due to cellular infiltration causing marked reduction in the visual acuity.
- Deep vascularization.
- Salmon patch appearance is typical of it.

Treat by systemic penicillin and topical cycloplegics and steroids (Fig. 18.5).

Tuberculosis

- It is usually unilateral and sectorial.

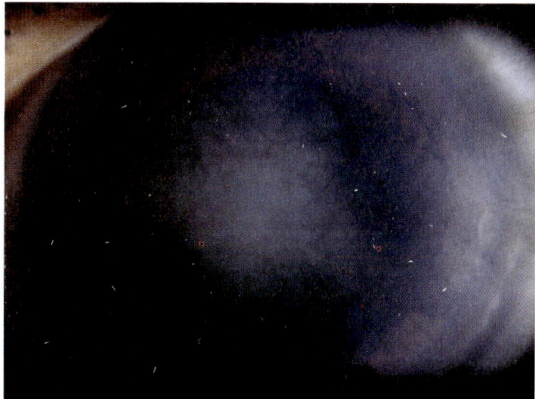

Fig. 18.5: Interstitial keratitis

- Cornea appears cloudy.
- Deep vascularization.

Treat with systemic anti-tubercular drugs and topical cycloplegics and steroids.

DISCIFORM KERATITIS

Disciform keratitis is characterized by a disk like opacity in the stroma of the cornea, often concentric in nature, usually following minor trauma or viral infection. The herpes is the most common cause. Most probably it is a manifestation of an antigen-antibody reaction, induced by the repeated entry of antigen into the sensitized stroma of the cornea.

Clinical Features

There is an interstitial haze in the cornea. The cornea appears rough and hazy. Slit lamp examination shows minute grey spots which takes up a shape of a disk, folds in the Descemet's membrane and few keratic precipitates. There is usually a clear space between the disk like opacity and corneal epithelium, though there may be some edema. Later, there is deep vascularization.

- There is always presence of irritation, pain, lacrimation, photophobia, circumciliary congestion and signs of mild anterior uveitis.
- The lesion remains localized. It may resolve rapidly. Usually it leaves a permanent scar in the cornea. It runs a long course, for months.

Management

- As the most common cause is a trauma, or viral infection, thus treat the case to eliminate the infection by proper antibiotics and antiviral drugs, locally.
- Due to its immunological reaction, it responds well to local steroids. Take care to eliminate the viral infection, before commencing the steroid therapy.

COGAN'S SYNDROME

Cogan's syndrome is characterized by a non-syphilitic interstitial keratitis associated with vestibule-auditory symptoms first described by Cogan.

Ocular Features

The interstitial keratitis is bilateral and presents with pain, photophobia, circumciliary congestion, dim vision, patchy infiltration of deep corneal stroma and mild uveitis.

Aural Features

There is vertigo, tinnitus and nerve deafness. The aural symptoms may precede or follow the onset of ocular features.

The etiology is unknown. The syndrome appears to be a part of a general hypersensitivity reaction affecting particularly the eye and ear due to factors such as Periarteritis nodosa, vasomotor disturbances, viral infection and also following intake of drugs and chemical poisons. It has been seen in association with diseases with infiltrative processes like sarcoidosis, Hodgkin's disease and mycosis pungoides.

KERATOCONUS

Keratoconus denotes—a non-inflammatory, bilateral, asymmetric ectasia of the cornea characterized by thining of the apical cornea and corneal scarring of obscure etiology. Usually it is bilateral though one eye may be more affected. It manifests at puberty.

It may be associated with numerous other ocular abnormalities such as retinitis pigmentosa, Leber's optic atrophy, vernal conjunctivitis, ectopia lentis, Congenital cataract, aniridia, Down syndrome and Marfan's syndrome.

Clinical Features

- Patient complains of gradual loss of vision, photophobia and monocular diplopia.
- It is almost invariably bilateral.
- It usually manifests at the puberty and more common in females.
- Most of the cases do not have a positive family history.
- Visual acuity is markedly reduced with distorted vision.
- There is dim vision with myopic astigmatism.
- Retinoscopy will reveal a scissor shadow.
- Refraction shows a high degree of irregular myopic astigmatism.
- Photo-keratoscopy shows compression of mires infero-temporarily-**Egg-shaped mires**.
- Keratometry will give high cylinders with oblique axis.
- Corneal sensation is diminished.
- There is a peculiar unusual glistening and lustre in the central area of the cornea.
- **Munson's sign:** There is an angular curve of the lower lid margin when the patient looks down.
- **Slit lamp** shows the following:
  i. Thinning of the cornea at the apex even to the extent that the pulse beat of the intraocular pressure may be clearly seen.
  ii. An endothelial reflex in the central portion of the cornea due to increased concavity of the posterior surface.
  iii. **Vogt's striae:** Vertical lines in the deeper layers of the stroma due to stretching phenomenon.
  iv. Increased visibility of the nerve fibres.
  v. **Fleischer's ring** at the base of the cone.
  vi. Ruptures in the Descemet's membrane.
  vii. Ruptures in the Bowman's membrane.

Management

Corneal Collagen Cross-linking

It is a new technique of corneal collagen cross-linking (CXL or C3R) by the photosensitizer riboflavin and ultraviolet type rays (UVA). It increases biomechanical strength of cornea and thereby arrests the progression of keratoconus. This is used only in cases in whom progression of keratoconus has been well documented.

Phakic IOLs

Phakic implants can be used to correct or reduce the refractive error.

Contact Lens

Contact lens improves the vision. The optimal correction can be provided by plain rigid gas permeable lenses.

Intacs

Intracorneal ring segments can be used to decrease astigmatism.

Full Thickness Keratoplasty

Once it is concluded that the condition is progressive then it is better to put a graft early rather than wait and allow the cornea to get damaged.

BAND-SHAPED KERATOPATHY (Girdle-Shaped opacity, Ribbon-Shaped Opacity, Band Keratitis, Zonular Opacity, and Trophic Keratitis)

Band-shaped keratopathy is characterized by the development of a grey-white band of opacity in the exposed part of the cornea in the palpebral aperture slightly below the middle of the pupil (Fig. 18.6).

Clinical Features

The first change is appearance of slight opacity at the level of Bowman's membrane in which dark round holes are seen by slit lamp examination. This change occurs initially near the periphery with a clear zone between the opacity and the limbus.

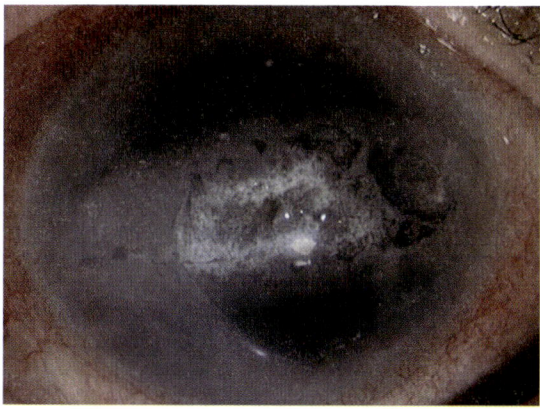

Fig. 18.6: Band-shaped keratopathy

- Gradually the opacity spreads towards the center resulting in an unbroken band across the cornea in the palpebral aperture.
- To begin with the opacity is situated below the epithelium. Later there are changes in the epithelium giving an appearance with many grey dots, holes and chalk like white crusts.
- There is deposition of calcium salts in the sub-epithelial space and on Bowman's membrane and superficial stroma as seen by slit lamp. The overlying epithelium is usually intact though it is irregular.
- Fluorescein stain shows staining of epithelium in a punctate manner.

There are Four Categories

Secondary to ocular disease: It is the most common type and is seen in case of uveitis, usually in old people with degenerated and soft eye. It may be seen in cases with Still's disease in children and following interstitial keratitis and glaucoma of long standing in adults.

Traumatic cases: It is rare but seen in the eyes which are exposed to a constant irritant such as mercury and calomel.

Constitutional: It may be seen in cases of hypercalcemia due to hyperparathyroidism or vitamin D poisoning in the treatment of sarcoidosis or osteoporosis.

Primary band-shaped keratopathy: It is rare and can be seen in young age and old age without any obvious cause in apparently normal eye.

Management

The best treatment is to provide a lamellar graft. There are no symptoms till the epithelium is intact. There is usually mild irritation with dim vision. The patient usually comes for cosmetic reasons. If no local etiological factor, then rule out systemic factors.

Chemical chelation is the mainstay of management.

Phototherapeutic keratectomy with an excimer laser.

SALZMANN'S NODULAR DEGENERATION

It is seen in cases with old phlyctenular keratits, trachoma, or interstitial keratitis. It is characterized by elevated sub-epithelial nodules in an opaque cornea or at the edge of a transparent cornea. The Bowman's layer is replaced by scar tissue and the epithelium is irregular. Keratoplasty is indicated.

ANTERIOR DYSTROPHY

Recurrent Corneal Erosion Syndrome

The important and common cause is trauma in the form of a scratch. A deficiency in the basement membrane or lack of hemidesmosomes attaching the basal cell layer of the corneal epithelium to the basement membrane plays an important role. It is more prevalent in diabetics and associated with Cogan's dystrophy and other corneal dystrophies.

- The patient awakes from the sleep with pain, lacrimation, photophobia and blurred vision.
- The recurrence can occur for months.
- Some patients respond well to topical artificial tears four times a day and an eye ointment at bed time.
- A severe case with recurrence may be treated by removing the entire epithelium and allowing regeneration of a new and stable epithelium.

Microcystic (Cogan's) Dystrophy

It is one of the most common dystrophy of corneal epithelium seen in clinical practice. It is characterized by dot like cysts, or linear lesions, or bleb like lesion, involving both the eyes. The pattern and the distribution of lesions show a change, if observed for a long time. About 10% cases develop recurrent corneal erosion syndrome usually after the age of thirty.

Reis-Buckler's Dystrophy

It presents in early childhood. It has an autosomal dominant inheritance. It is characterized by superficial ring-shaped opacities which appears like a honeycomb. Most cases develop recurrent erosions. It needs a grafting operation lamellar or penetrating to improve the vision.

STROMAL DYSTROPHY

Lattice Dystrophy

It presents with recurrent erosions during the end of first decade of life. It is characterized by branching spider like deposits of amyloid which interlace and overlap at different level within the stroma of cornea affecting central part and sparing the periphery. It is progressive and by the age of about thirty there is marked corneal haze with diminished corneal sensation, causing loss of vision thereby necessitating keratoplasty.

Granular Dystrophy

It is also a slowly progressive dystrophy presenting in the first decade of life. It is characterized by presence of discrete, crumb-like, white granules of hyline within the anterior stroma. The lesions spread deeper but leave the periphery. It is asymptomatic but some cases may develop recurrent corneal erosions. Patient usually complains of difficulty in night driving due to scattering of the light. A case with dim vision needs keratoplasty.

Macular Dystrophy

Though it is rare but affects vision much more. It is characterized by grey white opacities consisting of glycosaminoglycan. The corneal stroma in between the lesions is cloudy. In course of time the entire stroma gets involved including the periphery which differentiates it from other stromal dystrophies. Keratoplasty is the choice for providing vision.

POSTERIOR DYSTROPHY

Cornea Guttata

It is a common dystrophy characterized by focal accumulations of collagen on the posterior surface of Descemet's membrane giving an appearance of warts of Descemet's membrane. Specular microscopy shows dark spots when the lesions disrupt the regular endothelial mosaic pattern. In advanced cases it shows a beaten metal appearance. It occurs as a part of aging or as part of early Fuch's endothelial dystrophy. These lesions in the periphery are called as Hassall-Henle bodies.

Fuch's Endothelial Dystrophy

- It affects elderly females, more commonly.
- It is usually bilateral.
- It is slowly progressive.
- In early stage, the changes consist of cornea guttata which become numerous and spreads to periphery.
- Later endothelial decompensation causes edema of stroma.
- Later there is epithelial edema which results in bullous keratopathy causing pain.
- Edema and vascularization of stroma causes marked loss of vision.
- Keratoplasty provides relief and vision.

Posterior Polymorphous Dystrophy

It is a congenital dystrophy characterized by presence of vesicular geographical band-like opacities on the posterior surface of cornea. Later there is endothelial decompensation causing edema of the stroma and epithelium. There is marked loss of vision. Keratoplasty is indicated. Glaucoma may be associated with this so it is essential to examine the angle before planning for keratoplasty.

CORNEAL VASCULARIZATION

The cornea is invaded by blood vessels in a pathological state primarily as a defense mechanism against the disease or injury. It has a beneficial effect in resolving an inflammatory lesion. The invasion of cornea by blood vessels results in some loss of transparency and is the cause of opacification of graft due to development of antigen-antibody reaction by providing antibodies.

Clinical Examination

Focal illumination: The vessel wall reflect enough light to appear as a white streak.

Retro-illumination: The new vessels stand out as dark lines in a clear cornea. The vessels are easily visible in an opaque cornea.

Clinical Types

Superficial Vascularization

In superficial vascularization of cornea the vessels originates from the superficial limbal plexus by budding or loop formation and pass without interruption. The superficial vascularization can be Pannus, Fascicular and Equalet.

Pannus: An extensive superficial vascularization of cornea has been termed as a pannus. Pannus can be of four types:
- Pannus trachomatous.
- Pannus leprosus.
  Pannus phlyctenulosus.
- Pannus degenerativus.

Interstitial Vascularization

It is derived from the anterior ciliary arteries. The new vessels are straight and non-anastomosing. On examination the vessels appear to disappear from the view as they traverse the boundary between the cornea and the sclera. It can be of the following types:

Terminal loops: There is a growth of small loops which grow out from the limbus in a deeper plane.

Brush form: The vessels run in the substantia propria parallel and without any anastomosis giving an appearance of a brush.

Umbel form: A large vessel run far into the cornea and then breaks up into a star-shaped branches.

Network form: There is a free communication of loops to give an appearance of a network.

Interstitial arcades: These are derived from episcleral vessels and seen in the anterior portion of the cornea typically in the sclerosing lesions due to tuberculosis and leprosy.

Aberrant vessels: The vessels arise from episcleral vessels and traverse the stroma of the cornea in an irregular fashion.

Deep Vascularization

It is a rare phenomenon, occurring in interstitial keratitis of syphilitic origin when associated with uveitis. The vessels invade along the deepest layers of the stroma in front of Descemet's membrane.

Treatment: An early treatment results in reducing the opacification of cornea. An infective lesion should be treated by suitable antibiotic. Other treatments available are:
- Use of steroids locally and sub-conjunctivally.
- Peritomy.
- Superficial keratectomy.
- Lamellar corneal graft.
- Irradiation.

KERATIC PRECIPITATES

The deposition of material on the posterior surface of cornea is known as keratic precipitates. These can be seen clearly by slit lamp biomicroscopy, with direct illumination, retro-illumination and specular reflection. These vary in size, shape and distribution. The distribution depends on convection currents in the anterior chamber, gravity and changes in the endothelial cells. These may appear in a vertical line (Ehrlich-Tuck Line), fusiform shape, triangular shape, disseminated, centrally placed, peripherally placed and in irregular islets.

Physiological Precipitates

Cellular elements: These are seen on the endothelial surface of cornea. These are leucocytes circulating in the anterior chamber. These can be differentiated from pathological deposits by their slow amoeboid movements and absence of any tendency to agglutination.

Pigmented deposits: These are seen in old age—a senile change usually in people above the age of eighty. These are fine and adopt a triangular shape seen in the lower half of cornea.

Pathological Precipitates

Clinically, the most important is the deposition of cellular and fibrinous inflammatory precipitates popularly known as kp The appearance of these precipitates is preceded by bedewing of the corneal endothelium. Thereafter large aggregations of leucocytes and fibrin appear sometimes with pigment. These have been described under various names such as star map precipitates, mutton fat kp, plastic precipitates which have only a morphological value giving no etiological conclusion. As the inflammation subsides these may disappear completely or few may persist for years. The old precipitates appear thin, pale, translucent and show crenated edges (Fig. 18.7).

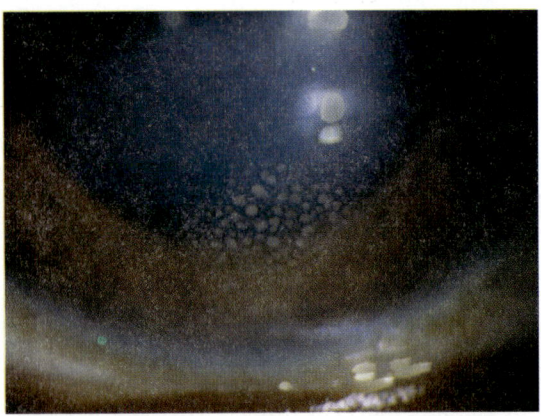

Fig. 18.7: Mutton-fat KP

CORNEAL STAPHYLOMA

Corneal staphyloma is an ectatic condition of the extensive corneal defect in which the uveal tissue gets incarcerated. It usually follows extensive corneal ulcer which has sloughed and cast off leaving an extensive corneal wound with incarceration of the iris. At this stage the iris is directly covered by the epithelium derived from the peripheral ring of the intact healthy cornea left after sloughing of the corneal ulcer. The citatrization may be rapid and dense so that it can withstand the intraocular pressure and the cornea becomes flat resulting in **applanatio corneae**. In some cases there may be rapid degeneration and shrinkage of the corneal scar tissue resulting in a contracted and shrunken scar-**Phthisis Corneae**. Most often the pseudo-cornea gives way to the raised intraocular pressure and bulges. The pseudo-cornea formed may be thick or thin. If the pseudo-cornea is thin, then the uveal tissue shines giving it a deep blue black color. The pseudo-cornea usually bulges as **Corneal staphyloma** and gives a bad cosmetic appearance. It is advisable to excise the eye and give an artificial eye.

CYSTOID CICATRIX AND FISTULA

The cystoid cicatrix and fistula result due to improper healing of a corneal scar. There is minimal scar tissue which is loosely arranged with spaces in between. The anterior wall may be formed by epithelium and the posterior wall by the pigment layer of the iris. As the scar is not dense and firm so it gives way to the normal intraocular pressure resulting in an ectatic citatrix of cornea. In some cases the aqueous percolates the iridic tissue and fill up the cystoid spaces in the scar forming bullae underneath it which is called as cystoid cicatrix In some cases the cicatrix may burst through the epithelium to form a corneal fistula. At this time the anterior chamber is lost or shallow and the intraocular pressure is low. The fistula heals quickly. With the normalization of intraocular pressure bleb is formed showing up in the white scar tissue. It may again burst and same cycle may be repeated several times until the development of an intraocular infection or hemorrhage. The fistula favors the down growth of the epithelium making the track permanent and angle of the anterior chamber and the anterior surface of the iris. It results in glaucoma.

KRUKENBERG'S PIGMENT SPINDLE

It is a condition in which the pigment derived from the uveal tract is deposited on the endothelium of the cornea in a shape of a vertical spindle. It may be a small or a large spindle. It is usually seen in the aged and mostly in the myopes and females. It is acquired in nature and pigment is derived from the uvea. Its presence has been associated with development of pigmentary glaucoma in later years and with diabetes also. A case with a Krukenberg's spindle must be watched for glaucoma diabetes and myopia.

BLOOD STAINING OF THE CORNEA

The blood staining of the cornea is due to absorption of the disintegrated products of the erthyrocytes which have broken down in the anterior chamber in a case of total hyphema typically associated with a raised intraocular pressure. Most likely the blood products enter the cornea through the damaged endothelium. The most common cause of blood staining of the cornea is the contusion of the eyeball. Clinically there is a wide spread staining of the corneal stroma involving entire cornea leaving a clear ring round the periphery. The cornea appears red rusty brown which later changes to greenish yellow or grey (Fig. 18.8).

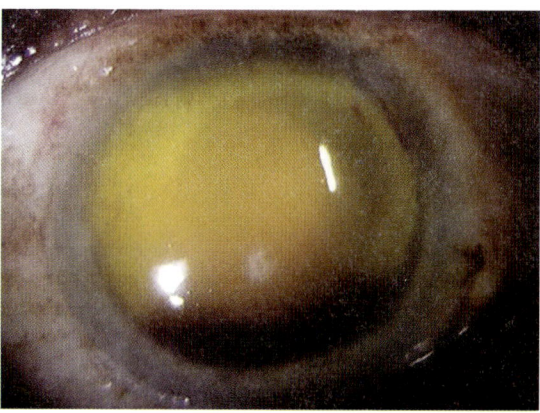

Fig. 18.8: Blood staining—cornea

There is no treatment of blood staining of the cornea. It can be prevented by an early treatment of total hyphema by evacuation and control of raised intraocular pressure. The eye is usually lost and needs excision if there is pain due to raised pressure.

VOGT'S WHITE LIMBAL GIRDLE

It is a common age-related degenerative condition of cornea. It is characterized by bilateral chalky white opacities involving temporal and nasal peripheral cornea. There may be clear zone of cornea between the opacity and limbus as in arcus senilis. Some case may not show any clear zone but has central prolongations.

WILSON'S DISEASE (Hepatolenticular Degeneration; Kayser-Fleicher Ring)

It is due to deficiency of the alpha-2 globulin ceruloplasmin and is characterized by deposition of copper in the tissue. The classical ocular manifestation is Kayser-Fleicher ring in the peripheral part of the cornea in the Descemet's membrane. Some patients may show a green "Sunflower" cataract.

POSTERIOR KERATOCONUS

It is a condition in which the anterior cornea does not protrude and the posterior cornea shows one or more excavations of varying size. There are no stress lines. There is irregular astigmatism. The condition is non-progressive.

KERATOGLOBUS

It is a rare condition of cornea characterized by thining and protrusion of the entire cornea. The cornea appears hemispherical and not like a cone as in keratoconus.

ROSACEA KERATITIS

The ocular manifestations include peripheral vascularization of cornea, thinning of cornea, punctate epithelial keratopathy, chronic blepharitis, and meibomitis. Rosacea is a common disease of skin of unknown etiology.

CORNEAL DEPOSITS

Corneal Deposits in Systemic Conditions

Chrysotherapy

Chrysiasis is the deposition of gold in the living tissue, occurring after a long treatment with administration of gold in cases of rheumatoid arthritis.

Cystinosis

It is a rare autosomal recessive inherited anomaly characterized by deposition of cysteine crystals, in the conjunctiva, cornea and retina.

Monoclonal Gammopathy

It occurs in association with multiple myeloma, lymphoma and Waldenström's macroglobulinemia. The corneal crystals deposition may be the earliest sign of the systemic disease.

Cornea Verticillata (Vortex Keratopathy)

It is characterized by symmetrical, bilateral greyish or golden corneal epithelial deposits in vortex fashion. It occurs in Fabry's disease and in cases who are on drugs such as chloroquine, amodiaquine, indomethacin, chlorpromazine and meperidine.

Fabry's Disease

Fabry's disease is a glycolipidosis due to a deficiency in the enzyme a-galactosidase A. The ocular manifestation include corneal verticillata and spoke-like lens opacities.

Mucopolysaccharidoses

It is a group of inborn errors of metaborism. The ocular features include corneal stromal infiltration, retinal pigmentary degeneration and optic atrophy. The systemic features include skeletal anomalies, mental retardation, and facial coarseness.

Endothelial Pigmentation of Cornea

- Congenital.
- Senile.
- Krukenberg's spindle.
- Pigmentary glaucbma.
- Turk's line.
- Trauma.

Blood Staining of Cornea

- Hyphema of long duration.
- Hyphema with raised intraocular pressure.
- Trauma causing severe hyphema.

Metallic Pigmentation of Cornea

- Copper (chalcosis).
- Keyser-Fleischer ring-associated with Wilson's disease.
- Intraocular foreign body of copper.
- Silver (argyrosis).
- It can occur from topical, and systemic use of silver salts.
- Gold (chrysiasis).
- It occurs from systemic use of gold.
- Iron (siderosis).
- Intraocular foreign body.
- Fleischer's ring is seen in cornea, in keratoconus, around the base of the cone.
- Hudson-Stahli line-seen at the junction of lower and middle third of cornea, as a horizontal line, related to exposure and trauma.
- Stacker's line-seen ahead of the head of pterygium.

Melanin Pigmentation of Cornea

- Epithelial melanosis.
- Congenital.
- Limbal melanoma.
- Limbal nevus.
- Stromal melanosis.
- Seen in ochronosis.
- Endothelial melanosis.
- Congenital.
- Krukenberg's spindle.
- Pigmentary glaucoma.
- Degenerative eyes.

19

A Case with
Scleral Lesions

History

Record the history with reference to the following:
- Any collagen disease (Rheumatoid arthritis, Sjögren's syndrome).
- Any metabolic disorder such as diabetes.
- Any history of tuberculosis anywhere in the system.
- Any history of repeated throat infection.
- Any history of gout.
- Any history of recent injury to the eyeball.
- Any history of recent conjunctivitis, keratitis or uveitis.
- Any history of herpes zoster.
- Any history of Wegener's granulomatosis.
- Any focal infection especially in nose, throat, teeth and genitourinary tract.
- Any history of retained foreign body in the eye.
- Any associated skin diseases like psoriasis and lichen planus.

CLINICAL EXAMINATION

The sclera is an accessible structure of the eye for complete clinical examination. However, it is not possible to examine the posterior sclera and the clinician has to diagnose on the presenting symptoms which are typical for inflammation of posterior sclera. Ophthalmoscopy does help to diagnose posterior staphyloma.

Inspection

- Lesion is unilateral or bilateral.
- Any proptosis of the eyeball.
- Any restriction of the movement of the eyeball.
- Any pain on the movement of the eyeball.
- Any chemosis of the conjunctiva.
- Congestion is localized or generalized.
- Congestion is superficial or deep.
- Nodule is diffuse, flat or raised.
- Any ischemic areas in the sclera.
- Any area of necrosis.
- Any raised area indicating staphyloma.
- Any healed scars in the sclera.

Ocular Movements

Conduct the ocular movements in all the direction and note if there is any restriction of the movement of the eyeball and any complain of pain during the movement. Retract the upper lid when patient is asked to look down and retract the lower lid when patient is asked to look up to expose the sclera.

Slit Lamp Biomicroscopy

A slit-lamp biomicroscopy provides more detail information about the lesion and vessels involved. While examining the sclera look for the following:
- Episcleral vessels are fine and superficial.
- Scleral vessels are deep and broad.
- Instillation of decongestant-phenylephrine 10%, one drop in the eye shall diminish redness markedly in episcleritis and almost no effect in a case of scleritis.
- Look for the structure of the scleral tissue at the site of the nodule.
- Conjunctiva moves freely over the nodule
- The nodule is flat or raised.

- Any areas of necrosis, ischemia or caseation in the sclera.
- Any healed slate color scars on the sclera.
- Look for aqueous flare and keratic precipitates to exclude any associated uveitis due to scleritis.

Test for Tenderness

Ask the patient to close the lids. Press the lid by finger over the nodule. Patient will complain of pain if there is tenderness.

Test for Foreign Body with Granuloma appearing as Nodule

Anesthetize the conjunctival sac. Feel the nodule with a blunt spatula for any foreign body embedded in the granuloma or projecting through the nodule especially if there is a history of foreign body.

Tonometry

It is essential to monitor the intraocular pressure during the disease process and essentially if on steroid therapy.

Ophthalmoscopy

It is helpful to detect posterior staphyloma and any other associated lesion in fundus.

Laboratory Investigations

- Complete blood picture.
- Complete urine examination.
- Serum uric acid estimation for gout.
- Serum levels of complement (C3), Immune complexes, rheumatoid factor (RF), antinuclear-antibodies (ANA) and LE cells for immunological survey.
- Fluorescent treponemal antibody absorption test (FTA–ABS). *Treponema pallidum* immobilization test, VDRL for syphilis.
- Mantoux test.
- X-ray chest, parnasal sinuses and orbit.
- X-ray sacro-iliac joints.

Clinical Features and Mangement

1. Episcleritis.
2. Anterior scleritis.
3. Posterior scleritis.

4. Scleromalacia perforans.
5. Ectasia and staphyloma.
6. Rheumatoid arthritis.
7. Systemic lupus erythematosus.
8. Polyartiritis nodosa.
9. Wagener's granulomatosis.
10. Blue sclera.

EPISCLERITIS

Episcleritis is a benign recurrent and self-limiting inflammation of episclera and overlying Tenon's capsule. It is regarded as hypersensitivity reaction to endogenous tubercular or streptococcal toxins. It is considered to be a collagen disorder. It has been associated with systemic diseases such as rheumatoid arthritis, Sjögren's syndrome, Wagener's granulomatosis, syphilis, herpes zoster, tuberculosis and focal infections.

Clinical Features

- It affects young adults and females more than males.
- It frequently affects both the eyes.
- Clinically, it may present as a localised redness which may appear flat or as a raised nodule usually near limbus. The nodule is hard, immovable and tender to touch. The conjunctiva over the nodule moves freely.
- There is mild congestion with mild ocular discomfort. Patient feels gritty and burning sensation. Patient may complain of foreign body sensation with mild pain, photophobia and lacrimation.
- On resolution it leaves a slate color scar on the sclera.
- The regular recurrence in a periodic manner has been labelled as Episcleritis Periodica Fugax.

Management

- Investigate the case to arrive at the etiological factor.
- Topical steroids help to resolve the malady within few days.
- Systemic non-steroidal anti-inflammatory drugs provide relief from pain and resolution.

ANTERIOR SCLERITIS

Scleritis is an inflammation of deeper layers of the sclera. It is a serious disease which may result in visual loss if not treated carefully and energetically. It is less common than episcleritis. It is usually bilateral and more common in females (Fig. 19.1).

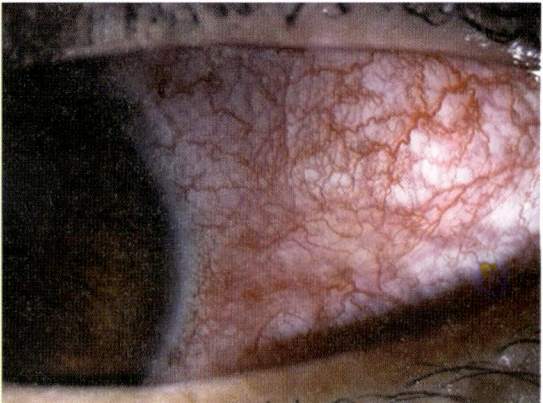

Fig. 19.1: Scleritis-nodule

Etiological Factors

Autoimmune Collagen Disorders

Such as Rheumatoid arthritis, Ankylosing spondylitis, Temporal arteritis, Polyarteritis nodosa, Sjögren's syndrome, Wegener's granulomatosis, Dermatomyositis Polychondritis, Lupus erythematosus and Scleroderma.

Endogenous Infections

Tuberculosis, syphilis, leprosy and sarcoidosis.

Viral Infections

Herpes simplex, herpes zoster and mumps.

Secondary infection from adjoining structures

Conjunctivitis, keratitis, uveitis and sinusitis.

Metabolic

Graves' disease, gout.

Miscellaneous Factors

Injury, irradiation, burns-acid, alkali and thermal.

Clinical Types if Anterior Scleritis

- Anterior diffuse non-necrotizing scleritis (Brawny scleritis).
- Anterior nodular non-nectrotizing scleritis.
- Anterior necrotising scleritis with inflammation.
- Anterior necrotizing scleritis without inflammation (Scleromalacia perforans).

Clinical Features

- The scleritis may be diffuse or in the form of a nodule.
- The scleritis may extend around the cornea as "Annular scleritis".
- The scleritis may extend on the cornea as "Sclerosing keratitis" with its angular or rounded apex towards the center of the cornea.
- The scleritis shows involvement of the cornea and uvea in the form of keratitis, iritis and anterior choroiditis.
- There is no ulceration or perforation.
- On resolution, the sclera becomes thin showing the underlying uveal tissue as bluish color area. This weak area is unable to withstand the normal intraocular pressure and shows an ectatic cicatrix "ciliary staphyloma".
- It is always associated with congestion, pain, lacrimation, photophobia and tenderness.
- The symptoms are severe in the necrotizing form with inflammation.
- The necrotizing form without inflammation is symptomless.

Management

- Systemic steroid therapy is necessary. Start with a high dose and taper it off with suppression of inflammation.
- Oral oxyphenbutazone, aspirin, salicylates and indomethacin to provide relief from pain and inflammation.

- Avoid local and subconjunctival steroids.
- Some cases may need immunosuppressive agents like methotrexate or cyclophosphamide.

POSTERIOR SCLERITIS

It is uncommon and difficult to diagnose. It give rise to following symptoms: proptosis, pain, diplopia, limitations of ocular movements, exudative retinal detachment, papilledema, edema of macula, and choroidal detachment. Treat similar to anterior scleritis.

SCLEROMALACIA PERFORANS

Typically, it affects females with long standing sero-positive rheumatoid arthritis. It is asymptomatic. There is a yellowish necrotic patch in the normal sclera showing the underlying uveal tissue. Perforation is rare unless there is trauma or raised intraocular pressure. There is no effective treatment. Repair of the patch can be attempted by a preserved homologous sclera.

ECTASIA AND STAPHYLOMA

Ectasia

Ectasia is a condition characterized by the stretching of the sclera without implicating the uvea. Ectasia may be total or partial.

Total ectasia: The typical example of total ectasia of the outer coat of the eyeball is seen in a case of a buphthalmos. The entire sclera stretches uniformly.

Partial ectasia: Partial ectasia occurs in ectatic coloboma, high myopia and in glaucoma as a cupping of the disk.

Staphyloma

Staphyloma is an ectatic condition of the outer coat (Sclera) of the eyeball in which the uveal tissue is incarcerated. Clinically there are four types of staphyloma:

Anterior ciliary staphyloma: It occurs in the region of the ciliary body where the anterior ciliary arteries penetrate.

Intercalary staphyloma: It occurs between the anterior extremity of the ciliary body and the limbus where the sclera is weak due to presence of the anterior ciliary veins and the canal of Schlemm.

The anterior staphyloma is obvious. It is usually heavily pigmented. Due to uneven thinning of the sclera the staphyloma appears as a lobulated dark blue color protrusions. It is difficult to distinguish the ciliary staphyloma from the intercalary staphyloma, yet the location of the anterior ciliary arteries helps. In the ciliary staphyloma, the anterior ciliary arteries emerge at the anterior border of the bulge and dark striae of the ciliary processes can be seen on transillumination. In the intercalary staphyloma, the anterior ciliary arteries emerge posteriorly.

Equatorial staphyloma: It occurs due to weakness of the sclera due to passage of vortex veins. It is localised. It is rarely diagnosed until surgery is undertaken for retina to expose the equatorial region. It gives rise to no symptoms.

Posterior staphyloma: It is seen in cases of high myopia, wherein the posterior pole bulges backwards. In fact it is an ectasia of the sclera.

Complication

Glaucoma: Glaucoma is a common complication of an anterior staphyloma.

Retinal detachment: Retinal detachment is common in an equatorial staphyloma.

Management

A glaucoma surgery in a case of anterior staphyloma is enough to retard or even stop the progress of the malady. For equatorial staphyloma, one can perform a scleral resection, or a buckling operation or a scleroplasty.

RHEUMATOID ARTHRITIS

Rheumatoid arthritis is a multisystem disorder. It typically affects women in the age group of 35 to 40. Most patients are positive for rheumatoid factor (sero-positive). The systemic manifestations includearthritis, subcutaneous nodules, vasculitis and occasional heart and lung disease. The ocular manifestations include keratoconjunctivitis sicca, peripheral keratitis, acute stromal keratitis, peripheral corneal guttering, keratolysis and sclerosing keratitis.

SYSTEMIC LUPUS ERYTHEMATOSUS

It is a multisystem disorder. The most common ocular manifestations include punctate epithelial keratopathy, keratoconjunctivitis sicca, scleritis, retinal phlebitis, anterior ischemic optic neuropathy and peripheral keratitis. The other systems involved are articular, skin, renal, blood, lungs, heart and central nervous system.

POLYARTERITIS NODOSA

Polyarteritis nodosa is a rare chronic necrotizing systemic vasculitis affecting medium sized and small arteries. The ocular manifestations include scleritis, choroidal vasculitis, retinal vasculitis, anterior ischemic optic neuropathy and peripheral keratitis. Keratitis may be occasionally a presenting feature of polyarteritis nodosa. Keratitis is unresponsive to topical steroids. A combination of steroids and cyclophosphamides may be beneficial.

WEGENER'S GRANULOMATOSIS

It is a very rare multisystem disease characterized by necrotizing granulomatous inflammations. The ocular manifestations include orbital involvement, retinal vasculitis, uveitis, scleritis, conjunctivitis and peripheral keratitis. The clinical features and management of peripheral keratitis are same as in polyarteritis nodosa.

BLUE SCLERA

The normal sclera is white and opaque so that the underlying uveal tissue is not visible. Thining of the sclera following its inflammation may show the underlying uvea as bluish coloration.

Blue sclera occurs as a part of clinical picture in the following: Osteogenesis imperfecta, Ehlers-Danlos syndrome, pseudoxanthoma elasticum, Marian's syndrome, and pseudo-hypoparathyroidism.

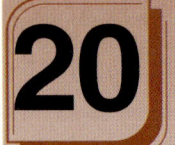

20

A Case with Abnormal Light Reflex of Pupil

History

Record the history with reference to the following:
- Any dim vision.
- Dim vision had been sudden or gradual.
- Dim vision accompanied by foggy vision.
- Any change in the appearance of the objects; look bigger or smaller or wavy.
- Dim vision from all the sides or from a particular side.
- Any associated symptoms with dim vision like photopsia, black spots, floating objects, shimmering light.
- Any ptosis.
- Enophthalmos.

3. Hemianopic pupillary reaction (Wernicke's reaction).
4. Hippus.
5. Ill-sustained pupillary reaction to light.
6. Argyll Robertson pupil.
7. Adie's pupil (tonic pupil).
8. Horner's syndrome (oculo-sympathetic palsy).
9. Pupillary pathway for light reflex.
10. Lesions of pupillary pathway and light reflex of pupil.
11. Clinical condition and pupil.
12. Pupil: some points to keep in mind.

CLINICAL EXAMINATION

Examination of the pupillary reaction should be done in dim illumination.

Size of Pupil

Ask the patient to look at Snellen test type. Examine the pupil by a dim light directed on the face from below so that pupils are seen in oblique illumination. Note the size of both the pupils and can measure with a millimeter rule. About 20% of population has a mild anisocoria. An anisocoria that varies with varying the illumination is pathological.

Clinical Features

1. Light reflex.
2. Swinging-flashlight test (Marcus Gunn pupil).

LIGHT REFLEX (Direct and Consensual)

The light reflex of the pupil should be elicited with a strong torch light. Ask the patient to look straight at a distance. Throw the light on the pupil of one eye. Observe the reaction of the pupil in the same eye and also in the opposite eye. Repeat the test by throwing the light in the opposite pupil and observe the reaction in both the eyes.

SWINGING-FLASH LIGHT TEST
(Marcus Gunn Pupil)

A bright light is thrown on one pupil and the reaction is noted. After two to three seconds the light is thrown on the opposite pupil. Repeat this swinging of light to and fro from one pupil to other and observe the reaction of the pupil in which the light is transferred. In a normal case the pupil on which the light is transferred shows constriction. In a normal case both the pupils will show constriction. If there is a lesion of one optic nerve thereby there is an afferent defect the pupil of that eye will show dilation on transfer of light instead of the constriction. This is due to afferent defect. The dilation of the pupil by withdrawing the light from the normal pupil outweighs the constriction produced by stimulating the diseased eye with optic nerve lesion. It may be earliest indication for optic nerve lesion like retrobulbar neuritis. The Marcus Gunn pupil is also seen in cases with extensive retinal pathology.

HEMIANOPIC PUPILLARY REACTION
(Wernicke's reaction)

The best method to elicit this reaction is to make the patient sit for slit lamp examination. Observe the reaction of pupil with beam of light reduced to a small spot. By moving the arm of slit lamp half of the retina can be stimulated. Watch the pupil reaction. Move the light to stimulate the opposite half of the retina and observe the pupil reaction. The pupil will show brisk reaction if the patient is normal. A case with an optic tract lesion will show a sluggish reaction on stimulating one half of the retina in comparison to the other half of the retina. As the light always diffuses from one half to the other the test is rarely unequivocal. It is more for an academic interest rather than clinical use.

HIPPUS

Hippus is a condition of oscillation of pupil. The oscillations are large and seen easily and independent of the light falling on the eye. This depends on the rhythmic activity of the nervous center. It is found in multiple sclerosis.

ILL-SUSTAINED PUPILLARY REACTION TO LIGHT

When a light is thrown on the pupil it contracts and then oscillates rapidly and finally settles down into a condition of contraction. There is a condition of pupil which shows lack of sustained contraction (ill-sustained) under the continued light on the pupil. This is due to diminished conductivity in the afferent pathway of the light reflex in optic neuritis. To elicit it throw the light on one eye and observe the reaction of the pupil. Throw the light on the other eye and observe the reaction of pupil. The pupil which shows ill-sustained contraction, i.e. the pupil will slowly dilate even in spite of keeping the light on the pupil is the affected eye with an optic nerve lesion. It is one of the earliest sign for optic nerve lesion if there is a definite dilation of pupil even with light on the pupil.

ARGYLL ROBERTSON PUPIL

It is due to neurosyphilis. It has the following features:
- Light-near dissociation. The pupil reacts briskly to near reflex and there is no reaction to light reflex. This is due to involvement of fibers of second neurone, i.e. between the pretectal nucleus and Edinger-Westphal nucleus.
- Both the pupils are involved but asymmetrically.
- To diagnose Argyll Robertson pupil the affected eye must have normal vision.
- Pupils are small and usually irregular in shape.
- Pupils dilate poorly with mydriatic.

ADIE'S PUPIL (Tonic Pupil)

It is frequently seen in females in the age group of 30 to 40 and usually follows a viral illness. It is unilateral in 80% of cases with following features.
- The pupil on the affected side is larger than the other eye.
- The light reflex is absent.
- The near reflex is present but slow and tonic.
- Accommodation is also slow on changing the focus from distance to near.
- Instillation of pilocarpine 0.125% in the affected eye causes constriction while the unaffected eye does not show change.

HORNER'S SYNDROME (Oculo-sympathetic Palsy)

It is due to interruption of sympathetic chain anywhere along its course. Features are as follows:

- Slight ptosis due to paralysis of Muller's muscle.
- Elevation of lower lid due to paralysis of smooth muscle attached to the inferior tarsal plate.
- An apparent enophthalmos due to narrow fissure caused by ptosis of upper lid and elevation of lower lid.
- Slight miosis. Reactions are normal to light and near reflex.
- Diminished sweating on the ipsilateral side of face.
- Heterochromia may be there.
- Increased amplitude of accommodation due to unopposed action of parasympathetic.

PUPILLARY PATHWAY FOR LIGHT REFLEX

There are four neurone arc.

First Neurone

The first neurone connects the retina to the pretectal nucleus in the midbrain. The light reflex is initiated from the retinal photoreceptors the rods and cones. The impulses from the temporal half of the retina passes uncrossed at chiasma and terminate in the ipsilateral pretectal nucleus. The impulses from the nasal half of the retina cross at the chiasma and pass up the optic tract of the opposite side and terminate in the contralateral pretectal nucleus.

Second Neurone

The second neurone connects each pretectal neclus to both Edinger-Westphal nuclei. Thus there is a double decussation of pupillary fibers one at chiasma and another in the pretectal area. This explains the direct and consensual light reflex. These fibers from pretectal nucleus to Edinger-Westphal nucleus can get damaged in syphilis and pinealomas resulting in the condition of light-near reflex dissociation.

Third Neurone

- The third neurone connects the Edinger-Westphal nucleus to the ciliary ganglion.
- The pupillary fibers are superficially located in the third nerve from the brainstem to the entry in cavernous sinus therefore any compressive lesion will give rise to a third nerve palsy with involvement of the pupillary reaction.
- The pupillary fibers occupy the central place in the third nerve when it passes through the cavernous sinus therefore any lesion here causes paralysis of the third nerve with sparing of a change in the pupillary reactions.
- In the orbit the pupillary fibers pass in the inferior division of the third nerve terminating in the ciliary ganglion via nerve to inferior oblique muscle.

Fourth Neurone

The fourth neurone connects the ciliary ganglion to the sphincter pupillae muscle. The fibers pass with the short ciliary nerves to terminate in the sphincter pupillae muscle.

LESIONS IN PUPILLARY PATHWAY AND LIGHT REFLEX OF PUPIL

Optic nerve lesion
- Direct light reflex is absent on the same side.
- Consensual light reflex is absent in the opposite eye.
- Direct light reflex present in the opposite side.
- Consensual light reflex is present on the same side.
- Near reflex is normal.
- There is unilateral amurosis (loss of vision).

Medial chiasmal lesion: There is bitemporal hemianopic paralysis of light reflex.

Lateral chiasmal lesion: There is binasal hemianopic paralysis of light reflex.

Optic tract lesion: There is contralateral hemianopic paralysis of light reflex (Wernicke's reaction).

Optic tract lesion in its proximal part (Beyond exit of pupillary fibers): The pupillary reactions are normal.

Lesion in superficial region of brachium and tectum: There is contralateral hemianopic paralysis of light reflex (Wernicke's reaction).

Lesion at the site of central decussation (Decussation in the Pretectal Area)
- There is bilateral paralysis of light reflex both for direct light reflex and consensual light reflex.
- Near reflex, lid reflex and psychosensory reflex present (It is a bilateral Argyll Robertson pupil).

Lesion affecting fibers between pretectal nucleus to Edinger-Westphal nucleus
- Direct and consensual light reflex absent on the same side (side affected) ipsilateral side.
- Direct and consensual light reflex present in the opposite eye or contralateral side. (It is unilateral Argyll Robertson pupil.)
- Near reflex intact.

A partial lesion like the above affecting fibers between pretectal nucleus to Edinger-Westphal nucleus but affecting only the constrictor fibers from the same side
- Direct light reflex is absent on ipsilateral side.
- Consensual light reflex is present on ipsilateral side.
- Direct and consensual light reflex present on the contralateral side.

Lesion of third nerve nucleus and supranuclear lesion: There is absolute paralysis of ipsilateral pupillary reaction.

Lesion of third nerve: There is absolute paralysis of ipsilateral pupillary reaction.

Lesion of ciliary ganglion
- The light reflex is abolished both ipsilateral.
- The near reflex is present (It is Argyll Robertson pupil).

CLINICAL CONDITION AND PUPIL

Optic Atrophy

Pupil is large and no reaction to direct light but consensual is present.

Optic Neuritis

Ill-sustained pupillary reaction or Marcus Gunn pupil.

Absolute Glaucoma

Direct and consensual both absent. The pupil is large and fixed.

Acute Glaucoma

Direct and consensual both light reflex absent. Direct and consensual both the light reflex absent. The pupil is large and fixed.

Third Nerve Paralysis

There is absolute paralysis of the papillary reaction. Direct and consensual both absent.

Paralysis of Third Nerve Fibers to Ciliary Ganglion

There is complete internal ophthalmoplegia. It occurs in syphilis, meningitis, encephalitis and trauma.

Irritation of Cervicle Sympathetic

There is unilateral dilation of pupil. It occurs due to lymph nodes, cervical rib, apical pleurisy and thoracic aneurysm.

Sympathetic Paralysis

There is constriction of pupil. It occurs in pontine hemorrhage.

Irtis

Small sluggish pupil.

Irritation of Third Nerve Centrally

Bilateral small pupil.

Horner's Syndrome

Small pupil.

PUPIL: SOME POINTS TO KEEP IN MIND

- In newborn the pupil is situated slightly to the nasal side of and below the center of cornea.
- The average diameter of pupil is about 4 mm.
- In Infancy the pupil is smaller than at birth.
- The pupillary reflexes appear at about the fifth month and are active by sixth month.
- The pupil is at its greatest diameter at adolescence.
- The pupil becomes smaller with advancing age.
- Myopes have larger pupil than hypermetropes.
- Many normal persons have slight difference in the size of pupil. It is physiological anisocoria.
- Mydriatics and cycloplegic drugs are more effective on blue iris than on brown iris.
- Pupil controls the amount of light entering the eye.
- Pupil may be dilated due to dim illumination, myopia and use of sympathomimetic drugs topically.
- Pupils may be constricted due to bright illumination, syphilis of central nervous system and use of para-sympathomimetic drugs topically and narcotics.
- A tonic pupil of Adie dilates well with atropine. But Argyll Robertson pupil does not dilate well with atropine.
- If the pupil is enlarged due to sympathetic irritation then;
  - Pupil constricts due to light and accommodation.
  - Pupil constricts to eserine.
  - Pupil dilates well to atropine.
- If the pupil is constricted due to sympathetic palsy then Pupil constricts to light and accommodation. Pupil constricts to eserine. Atropine is relatively inactive to cause dilation.
- If the pupil is enlarged due to paralysis of third nerve then Pupil does not react to light and accommodation. Atropine cause further dilation of pupil. Pilocarpine causes constriction if lesion is proximal to ciliary ganglion.
- If pupil is small due to irritation of third nerve then atropine causes greater dilation.

21

A Case with Leukocoria in a Child

History

Record the history with reference to the following:
- Age of the child at the time of noticing white reflex from the pupil.
- Any other sibling has a white reflex from the pupil.
- Any history of prematurity.
- Any history of low birth weight.
- The white reflex is unilateral or bilateral.
- Any other symptoms.

CLINICAL EXAMINATION

Inspection

Inspect the child in day light and also with a torch light. Observe the reflex from the pupil whether occupying the complete pupil or coming from a quadrant. Note its color-white, grey-white or pinkish-white. Observe for any squint.

Retonoscopy

Observe the corneal reflex to assess the squint if any. Observe the reflex from the pupil. Assess the state of refraction of both the eyes.

Direct Ophthalmoscopy

Observe the reflex. By changing the lens in the disk observe and assess the condition of the fundus and ocular media. Observe for any vitreous pathology especially floaters and condition of lens. If any change is noticed then draw a diagram and make a note of it for follow up assessment.

Indirect Ophthalmoscopy

The examination should be performed with full mydriasis using a scleral indentation to examine the extreme periphery.

Slit Lamp with Fundus Contact Lens

It helps to examine the central and peripheral fundus under high magnification. It helps to examine the vitreous in detail.

Clinical Features and Management

The following maladies are the most important diagnostic consideration in a child with leukocoria- a white, grey-white, pink-white or yellow-white reflex from the pupil.
1. Retinoblastoma.
2. Persistent hyperplastic primary vitreous.
3. Exudative retinopathy of coats (Coats' syndrome).
4. von Hippel-Lindau angiomatosis.
5. Retinopathy of prematurity (retrolental fibroplasia).
6. Endophthalmitis due to toxocariasis.
7. Endophthalmitis due to cysticercosis.
8. Fundus coloboma of choroid.
9. Incontinentia pigmenti (Bloch-Sulzberger syndrome).
10. Prenatal and infantile trauma causing vitreous hemorrhage.

RETINOBLASTOMA

Incidence

- It is most common primary malignant intraocular tumor of childhood occurring 1 in 20,000 live births.

- It is bilateral in about 25 to 30% cases although one eye is affected earlier and more extensively than the other.
- There is no sexual predilection.
- In most cases it manifests prior to the age of three.

Genetics and Heredity

Retinoblastoma gene identified as 14 band on the long-arm of chromosome 13 (13q14) is a *cancer suppressor or antioncogenic gene.* Inactivation of this protective gene by two mutations (*Knudson's two hit hypothesis)* is the causative factor for occurrence of retino-blastoma. Retinoblastoma may manifest as hereditary or sporadic form.

Clinical Features

The most important aspect is to examination of both the eyes under full mydiasis and anesthesia to group the tumor and plan treatment accordingly (Figs 21.1 and 21.2).

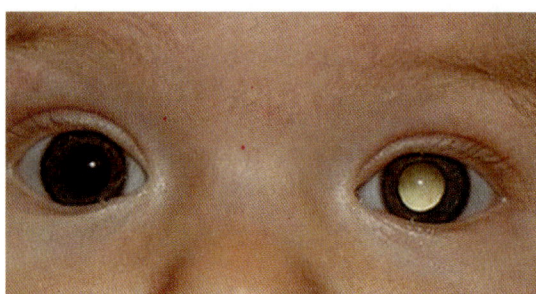

Fig. 21.1: Leukocoria due to retinoblastoma

Quiescent Stage

- Yellowish-white pupillary reflex or leukocoria or amaurotic cat's eye appearance draws the attention of parents.
- The child may be brought with and for convergent squint, low vision or nystagmus.
- Endophytic retinoblastoma-ophthal-moscopy and fundus contact lens examination the tumor appears as a white or pink color mass with fine vessels and small hemorrhage on the surface. Sometimes large nutrient vessels may be seen.

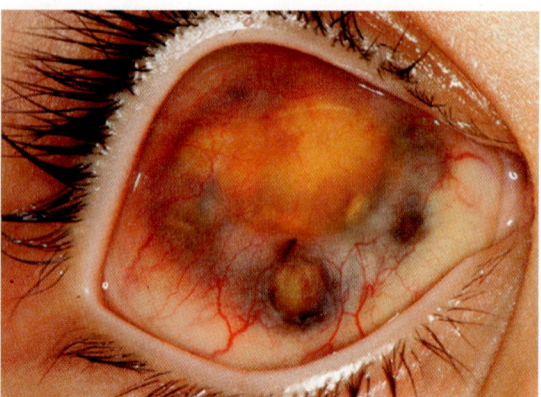

Fig. 21.2: Retinoblastoma glaucomatous stage

It may appear glistening white-typical "cottage cheese" appearance if there is calcification.

- Exophytic retinoblastoma-ophthalmos-copy shows exudative retinal detachment.
- The cases with vitreous hemorrhage, retinal detachment or an inflammatory reaction need other tests to arrive at the conclusive diagnosis.

Glaucomatous Stage

In later stage child may present as a case of buphthalmos or proptosis. The intraocular pressure is high. This stage is characterized by severe pain and redness.

Extraocular Extension

The globe bursts through the sclera usually at the limbus or near the optic disc. There is rapid fungative growth that involves extraocular tissue.

Distant Metastasis

The metastasis occurs in preauricular and other lymph nodes and direct extension through optic nerve. The common sites for metastases are skull, orbit, long bones, viscera, spinal cord and lymph nodes.

INTERNATIONAL CLASSIFICATION OF RETINOBLASTOMA

Group A	Small tumor less than 3 mm.
Group B	Large tumor more than 3 mm.

Group C   Focal seeds of tumor-subretinal and or vitreal less than 3 mm from retinoblastoma.

Group D   Diffuse seeds of tumor-subretinal or vitreal more than 3 mm from retinoblastoma.

Group E   Extensive tumor-occupying more than 50% of globe or associated complications.

Investigation

- Complete blood picture, ESR and hemoglobin.
- Bone free X-ray of the globe for any calcification.
- B-scan ultrasonography for presence of calcification.
- CT scan for involvement of optic nerve, orbit, pineal or central nervous system.
- Aqueous humour paracentesis for enzyme assay and cytology. An aqueous to plasma Lactate dehydrogenase ratio of greater than 1.0 is suggestive.
- ELISA test to exclude toxocariasis.
- Fine needle biopsy may be required when there is doubt about the diagnosis.
- *Metastatic workup:* Metastatic workup includes bone scan, cerebrospinal fluid analysis, bone marrow aspiration and analysis and whole body CT/MRI when required.

Management

- Cabalt plaque irradiation is good for a small tumor.
- Photocoagulation with xenon arc is indicated in small posterior tumors not involving the optic nerve and macula.
- Cryotherapy is useful for small anterior peripheral tumors. Cryo should be repeated at least three times.
- Laser photocoagulation is useful for posterior small tumors away from macula.
- Radiotherapy with an external beam is useful for cases with medium or large tumors.
- Systemic chemotherapy is indicated in cases with metastasis.
- Enucleation with care to take a long piece of the optic nerve is the treatment of choice

in advanced cases with poor vision. The involvement of the optic nerve indicates metastasis.

- Histopathology of enucleated eye is a must to assess the prognosis. A well differentiated tumor shows rosettes. The mortality is about 8% in cases showing rosettes. A highly undifferentiated tumor has a mortality of 40%.
- Rarely spontaneous regression with shrinkage of the eyeball may occur due to necrosis followed by calcification. Role of immunological phenomenon has been thought of.

PERSISTENT HYPERPLASTIC PRIMARY VITREOUS

This condition is the result of failure of regression of the embryonic hyaloid vascular system. Clinically, it presents with a white reflex from the pupil. On examination, there is whitish pinkish mass behind the lens.

Clinical Features

- It is unilateral in about 90% of cases.
- There is no history of premature birth, low birth weight or having received any prenatal oxygen.
- A white reflex from the pupil is the most common presenting sign.
- Patient may be brought for squint or nystagmus.
- It is characterized by the presence of:
  - A retrolental funnel-shaped mass of fibrovascular tissue which gives rise to white reflex. It may vary in size from a small plaque just nasal to center (**Mittendorf's dot**) to a complete plaque covering of the posterior lens surface. The mass is usually grey or pink.
  - Identification of hyaloid artery confirms the diagnosis. The hyaloid artery may be patent or occluded. Usually it is represented by vascular remnant that extends from the mass into the vitreous cavity.
  - The mass is vascular and repeated hemorrhages within the mass, vitreous and perilenticular space is common.

– The lens is clear to begin with but becomes cataractous due to rupture of posterior capsule. It may lead to swelling of the lens and secondary glaucoma of angle closure type.

– Vitreous organization may be seen at various stages of fibrosis.

Management

Closed intraocular microsurgical technique as lensectomy and vitrectomy is useful to restore some useful vision.

EXUDATIVE RETINOPATHY OF COATS (Coats' Syndrome)

Clinical Features

- It is non familial.
- It is unilateral and primarily affects infants and children.
- It is more common in boys than girls.
- It is a condition with severe form of retinal telangiectasia-(idiopathic congenital vascular malformation).
- It presents as a case with white reflex from the pupil (leukocoria), strabismus or loss of vision.
- It is characterized by
  - Large areas of intra and sub-retinal exudates and hemorrhages with over-lying dilated and tortuous vessels with small aneurysms at the posterior pole and around the optic disk.
  - Majority of cases develop exudative retinal detachment, a retrolental mass, cataract, rubeosis iridis, uveitis, glaucoma and eventually phthisis bulbi.

Coat's Syndrome has been Classified in Five Stages

Stage I: Telangiectasia only
Stage II: Telangiectasia and exudates without and with foveal involvement
Stage III: Retinal detachment-shallow or total
Stage IV: Total retinal detachment with glaucoma
Stage V: Total blindness

Management

An early diagnosis and management with laser or cryotherapy may prevent the progress of the disease process and save some useful vision. Control the intraocular pressure.

IntravitrealVEGF inhibitors—may be helpful.

VON HIPPEL-LINDAU ANGIOMATOSIS (Retinal capillary hemangiomas, Angiomatosis retinae)

The retinal capillary hemangiomas if associated with systemic lesions then it is referred as the von Hippel-Lindau syndrome. It is one of the phacomatoses.

Clinical Features

- There are multiple lesions in the retina.
- The lesion may be small red nodule or a large orange-red color tumor.
- It is supplied by large feeder vessels which are tortuous.
- Hard exudates are seen in the surrounding retina and also in other parts of the fundus.
- Later retinal detachment develops.

Systemic

- All patients with retinal lesions must be referred for neurological examination.
- Hemangioblastomas may involve the cerebellum, medulla, pons, and spinal cord.
- Patient may show cysts of kidneys, liver, ovary and lungs.
- Patient may show the rare findings of hypernephroma, phaeo-chromocytoma, and polycythemia.
- Skin lesions are absent.

Management

Treat the tumor mass with laser or cryotherapy early to save the useful vision. Photodynamic therapy and anti-VEGF therapy may be helpful. Vitrectomy may be considered.

RETINOPATHY OF PREMATURITY
(Retrolental fibroplasia)

Retinopathy of prematurity is a vaso proliferative malady affecting the avascular retina of premature infants with abnormal retinal neovascularization

Clinical Features

- It affects premature infants who have received oxygen.
- Infants with gestation period of less than 37 weeks are at more risk.
- Infants with birth weight less than 1300 gm are at more risk.
- It is a trilateral disease.
- The eyes are of normal size at birth.
- Retrolental membrane is not present at birth and develops later and gives rise to white reflex.
- There is peripheral neovascularization, vitreous hemorrhage and later proliferative retinopathy.
- There may be a funnel shaped total tractional retinal detachment.
- There may be retrolental fibrovascular sheets.

Management

- Prophylaxis is the real need to save the eye with useful vision. The premature newborns should not be placed in incubators with oxygen concentration of more than thirty percent.
- Regular screening in the early stage is rewarding.
- Cryotherapy to ablate the vascular immature retina.
- Scleral buckling with vitrectomy for tractional detachment.
- Vitamin E—the role is not clear.

ENDOPHTHALMITIS DUE TO TOXOCARIASIS

Clinical Features

- It is caused by the roundworms of cats (toxocara cati) and dogs (toxocara canis).
- Humans get infected by use of contaminated food by the ova which are shed in dogs and cats faeces.
- Clinically ocular infestation can present as; toxocara chronic endophthalmitis, posterior pole granuloma or peripheral granuloma.
- Patient presents with a white reflex from the pupil, squint or loss of vision.
- The white reflex is due to vitreous abscess.
- The diagnosis is based on the clinical picture, history, eosinophilia and if possible a toxocara specific larval antigen immunodiagnostic test.

Management

- The aqueous humor lactic acid dehydrogenase assay which is higher in retinoblastoma may be useful.
- ELISA blood test.
- Steroids given systemic and periocular is the only treatment available.
- Pars plana vitrectomy in cases of endophthalmitis and vitreous bands may help to save some vision.

ENDOPHTHALMITIS DUE TO CYSTICERCOSIS

Cysticercus cellulosae, the larval stage of the pork tapeworm—*Taenia solium*, may cause an intravitreal abscess to give rise to a white reflex from the pupil. A living worm induces minimum reaction. A dead worm induces severe reaction.

FUNDUS COLOBOMA

A typical fundus coloboma appears as an oval defect in the retina and choroid with its apex towards the optic disc. The optic disk may be or may not be included in it. The surface is depressed with irregular margins and few vessels are seen over the surface. The central vision is diminished. On examination with a torch light or retinoscopy there is a white grey reflex in the lower part of the pupil. The appearance of white reflex depends on the size of the coloboma.

INCONTINENTIA PIGMENTI
(Bloch-Sulzberger Syndrome)

This is a rare skin disorder affecting female infants. It is characterized by recurrent vesiculobullous dermatitis which causes irregular patches of hyperpigmentation on the trunk and extremities. About one-third cases show ocular findings. The patient presents with a white reflex from the pupil. This is due to a retrolental mass of detached retina and fibrous tissue.

PRENATAL AND INFANTILE TRAUMA CAUSING VITREOUS HEMORRHAGE

Trauma forms an important cause of visual loss in infants. The trauma results in vitreous hemorrhage. The organised vitreous hemorrhage assumes a white pale or pink color. It mimics retinoblastoma by a white reflex from the pupil. The history of trauma may not be available. One has to rely on the clinical examination and presence of organized fibrous mass in the vitreous.

22

A Case with Uveal Lesions

History

Record the history with reference to the following:
- Pain.
- Redness.
- Photophobia.
- Lacrimation.
- Floaters.
- Positive scotoma.
- Dim vision.
- Acute or insidious onset.
- Systemic disease.
- Spots of vitiligo on the body.
- Poliosis.
- Any trauma.

CLINICAL EXAMINATION

Visual Acuity

Visual acuity should be evaluated with proper refraction and pin hole test on the first examination and on follow up visits. It gives a fair idea whether there is progress or deterioration of the disease process.

Slit Lamp Biomicroscopy

Corneal Scar

A faint thin nebular type may indicate occurrence of herpes simplex.

Keratic Precipitates

Keratic precipitates are typically seen in a triangular form in the lower part of corneal endothelium (Fig. 22.1). This is due to convection current in the aqueous humor.

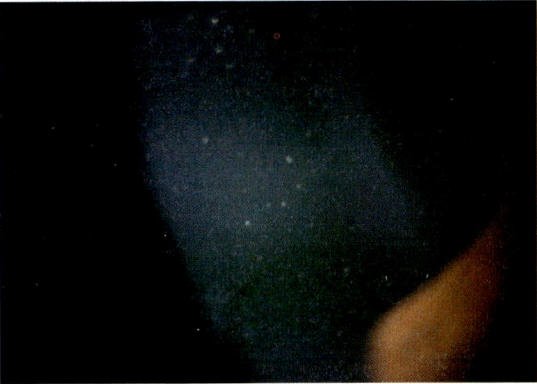

Fig. 22.1: Keratic precipitates

Keratic precipitates are composed of chronic inflammatory cells such as macrophages, lymphocytes and plasma cells. Keratic precipitates are best seen by retro-illumination method of slit lamp biomicroscopy. In retro-illumination, the cornea is illuminated by the light reflected from the iris and fundus.

- In acute anterior uveitis the corneal endothelium gets covered by hundreds of small keratic precipitates.
- Small keratic precipitates are characteristic of herpes zoster and Fuch's uveitis.
- Medium size keratic precipitates are seen in acute and chonic anterior uveitis.
- Large and waxy keratic precipitates are typical of a granulomatous uveitis and are called as **mutton-fat** keratic precipitates. These are composed of epitheloid cells and mononuclear macrophages.

- Fresh keratic precipitates are white and round in shape.

- Old keratic precipitates are shrunken and pigmented.

Aqueous Flare

The aqueous humor appears optically empty to the passage of light by a slit lamp beam. A visible beam of light indicates that the aqueous humor is plasmoid in nature and thus gives an aqueous flare. Direct the slit lamp beam at an oblique angle to the plane of iris, and use a short 2 mm slit for grading cells and flare. Make a note of it and use it for comparison on follow up to assess the progress of the disease. An intense flare and suspended cells not showing any movement indicates that there is marked fibrin in the aqueous.

Cells in Aqueous

The presence of cells in the aqueous indicates active inflammation of the iris and ciliary body. These cells are white and should be distinguished from brown pigmented cells which are uveal tract cells and usually do not indicate any inflammtory activity. To see and count the cells use a three millimeter long and one millimeter width slit. The cells are usually moving. If the cells are suspended then it indicates that there is fibrin in the aqueous. The cells are counted in the beam. Larger the number of cell count more severe or active is the disease process.

Iris Nodules

The nodules on the iris indicate a granulomatous inflammation. The nodules have been observed in severe non-granulomatous uveitis also.

Koeppe's Nodules

Koeppe's nodules are at the pupillary border. These are gray, translucent and lie in the posterior layer of iris (Fig. 22.2). It has been suggested that iris movement causes the cellular infiltrates to clump together beneath the pupillary margin and appear as Koeppe's

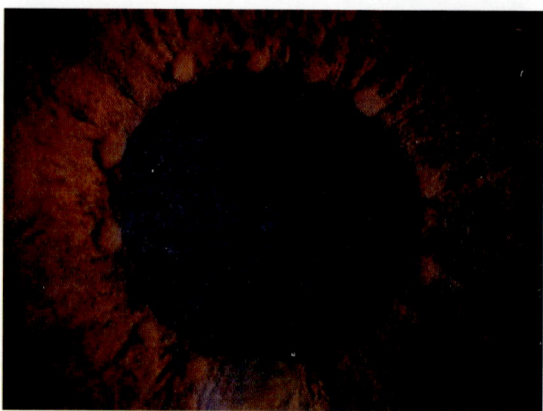

Fig. 22.2: Koeppe's nodules

nodules. This may account for their frequent presence.

Busacca's Nodules

Nodules on the anterior surface of iris are called as Busacca's nodules. These indicate a granulomatous type of inflammation. These are less common.

Iris Atrophy

Iris atrophy is an important clinical feature of Fuch's uveitis syndrome and occurs as sequelae to herpes simplex and herpes zoster uveitis.

Rubeosis Iridis

Rubeosis iridis is a condition of neovascularization of iris. It is seen in chronic anterior uveitis and in Fuch's uveitis. It can encroach on the angle of the anterior chamber producing rise of intraocular pressure.

Posterior Synechia

An adhesion between the anterior lens surface and the iris is known as posterior synechia. Posterior synechia develops easily in a case of uveitis. One of the important aspect of treating a case of uveitis is to prevent the formation of posterior synechia by keeping the pupil dilated. If synechia has developed then every effort should be made to break the synechia by using atropine or phenylephrine hydrochloride topically or even subconjunctivally with caution in a cardiac case. In severe acute cases the exudates may cover the pupil resulting in a condition of "occlusion of pupil". A 360° synechia may result in a condition of 'seclusion of pupil', preventing the passage of aqueous from the posterior to anterior chamber. This leads to a forward bowing of the iris (iris-bombe).

Peripheral Anterior Synechia

The exudates may result in formation of adhesion between the peripheral iris and posterior surface of cornea at the angle resulting in peripheral anterior synechia. It tends to increase the intraocular pressure. It can be prevented by early treatment of uveitis with steroids. To examine the angle of anterior chamber a gonioscopy is performed.

Anterior Vitreous

Examine the anterior vitreous for cells. Presence of cells in the anterior vitreous indicates involvement of ciliary body.

Lens Opacity

A patient of iridocyclitis develops posterior sub-capsular cataract. It can be examined by slit lamp. The cataract gives an appearance of bread crumbs with polychromatic luster. It is likely to cause dim vision. In some cases the cataract may gradually progress to mature cataract. Treat it by surgery.

Three Mirror Contact Lens

- Examine the angle of anterior chamber for peripheral anterior synechia and neo-vascularization, and study the angle whether narrow or wide.
- Examine the posterior fundus specially macula for any evidence of cystoid macular edema which occurs as a complication of anterior uveitis and is responsible for marked loss of vision.
- Examine the periphery of fundus for any evidence of pars planitis.

- Examine the posterior vitreous for vitreous opacities which may be fine, thick, strings or floaters moving freely in the vitreous with the movement of the eyeball.
- Examine the fundus as a whole for any evidence of choroiditis, fresh or healed.

Ophthalmoscopy

It is important to examine the fundus in each case of uveitis whether it is anterior or posterior uveitis. Fundus should be examined by direct and indirect ophthalmoscopy.

- Look for any evidence of choroiditis. A patch of choroiditis appear as a yellow gray patch with indistinct margins. A healed patch appears white with clear margins and pigmentation around it. The retinal vessels cross over the patch. Patient may have few focal lesions or it may be diffuse choroiditis.
- Look for macula for any evidence of edema, cyst, hole, pigmentation, exudation, and any degenerative changes.
- Look for the optic disk for papillitis or optic atrophy.
- Assess the clarity of the fundus. If not clear then there are vitreous opacities. To grade the clarity look for optic nerve head, retinal vessels, and normal reflex of the retinal nerve fibers. Looking at these three landmarks, one can make a note about the haze of the vitreous which shall later help to assess the progress.

Tonometry

Intraocular pressure must be recorded on the first visit and later on each subsequent visit as long as the patient is under treatment. There is tendency for intraocular pressure to rise. In early stage of uveitis it is due to formation of plasmoid aqueous. In later stage it is due to block in the passage of aqueous due to pupillary block or block at the angle of anterior chamber. In chronic cases the intraocular pressure may be low. A low pressure is a bad omen indicating that the ciliary processes have become atrophic.

Ultrasonography

It is helpful in the cases where in the fundus examination cannot be done due to either vitreous haze or lens opacities. It is helpful to diagnose a case with tumor or exudative detachment.

Fluorescein Angiography

It is very helpful in the diagnosis of macular pathology due to uveitis specially when there is dim vision more than that can be explained by vitreous haze or lens opacity. Documentation in the form of photographs is helpful for follow-up.

Electroretinogram

It helps to differentiate a case of choroiditis with a degenerative condition of retinitis pigmentosa.

Laboratory Investigations

An extensive laboratory test to find out the cause has been futile.

The following test can be done in a case depending on the clinical diagnosis. Other tests are conducted depending on the requirement for an individual case.

- Complete blood picture.
- Urine examination—Routine, culture and sensitivity.
- Stool examination for cysts and ova to rule out parasitic uveitis.
- Blood sugar—fasting and post-prandial.
- Serological tests for syphilis, toxoplasmosis and histoplasmosis.
- Tests for antinuclear antibodies, Rh factor, LE cells, C-reactive proteins.
- Skin tests-tuberculin test, Kveim's test and toxoplasmin test.

X-ray

X-ray of chest done in every case shall be fruitful. X-ray of sacroiliac joints for a case of spondylitis.

CLASSIFICATION OF UVEITIS

The term Uveitis covers inflammation of the uveal tissue only. There is a close relationship between three distinct parts of the uveal tissue-iris, ciliary body and choroid, therefore the inflammatory processes tends to involve the uvea as a whole. There is always some associated inflammation of the adjacent structures such as cornea, sclera, vitreous and retina.

1. *Anatomical classification*
   - **Anterior uveitis**
     Iritis, anterior cyclitis, iridocyclitis
   - **Intermediate uveitis**
     Posterior cyclitis
     Pars planitis
     Hyalitis
     Basal retinochoroiditis
   - **Posterior uveitis**
     Choroiditis
     Chorioretinitis
     Retinochoroiditis
     Neurouveitis
   - **Pan uveitis**
     The international uveitis study group has recommended that the classification based on anatomical location be followed.
2. *Clinical classification*
   - Acute uveitis.
   - Chronic uveitis.
3. *Pathological classification*
   - Granulomatous uveitis.
   - Non-granulomatous uveitis.
4. *Etiological classification (Duke Elder's)*
   - **Infective uveitis:** It can be exogenous, secondary or endogenous
     It can be due to bacterial, viral, fungal, parasitic or rickettsial infective uveitis.
   - **Allergic or hypersensitivity linked uveitis:** It can be due to microbial, anaphylactic, atopic, autoimmune or HLA-associated uveitis.
   - **Toxic uveitis:** It can be due to endotoxins, endocular toxins or exogenous toxins.
   - **Traumatic uveitis:** It can be due to direct trauma, irritative effect, retained intraocular foreign body and sympathetic ophthalmia.
   - **Non-infective systemic disease uveitis:** Such as sarcoidosis, rheumatic and rheumatoid arthritis, diabetes, gout, etc.

- **Idiopathic uveitis**: It can be specific or non specific uveitis.

Clinical Features and Management

1. Anterior uveitis.
2. Posterior uveitis.
3. Pars planitis.
4. Herpes simplex uveitis.
5. Herpes zoster uveitis.
6. Phacoanaphylactic uveitis.
7. Phacotoxic uveitis.
8. Ankylosing spondylitis.
9. Reiter's syndrome.
10. Behcet's syndrome.
11. Vogt-Koyanagi-Harada's syndrome.
12. Glaucomatocyclitic crisis.
13. Sarcoidosis uveitis.
14. Acquired syphilitic uveitis.
15. Tubercular uveitis.
16. Leprotic uveitis.
17. Toxoplasmosis uveitis.
18. Toxocariasis.
19. Onchocerciasis.
20. Presumed ocular histoplasmosis syndrome.
21. Candiasis.
22. Fuchs uveitis syndrome.
23. Juvenile chronic iridocyclitis.

ANTERIOR UVEITIS

Clinical Features

- Main symptoms are pain, redness, lacrimation, photophobia, blepharospasm and dim vision.
- Mild lid edema.
- Narraow or irregular pupil.
- Circumciliary congestion.
- Keratic precipitates and aqueous flare.
- Cells in the aqueous and anterior vitreous
- Iris may show atrophic patches, nodules, synechia.
- Fundus examination may reveal macular edema.
- Gonioscopy may show blocked angle due to synechia.
- Intraocular pressure may be raised.

Management

- Use mydriatics and cycloplegic to keep the pupil dilated and to break the synechia if any. These helps to prevent synechia, keep pupil dilated and give comfort to the patient by reducing inflammation and congestion of Iris.
- Use steroids-topically, sub-conjunctivally, periocular injection and systemic. Start with a higher does and taper off gradually.
- Suitable antibiotic to cover up for endogenous infection which may be responsible for uveitis. Change the antibiotic if the investigations or laboratory report is suggestive.

POSTERIOR UVEITIS

Clinical Features

- Main symptoms are floaters in front of the eye and dim vision if the lesion is central.
- A positive scotoma in early stage.
- Vitreous shows opacities which may be fine, thick or stringy.
- Ophthalmoscopy show patches of choroiditis which may be in active, healing or healed stage. A whitish yellow patch with pigments around it and retinal vessels crossing over it is typical finding of a healed patch of choroiditis.

Management

- Use suitable antibiotic to cover up an endogenous infection.
- Use steroids-systemic and in the form of periocular injection.
- Use mild cycloplegics to prevent formation of synechia which are likely to occur as there is always some silent anterior uveitis associated with posterior uveitis.

PARS PLANITIS

Clinical Features

- Main symptom is floaters and in some cases dim vision if there is involvement of macula.
- Cells in the aqueous.
- Few keratic precipitates.
- No posterior synechia.
- Cells in the anterior vitreous.
- Small gelatinous exudates appear known as snowballs or cotton balls.

- Posterior vitreous detachment is common.
- On indirect ophthalmoscopy there is presence of grey white plaque involving the inferior pars plana. This plaque is known as snow-banking.
- Main complications are cystoid macular edema, cataract and tractional retinal detachment.

Management

- Clinical course is variable. It may be low grade self-limiting process or a chronic course lasting few years.
- Visual prognosis is good.
- Treat by periocular injection or posterior sub-tenon injection of methylprednisolone repeatedly. Some cases may need systemic steroids for a short duration followed by injection.

HERPES SIMPLEX UVEITIS

A superficial dendritic ulcer of herpes simplex is almost always associated with mild anterior iritis. Severe iritis has been observed with deep herpetic keratitis. The iritis is probably due to simple axon reflex and may be also due to immune mechanism. Topical steroids give a good response which favors an immune nature of the iritis. Look for hyphema, iris atrophy and some corneal signs in a case of herpes simplex. A careful examination of cornea may reveal nebular opacities especially by the sclerotic scatter method of examination by slit lamp biomicroscopy. The iris atrophy in herpes simplex tends to affect small areas and nearer to the pupil than in herpes zoster wherein the atrophic area is large and close to root of the iris.

HERPES ZOSTER UVEITIS

The involvement of the eye is about 85% in the cases with involvement of the nasociliary nerve. The iritis often follows soon after involvement of the cornea. On examination, there is diminished corneal sensation, corneal opacities, and iris atrophy. Some case may show hyphema and raised intraocular pressure. There is severe pain in the eye with marked circumciliary congestion. Treat by topical steroids and cycloplegics with carbonic anhydrase inhibitors if required. Refer the case to neurologist.

PHACOANAPHYLACTIC UVEITIS

It is an autoimmune reaction to lens protein. It occurs after an injury to the lens capsule or after an extracapsular cataract surgery. Treat by steroids and removal of any lens matter left behind.

PHACOTOXIC UVEITIS

Clinically it is less intense than the phaco-anaphylactic endophthalmitis. It is probably due to low grade immunologic reaction to lens protein.

ANKYLOSING SPONDYLITIS

Clinical Features

- It is a chronic inflammatory arthritis of unknown cause affecting axial skeleton.
- Usually affects males between 20 and 40 years of age who are positive for HLA-B27.
- Keratic precipitates are small and dusting the corneal endothelium.
- Cells in the aqueous and aqueous flare.
- Fibrinous exudates in anterior chamber which leads to formation of posterior synechia, seclusio pupil, iris-bombe.
- Raised intraocular pressure.
- It becomes a chronic uveitis in course of time.
- Uveitis is usually acute, recurrent and non-granulomatous.
- Uveitis may precede or follow the diagnosis of ankylosing spondylitis. No correlation with joint involvement.

Investigation

- X-ray of the sacroiliac joint is a must in a young adult with acute unilateral uveitis whether there is presence or absence of low back ache. X-ray is positive before the patient is symptomatic.
- Tissue typing for HLA-B27. A positive test

confirms the diagnosis even though the X-ray may be normal.

Management

- Treat by topical steroids and cycloplegics.
- A periocular injection of steroid is helpful.
- Case must be under treatment of a rheumatologist.

REITER'S SYNDROME

Reiter's syndrome consists of a triad of urethritis, conjunctivitis and sero-negative arthritis.

Clinical Features

- It is of unknown etiology.
- It affects young people and most of them are positive for HLA-B27. Thus it has a strong relationship with ankylosing-spondylitis. Most of the cases develop ankylosing-spondylitis in course of time.
- The disease may present as non-specific urethritis following post sexual contact, an attack of dysentery and an attack of arthritis affecting knee, ankle and Achilles tendon.
- Uveitis is acute and unilateral affecting iris and ciliary body-iridocyclitis.
- Conjunctivitis may be associated with punctate epithelial or sub-epithelial keratitis.
- Along with arthritis there may be peri-ostitis causing a calcaneal spur.
- Chlamydiae have been recovered from the cases of Reiter's syndrome. Other organisms and viruses have also been implicated.
- Syphilis may be associated so perform an FTA-ABS Test.

Management

- Tissue typing for HLA-B27 is helpful.
- X-ray of knee, ankle and feet.
- Uveitis to be treated by topical and periocular injection of steroids.
- Cycloplegics topically helps to prevent many complication of uveitis.

- Some may need systemic steroids.
- Treat syphilis if FTS-ABS test is positive.
- Treat urethritis and conjunctivitis with topical and systemic antibiotics.

BEHCET'S SYNDROME

Clinical Features

It is a disease of unknown etiology. Both the virus and immunologic factors have been thought of and proposed. It affects young people. Patient is positive for HLA-B51

It is a multisystem disease and manifests with following:

- Recurrent oral shallow ulcers which are painful with central yellow necrotic base. These occurs in crop and involves the tongue, lips, gums and buccal mucosa.
- Gential ulcers which begin as vesicles and later ulcerate are more painful in male than in female.
- Skin lesions appear in the form of pus-tules, furuncles and erythema nodosum.
- Neurologic disorders may be non-locali-zing thus suggest multiple sclerosis.
- Anterior uveitis (iridocyclitis) may be unilateral or bilateral and acute in onset with hypopyon is characteristic ocular feature.
- Ophthalmoscopy may show varied lesions like cystoid macular edema, periphlebitis, retinal central vein occlusion and optic atrophy.
- Poor visual prognosis. Acute iridocyclitis becomes chronic and associated vasculitis may lead to blindness.

Management

- Anterior uveitis responds to steroids topically and periocular injection and cycloplegics.
- Systemic steroids may be needed in most cases.
- Some cases who do not respond to steroids may need immunosuppressive drugs under the supervision of a physician who will treat and look after the other systemic problems like genital and mucosal ulcers, skin lesions and neurological lesions.

VOGT-KOYANAGI-HARADA'S SYNDROME
(Uveomeningitis syndrome)

Clinical Features

- It is a condition of uveitis with meningeal signs of headache and neck stiffness. Meningeal symptoms may be latent. Spinal fluid examination often shows lymphocytosis in early acute phase.
- Patient presents with dim vision, headache, tinnitis, vertigo, and nausea.
- It is of unknown etiology.
- Clinically and immunologically it is similar to sympathetic ophthalmitis.
- It affects pigmented people more and has an increased prevalence of HLA-B22.
- Positive for HLA-DR4 and DW15.
- A viral etiology has been postulated but unproved.
- Histlopathologic study has revealed Dalen-Fuchs nodules.
- Fluorescein angiography shows sub-retinal leak.
- To label a case as a Vogt-Koyanagi-Harada's syndrome; three of the following four signs must be present:
  1. Meningeal signs of headache and stiff neck.
  2. Skin lesions of alopecia, poliosis and vitiligo.
  3. Anterior uveitis usually bilateral and granulomatous type. On examination there are keratic precipitates and posterior synechia.
  4. Posterior uveitis with diffuse choroiditis and/or exudative retinal detachment.

Management

- Treat the anterior uveitis vigourously with steroids topically, sub conjunctivally, periocular injection and systemically with a high dose and taper gradually. Anterior uveitis often leads to cataract, glaucoma and thick posterior synechia jeopardizing the visual outcome which is otherwise good with posterior uveitis.
- Use cycloplegics for a sufficient long time to prevent complication of synechia.

- Exudative retinal detachment settles down spontaneously or with the help of steroids with good visual acuity. The fundus shows a mottled appearance with poliferation of pigment epithelium on settlement of retina. It needs patience from patient and treating eye physician.

GLAUCOMATOCYCLITIC CRISIS (Posner-Schlossman Syndrome)

Clinical Features

- It is a condition of recurrent attack of secondary open angle glaucoma with mild anterior uveitis.
- It affects young adults 40% of whom are positive for HLA- BW54.
- During the attack the intraocular pressure may rise to 40–60 mm Hg.
- Patient may see halos and complain of blurring of vision but no pain.
- During attack there may be aqueous flare, few pigmented keratic precipitates, epithelial edema of cornea, hetero-chromia, but no posterior synechia.
- In between the attacks the eye is normal with normal intraocular pressure, normal visual fields and normal optic disk.
- Usually unilateral but 50% patients have bilateral involvement.

Management

- These patients have high incidence of associated diabetes so check for blood sugar.
- During attack control the intraocular pressure by medical therapy—topical timolol maleate and systemic carbonic anhydrase inhibitors.
- To control inflammation—use topical steroids with care as many of these patients may be steroid responders. Most of these cases have open angle glaucoma.

SARCOIDOSIS-UVEITIS

Clinical Features

- Sarcoidosis is multi-system granulomatous disorder of unknown etiology. It affects young adults and presents with bilateral hilar lymphadenopathy, pulmonary infiltration, skin and ocular lesions.

- X-ray chest-shows bilateral hilar fullness and later followed by reticulonodular infiltrates leaving pulmonary fibrosis.
- There may be an acute onset with erythema nodosa.

Ocular lesions may be
- Sarcoid plaques on the skin of the eyelids.
- Sarcoid granuloma of the lid margin.
- Granulomatous infiltration of lacrimal gland.
- Episcleritis.
- Acute iridocyclitis.

Chronic iridocyclitis with Koeppe's and Busacca's nodules on iris, with mutton-fat keratic precipitates.

Ophthalmoscopy Shows

Peripheral retinal periphlebitis. Periphlebitic nodules due to perivascular accumulation of granulomatous tissue (Candlewax drippings).
- Retinal granulomas.
- Venous occlusion.
- Choroiditis patches.
- Vitreous haze.

Diagnostic Tests

- *X-ray chest:* shows hilar lymphadenopathy and nodular infiltration.
- Biopsy-showing histologic evidence of non-caseating granulomas. Lung biopsy by the tracheobronchial fiberoptic technique is accurate in 90% of cases.
- *Kveim-Slitzbach test:* An intradermal injection of saline suspension of sarcoid tissue (antigen) obtained from the spleen of the patient with active sarcoidosis shall induce a granulomatous reaction seen four weeks later on biopsy.
- Angiotensin converting enzyme (ACE) shows raised level.
  The normal serum level of Angiotensin converting enzyme is 12–35 nmol/min per ul in men and 11–29 nmol/min per ul in women. It is elevated in patients with active sarcoidosis.
- Gallium -67 scan of head, neck and thorax. There is an increased uptake of gallium in patients with active systemic sarcoidosis.
- Hypercalciuria is common.

Management

- Topical and periocular steroids.
- Systemic steroids mainly in posterior segment involvement
- Laser photocoagulation in neovascularization
- Topical cycloplegics to prevent formation of synechia.
- Refer the case to Physician.

ACQUIRED SYPHILITIC UVEITIS

Syphilis is a chronic infection caused by a spirochaete *Treponema pallidum* acquired by venereal infection.

Clincial Features

- Uveities is usually acute and becomes chronic.
- It may be granulomatous or non-granulomatous.
- Chorioretinitis occurs in about 50% cases and may be multi-focal or diffuse.
- It may cause neuroretinitis which may lead to optic atrophy.
- Some cases may show peri-phlebitis and peri-arteritis
- In healed stage the fundus shows extensive pigmentary changes like that of retinitis pigmentosa.
- Patient may complain of night blindness

Diagnostic Test

- FTA-ABS (Fluorescent Treponemal Antibody Absorption) blood test. It is the most specific test today. It becomes positive in early stage of disease and remains positive for rest of the life. It is read as reactive, weakly reactive or non-reactive. It does not indicate clinical activity of the disease. It may give false positive results in a case who had a smallpox vaccination, atypical pneumonia and in narcotic addicts.

- VDRL (Venereal Disease Research Laboratory) test. It is a non-specific test useful for screening. It becomes positive early. It also becomes negative following anti-syphilitic treatment. It becomes negative after many years. It decreases with treatment so useful in following the treatment response.

Management

- Use topical steroids and cycloplegics.
- Some cases may need periocular steroids
- Treat syphilis by penicillin or erythromycin if sensitive to penicillin.
- VDRL test shall help to study the response.
- Refer the case to Skin and VD Department.

TUBERCULAR UVEITIS

Tuberculosis is a chronic granulomatous infection caused by *bovine or human tubercle bacilli.* Bovine tubercle bacilli causes tuberculosis by drinking milk from infected cattle. Human tubercle bacilli spread by droplet infection.

Clinical Features

- Granulomatous type of anterior uveitis showing koeppe nodules, synechia, and mutton fat keratic precipitates.
- Choroiditis which may be focal or diffuse.
- Vasculitis (Eales' disease).

Diagnostic Test

- *Sputum examination:* Examine sputum for acid fast bacilli.
- *X-ray chest:* A positive X-ray finding is of significance. A negative X-ray chest does not exclude tuberculosis.
- *Tuberculin test:* A negative test is helpful to an extent to exclude tuberculosis as a cause. A positive test unless strongly positive does not help.
- *Isoniazid test:* A good response to isoniazid 300 mg daily for three weeks is suggestive of tubercular infection.

Management

- Instill topical steroids and cycloplegics.
- Inject periocular steroid if needed.
- Treat tuberculosis by systemic administration of anti-tubercular drugs
- Isoniazid 300 mg daily for 12 months.
- Rifampicin 450 to 600 mg daily in a single dose before breakfast—for 12 months.

It is advisable to refer the case to Physician to treat tuberculosis.

Assess the progress of the uveitis by clinical judgment, laboratory and radiological investigations.

LEPROTIC UVEITIS

Leprosy (Hansen's disease) is known for causing ocular complications. The causative organism is *Mycobacterium leprae.* It has an affinity for skin, peripheral nerves and the anterior segment of the eye. Leprosy manifests in lepromatous or tuberculoid form. Uveal involvement is more common in the lepromatous form of leprosy.

Clinical Features

Anterior segment lesions include the following

- Madarosis.
- Keratitis.
- Lagophthalmos.
- Conjunctivitis.
- Scleritis.
- Episcleritis.
- Uveitis.

It may occur as acute iritis (non-granulomatous) or chronic iritis (granulomatous) form.

Slit lamp examination will show the "iris pearls" at the pupillary margin, nodular lepromata and atrophy of the iris with formation of holes in the iris.

Management

- Topical steroids and cycloplegics.
- Treat leprosy by systemic therapy-Dapsone 50–100 mg daily.

- Patient needs a regular follow up and treatment for long time.
- Refer the case to Dermatologist for treatment.

TOXOPLASMOSIS

Toxoplasmosis is caused by an intracellular protozoan parasite—"*Toxoplasma gondii*". The cat is the definate host for the parasite. The mice, cattle, sheep, pigs and humans are intermediate host. Humans get infected by ingestion of undercooked meat of the intermediate host animal and by ingestion of cysts. The flies, cockroaches and the dirt contaminate the food by transfer of cysts onto food. The parasite may pass through the placenta to infest the fetus if acute toxoplasmosis occurs during pregnancy. If the mother is infested before pregnancy the fetus will not be affected.

Clinical Features

A case of congenital toxoplasmosis shows triad of
- Convulsions
- Bilateral healed punched out pigmented chorioretinal scar at the macula.
- Intracranial calcification seen in X-ray skull.

A case of recurrent toxoplasmic retino-choroiditis shows
- Granulomatous or non-granulomatous anterior uveitis.
- Hazy vitreous due to vitritis.
- Satellite lesions adjacent to the old healed scar is the most common fundus finding.
- Retinitis which may be a solitary lesion or a multifocal usually affects the post equatorial area. Active retinitis appears as a yellow white lesion with blurred margins.
- The lesion heals leaving a clear cut atrophic scar with pigmentation around it.
- There is loss of vision due to involvement of fovea, papillomacular bundle and optic nerve.
- Retinal neovascularisation and tractional retinal detachment occurs as rare sequelae.

Laboratory Tests
- Indirect fluorescent antibody test
- Hemagglutination test
- ELISA test.

Management
- Steroids to be given topically, periocular injection and systemic also if needed.
- Drugs acting against *Toxoplasma gondii* such as Clindamycin, Spiramycin, Sulfadiazine or Pyremethamine.
- Laser and cryopexy have been used in front of an advancing lesion to save the macula.

TOXOCARIASIS

Toxocariasis is an infestation caused by roundworms of cats —*Toxocara catis* and dogs— *Toxocara canis*. Humans get infected by ingestion of food contaminated with ova which are shed in dog's and cat's faeces and also due to close contact with puppies. Clinically it can cause ocular toxocariasis.

Clinical Features
- The common ocular unilateral lesions are: Chronic endophthalmitis, posterior pole granuloma and peripheral granuloma.
- Other less common lesions include Pars planitis, anterior uveitis, optic papillitis, vitreous abscess and retinal tracks.
- Vision is markedly affected in endophthalmitis and posterior granuloma.
- It usually leads to retinal detachment, cyclitic membrane, cataract and macular edema affecting the vision markedly.
- Diagnosis by typical clinical picture and ELISA test

Management
- A quiet eye with granuloma needs no treatment.
- Treat endophthalmitis with steroids, systemic and periocular.
- Antihelminthic drugs are of no value in treating a case of endophthalmitis.
- Pars plana vitrectomy is indicated in endophthalmitis, cyclitic membrane and vitreoretinal traction.

- As a prophylaxis—puppies should be dewormed with piperazine, at regular intervals and avoid close contact of children with puppies.
- Chronic endophthalmitis occurs usually in children so differentiate from retinoblastoma, Coats' disease and fungal endophthalmitis.

ONCHOCERCIASIS

Onchocerciasis is due to infestation with *Onchocerca volvulus*—a filarial nematode worm. It is transmitted to humans by the bite of black fly (sandfly) *Simulium damnosum*. It is endemic in tropical Africa and Central and South America. The usual ocular infection results in conjunctivitis and keratitis causing blindness in millions in that region. Microfilariae are mobile and can reach the eye. It can pass into the anterior chamber and cause chronic iridocyclitis. Microfilaria can be seen swimming in the anterior chamber and vitreous. A severe inflammation follows the death of organism.

Clinical Features

- A low grade of iridocyclitis.
- A microfilaria seen swimming in the aqueous.
- Localized atrophy of iris.
- Chorioretinitis with pigmentation is seen.
- Presence of a skin nodule and its biopsy helps in the diagnosis.
- There is eosinophilia.

Management

- Excise the nodule if present to avoid further dissemination of microfilaria.
- Hetrazan (diethylcarbamazine citrate) 100 mg four times a day for 10 to 14 days orally.
- Antihistamines and steroids to reduce the side effects caused by the massive death of the organisms.
- In endemic zone 50 mg daily of hetrazan provides cover.

PRESUMED OCULAR HISTOPLASMOSIS SYNDROME

Histoplasmosis is a fungal infection caused by *Histoplasma capsulatum*. The infection is acquired by inhalation and the organism pass via blood stream to the spleen, liver and to choroid resulting in multiple foci of granulomatous inflammation.

Clinical Features

The fundus examination shows the following lesions.
- Multiple atrophic choroidal spots.
- Peri-papillary atrophy.
- Hemorrhagic disciform maculopathy
- Vitreous is never involved.
- Patient reports to the ophthalmologist for the loss of vision with complain of metamorphopsia, loss of central vision and a positive scotoma.
- Slit lamp biomicroscopy with fundus contact lens shows the elevation of macula.
- Fluorescein angiography is helpful in detecting early macular lesions.

Management

- Clinical diagnosis is supported by Histoplasmin skin test but not confirmed.
- In all cases with macular lesions the argon laser photocoagulation is the treatment of choice.
- Steroids in the desperate cases in which photocoagulation is contraindicated.

CANDIDIASIS

Candidiasis is caused by *Candida albicans*—a yeast like fungus. It is frequently present in the human skin, mouth, gastrointestinal tract and vagina. It can acquire pathogenic properties in the following three main groups of patients and may result in ocular involvement.
- Drug addicts acquire the disease through the use of non-sterile needles and syringes.
- Patients with long-term indwelling catheters.

- Patients with decreased immunity, due to AIDS, malignancy, and on long term use of steroids, antibiotics and cytotoxic agents.

Clinical Features

Anterior uveitis is common and is associated with hypopyon. Multifocal retinitis with hemorrhages and heal with faint glial scar. Vitreous may show floating white-puff ball-or-cotton ball colonies.

Advanced cases may show a vitreous abscess. Later there may be tractional retinal detachment due to vitreous fibrosis.

Management

- Topical cycloplegics and antifungal.
- Systemic antifungal drugs like Keto-conazole, Flucytosine or amphotericin-B.
- Para plana vitrectomy—In severe cases with vitreous abscess or endophthalmitis.

FUCHS UVEITIS SYNDROME
(Fuchs Heterochromic Uveitis)

Fuch's uveitis syndrome is a unilateral chronic non-granulomatous anterior uveitis with an insidious onset. It affects young adults. It is usually asymptomatic. Some patients may complain of vitreous floaters, dim vision or change in the color of the eye.

Clinical Features

- Iris heterochromia
- Iris may show Koeppe's nodules occasionally.
- No posterior synechia.

- Keratic precipitates are small round grey-white and scattered throughout the corneal endothelium and never become pigmented.
- Pupil of the affected eye is irregular and larger than the fellow eye. It is due to atrophy of iris sphincter.
- There is minimal aqueous flare and cells.
- Vitreous may show few cells and opacities.
- Early cataract formation causing loss of vision.
- Glaucoma occurs in these cases and is the cause for loss of vision.

Management

- Topical steroids help to control the transient acute symptoms.
- Prolonged use of steroids is of no help and is likely to produce cataract and glaucoma.
- Cycloplegics are not required as there is no posterior synechia.
- A regular check up for raised intraocular pressure is essential.
- Glaucoma is open angle type.
- If there is a cataract then operate. Good response to cataract surgery.

JUVENILE CHRONIC IRIDOCYCLITIS

Juvenile chronic iridocyclitis is associated with juvenile chronic arthritis in most cases. About 75% of cases are girls. The malady is insidious and asymptomatic. Usually the patient is brought when there is a white reflex from the eye due to formation of cataract or a white patch on the cornea due to band keratopathy. The eye is lost if not diagnosed early.

23

A Case with Lens Opacity

History

Record the history with reference to the following:
- Age at which the lens opacity was noticed.
- Dim vision is gradual or sudden.
- Vision is better in bright light or dim illumination.
- Frequent change of glasses.
- Seeing halos.
- Any history of diplopia or broken image.
- Black spot in the field of vision.
- Any change in color values.
- Occupation—exposed to heat as working on furnace.
- And history of trauma even mild.
- Any past eye ailment like detachment of retina, diabetes, uveitis or night blindness.
- Any associated systemic disease.
- If the patient is an infant then ask about history of maternal infection, viral fever, rubella, toxoplasmosis during pregnancy.
- Mental retardation in a child.

CLINICAL EXAMINATION

A thorough examination of the eye and system is essential in every case of cataract irrespective of the age and etiological factor. In a case of a child or an infant general anesthesia should be used to examine the eyes. After initial examination of the external eye the lens must be examined under full mydriasis and cycloplegic with slit lamp bio-microscopy.

Visual Acuity

Assess the visual acuity of a case and make a record of it for follow up examination. If there is no hand movements then test for perception of light and projection of light from four quadrants repeating it before making final conclusion.

Torch Light

An examination by simple pen torch light will give an idea about lens opacity as there is a grey shadow from the pupil when the light is thrown on the eye from any direction.

Pupillary Reaction

A normal pupillary reaction indicates good prognosis. A Marcus Gunn pupillary reaction indicates a poor prognosis. A case with abnormal pupillary reaction must be further investigated to evaluate the prognosis.

Retinoscopy

A clear red reflex rules out any lens opacity. Usually the lens opacities appear black in form of spots, spokes, dots, in the red back ground. No red reflex is seen if there is complete lens opacity.

Ophthalmoscopy

- Fundus appears hazy if there is lens opacity in capsule or nuclear opacity.
- Lens opacity appear as black spots, spokes or dots, in the red backgound.

- There is no red reflex if there is a complete lens opacity.

Indirect Ophthalmoscopy

In early cases of lens opacity indirect ophthalmoscopy gives a better view of fundus. Wherever possible it is rewarding to examine the fundus and note the finding.

Slit Lamp Biomicroscopy

Examine the case with full mydriasis and short duration cycloplegic like tropicamide or cyclopentolate hydrochloride for better evaluation.

- Diffuse light is useful to survey the anterior and posterior lens surface and large opacities of the lens.
- Retroillumination is required for viewing anterior capsular changes.
- Direct illumination provides a clear view of opacities in the posterior capsule and posterior cortex.
- Specular reflection allows view of elevations and depressions and opacities of the anterior lens capsule. These appear as dark spots in the area of specular reflection.
- Direct focal illumination is used to examine the "zones of discontinuity". The zones of discontinuity are composed of anterior and posterior surfaces of the following structures which are concentric to one another; capsule, line of disjunction, adult nucleus, infantile nucleus and fetal nucleus. The fetal nucleus contains anterior and posterior Y-sutures. With the age many zones of discontinuity are added peripherally in the adult nucleus representing lenticular growth.
- The sub-capsular clear zone is a true zone which lies between the capsule and the line of disjunction. Obliteration of this zone is one of the earliest sign of cataract formation.
- The zones of discontinuity appears as bright stripes in a narrow and oblique beam of slit lamp concentric to one another. It is due to change in the refractive index of each zone or each layer of the lens.

- Examine the cornea for corneal dystrophy.
- Examine the conjunctiva for keratoconjunctivitis sicca.
- Look for iris atrophy, rubeosis, iridodonesis, synechia and persistent pupillary membrane.

Gonioscopy

Gonioscopy is essential in cases of complicated cataract, secondary cataract, cataract associated with close angle glaucoma, pigmentary glaucoma, exfoliation syndrome, and traumatic cataract. This will give information about the chamber angle and so better planning of cataract surgery.

Tonometry

It is essential to record the intraocular pressure in every case of lens opacity, irrespective of age of the patient, morphology of the cataract and its stage of maturation and etiological factor.

Field of Vision

In early case with good visual acuity and associated glaucoma a record of field shall be helpful to evaluate the prognosis and planning the surgery. In a patient with reduced vision the confrontation test may be employed.

Special Investigation in a Case with Mature Cataract

Special investigation shall be useful only when the case shows a normal pupillary reaction and good projection and perception of light. These tests are meant to assess the retinal function where the history is unreliable and suggestive of some pathology in the posterior segment of the eye. The electroretinography, electrooculography, visually evoked potential and ultrasonography are helpful in evaluation of a case with suspected posterior segment pathology.

Systemic Examination

- It is essential to conduct a thorough systemic examination to assess the general health status.

- There are many syndromes associated with cataract thus a systemic check up shall help to identify the syndromes.
- General health has an important role in the success of the surgery.

Dental Check Up

As most of the patients are elderly past 6th decade some dental problem is likely to be there. Take care to diagnose and treat any septic focus prior to surgery.

Electrocardiogram

A preoperative electrocardiogram is a must in any case taken for surgery particularly when there is a chance for general anesthesia. It informs about the heart function and thus proper care can be taken during surgery if there is any problem. A vaso-vagal reflex is known to occur during surgery on the eye.

X-ray Chest

It should be included as a part of routine checkup.

Laboratory Investigations

- Complete blood picture.
- Blood sugar— fasting and post prandial.
- Complete urine examination.
- Other test like serum electrolytes, serum cholestrol, etc. as per need in a particular case.

Special Laboratory Investigations

- TORCH test for intrauterine infection of toxoplasmosis, rubella, cytomegalo virus and herpes virus.
- Galactosemia.
  Urine test for reducing substances, Red blood cell transferase and galactokinase levels.
- Hypocalcemic syndrome.
  Serum calcium and phosphate levels and X-ray skull.
- Lowe's syndrome.
  Urine chromatography for the amino acids.

Clinical Features and Management
1. Agerelated or senile cataract.
2. Traumatic cataract.
3. Toxic cataract.
4. Complicated cataract.
5. Metabolic cataract.
6. Maternal infection causing cataract.
7. Dermatogenic cataract.
8. Congenital cataract.
9. Developmental cataract

AGE-RELATED OR SENILE CATARACT

Any opacity in the lens is known as *Cataract.*

The lens is a transparent structure. The transparency is disturbed due to degenerative process resulting in opacification of lens fibers. Any factor, physical or chemical, that disturbs the critical intracellular or extracellular equilibrium of water and electrolytes or deranges the colloid system within the lens fibers induces opacification of the lens.

Senile cataract is the most common type of acquired cataract affecting males and females equally and usually above 60 years of age. The condition is bilateral but one eye gets affected earlier than the other.

The senile cataract manifests as:
- Sub-capsular cataract.
- Cortical cataract.
- Nuclear cataract.

It is common to find the above mentioned forms of senile cataract co-existing in the same eye. The cortical cataract is predominant in acquired senile cataract-age-related cataract.

Sub-capsular Cataract

These opacities are seen as brown granules and cysts in the posterior and anterior sub-capsular region. Patients with sub-capsular posterior cataract suffer much from the glare of bright sun light and head lights of automobiles. Their near vision is disturbed more than the distance vision. It affects the people in the age group of 6th to 8th decade. It is easily diagnosed by slit lamp examination.

Cortical Cataract

Cortical cataract evolves due to hydration followed by coagulation of proteins

In cortical cataract, the lens opacity involves, anterior, posterior and equatorial cortex. There are wedge-shaped opacities, with clear lens in between. The apices are towards the center. The patient complains of uniocular polyopia or seeing more than two images. He needs a frequent change in his glasses. His dim vision and polyopia is due to sectorial alteration in the refractive index of the lens. This stage of cataract can be easily diagnosed by plane mirror examination, ophthalmoscopy and slit lamp bio-microscopy. The wedge-shaped opacities appear black against the red background of the reflex from the fundus. Patient can be helped by advice about using bright illumination and change of glasses. In course of time the entire cortex becomes opaque.

Nuclear Cataract

Nuclear cataract evolves due to an increased sclerosis (optical density) of the lens nucleus with aging.

This sclerotic process renders the lens inelastic and hard that decreases its ability to change its shape in the act of accommo-dation. These changes begin centrally and spread peripherally. These changes are accompanied by an accumulation of yellow-brown pigment urochrome which may represent an oxidation product of either aromatic amino acids or lipids. The pigment absorbs its complimentary color the blue light which results in relative increase in transmission of red-yellow light perceived by the patient. It causes change in the color values and affects paintings of painters. The excess sclerosis results in formation of a brown or a black nucleus (**cataract brunescens and cataract nigra**). The process of sclerosis is very slow taking years for maturation. The process of sclerosis is associated with increase in refractive index of the lens nucleus which induces myopia. It is because of this induced myopia, the elderly patients with nuclear cataract are able to read and write again without the help of their near glasses. This natural phenomenon is known as a **second sight of aged.** It is seen in the cases of nuclear cataract. Patient becomes myopic due to increase in the refractive index of the lens nucleus and also with increased spherical aberration. These patients are able to read again without near spectacles and so this regain in the near sight is referred as second sight of the aged. They do suffer from loss of distance vision to 6/36 or less and that is enough for them for their normal work at that age of retired life. Treat by prescribing glasses or cataract operation with capsular implant.

Symptoms

- Glare.
- Uniocular diplopia.
- Colored halos.
- Change in color perception.
- Black spot in the field of vision.
- Secod sight of aged.
- Vision is blurred, distorted or misty.
- Dim visual acuity.
- Slit lamp biomicroscopy shall reveal the morphology of lens opacity.

Stages in Maturation of Senile Cortical Cataract

I. Immature Cataract (Incipient Cataract)

The cataract is immature if there are clear zones in between the opacities of lens as seen by slit lamp. Patient complains of dim vision in dim illumination and polyopia. Advice about using bright illumination and frequent change of glasses shall be helpful to patient.

II. Mature Cataract

The entire cortex is opaque. There is no red reflex on plane mirror examination or ophthal-moscopy. Surgery is the only choice to give him vision.

III. Intumescent Cataract

The lens is swollen due to imbibing of fluid. It can occur during immature or mature stage of cortical cataract. The anterior chamber is shallow, the iris lens diaphragm is pushed forward, and may induce block of the angle which may precipitate an attack of secondary glaucoma.

IV. Hypermature Cataract

The lens becomes smaller and the capsule of the lens appears wrinkled. This is due to leakage of water from the lens. The anterior chamber is deep.

V. Morgagnian Cataract

The cortex has become liquefied. The small nucleus sinks to the bottom of lens capsule. On examination the lens nucleus gives a yellow convex line in the lower part of pupil while the upper part of pupil appears milky white. The lens may subluxate or even dislocate easily at this stage.

Complications of Cortical Cataract during Maturation

- Phacolytic glaucoma.
- Phaco-antigenic uveitis (phacoanaphylaxis).
- Phaco-morphic glaucoma.
- Pseudo-exfoliation.

Phacolytic Glaucoma

Phacolytic glaucoma is a complication of a mature cataract. The lens capsule is intact. The lens proteins leak out through the permeable lens capsule and invoke a macrophagic response. The macrophages ingest the lens material and get deposited on the lens capsule, iris and trabecular meshwork. This results in the obstruction to the outflow of aqueous which manifests as secondary glaucoma.

Clinical Features

- Presence of mature cataract with pain and redness.
- Aqueous flare is seen in the beam of slit lamp.
- Raised intraocular pressure.
- Gonioscopy may show deposition of macrophages in the trabecular meshwork.
- Slit lamp examination will show deposition of macrophages on lens capsule and iris.

Treatment

- Reduce intraocular pressure by systemic carbonic anhydrase inhibitors.
- Early and planned cataract surgery.

Phaco-antigenic Uveitis

It is a granulomatous inflammation of uvea due to release of lens proteins through a ruptured lens capsule due to trauma or following extracapsular extraction of cataract. Phaco-antigenic uveitis occurs only in few cases following rupture of lens or extracapsular cataract extraction. This unpredictability of phaco-antigenic uveitis occurring in few cases may be possibly related to the innate nature of an individual's immune system as determined by immune response genes.

Clinical Features

- History of trauma or surgery on lens.
- Gradual increase in pain and redness.
- Lens matter may be visible in anterior chamber on slit lamp.
- Intense circumciliary congestion.
- Raised intraocular pressure.
- Aqueous flare is seen on slit lamp.

Treatment

- Systemic and topical steroids if lens remnants are few and small.
- Surgical removal of the lens matter whether due to trauma or left after extracapsular cataract extraction.

Phacomorphic Glaucoma

This occurs due to intumescence of the lens during the maturation of a cortical cataract. The clinical picture is similar to that of primary angle closure glaucoma.

Clinical Features

- The cataract is immature or mature.
- The anterior chamber is shallow.
- The iris lens diaphragm is pushed forward.
- Intense circumciliary congestion.
- Cornea may show mild edema.
- Intraocular pressure is raised.
- Gonioscopy may show peripheral anterior synechia.

Treatment

- Cataract extraction.
- Supportive therapy to reduce intraocular pressure and inflammation of the eye.
- Cataract extraction with trebeculectomy if gonioscopy show peripheral anterior synechia.

Pseudo-exfoliation

Pseudo-exfoliation syndrome is a bilateral condition affecting elderly people with cataract. There is a deposition of grey material on the lens capsule, ciliary zone, iris, trabecular meshwork and pupillary margin. Histologically the material is found in the basement membranes of the ciliary body, iris and lens epithelium. Its nature and origin is unknown. A current theory is that the pseudo-exfoliation syndrome represents a systemic basement membrane disease. Its clinical importance is that more than 30% of the affected people develop open angle glaucoma. Clinically grey amorphous material is seen on the lens capsule in the pupillary region. It is frequently seen at the pupillary margin. On dilation of pupil the material can be seen along the pre-equatorial region of the lens. A regular check up for intraocular pressure is needed to diagnose glaucoma early. Treat by removal of lens.

Management

The best management of lens opacity (cataract) is phacoemulsification with intraocular lens implant.

Types of Intraocular Lenses

Anterior chamber lenses: Anterior chamber lens lies entirely in the anterior chamber in front of iris. The lens gets fixed by its haptics supported against the scleral spur in the angle of anterior chamber. There are many designs of anterior chamber lens available. Each surgeon has his own choice. The most popular anterior chamber lens is the mark VIII and IX of choice.

Iris supported lenses: The iris supports the lens. It is important that the iris has a good structural integrity. There are many designs but the basic principal is same.

Posterior chamber lens: These lenses lie behind the iris. The flexible haptics are inserted into the ciliary sulcus a groove between the root of the iris and the ciliary body. These have been introduced recently. The follow up will enable to assess their place in the intraocular implant surgery. In some posterior chamber lenses the optics and haptics lie in the same plane while in others the haptics are angled slightly anteriorly enabling easier insertion into the ciliary sulcus and allowing for a greater separation between the pupil and optics.

Capsule-fixated lenses: The intraocular lens is fixed in the lens capsule of the patient. A planned extracapsular cataract extraction is performed. The lens is placed in the capsular bag with haptics of lens between the anterior and posterior capsule in periphery. It provides good capsular fixation. It is the most widely accepted mode of management of cataract.

Aphakic correction

It can be corrected by three methods
- Spectacles.
- Contact lenses.
- Intraocular lens.

Spectacle correction: Spectacle correction causes the following problems
- There is about 30% magnification of the objects seen.
- The objects seem closer to the patient than its actual position. It gives problem in day-to-day function.
- Distortion of objects due to spherical aberration.
- The field of vision is limited by the size of lens and due to prismatic effect on light rays entering the edge of the lens.
- Small movement of spectacle causes change in the effective dioptric power of the lens so disturbs the vision. Some patients learn to take advantage of this phenomenon, and learn to read and write with distance glasses by moving the spectacle forward on the nose.

Contact lenses: Contact lenses help to solve many problems of spectacles. Optically the contact lens is better than spectacles. There are practicle problems in the use of contact lens.

- There is about 8% magnification of the objects seen.
- There is full field of vision and little distortion of objects.
- These are not suitable for very young and very old patients as they are not able to handle these lenses.
- These are unsuitable in a dry, dusty and smoky environment.

Thus contact lenses offered few advantages over spectacles but at the same time offered problems. A large number of aphakic patients are unable to use contact lenses.

Intraocular lenses: Intraocular lens has corrected all the optical problems faced by the patient with the use of spectacles or contact lenses.

- There is no magnification or very little.
- There is no distortion.
- There is full field of vision.
- Small optical aberration.

Intraocular lens provides good vision all the time. With the improvement in the surgical technique, appliance available, and quality of the lenses, an implantation of an intraocular lens is very safe. The patient is almost normal for his distance vision and uses near glasses as he used to wear before the surgery. The only complication is posterior capsule opacification. This opacification can be easily treated by Nd: YAG Laser capsulotomy.

Neodymium: YAG Laser capsulotomy: Posterior capsule opacification is most common cause of visual loss. The most common indications for its use are the cases who develop opacity of the posterior capsule as a late complication following an uncomplicated extracapsular cataract extraction. The opacification of the posterior capsule is due to either residual sub-capsular plaque or capsular fibrosis. It causes gradual dim vision in the eye which had a good vision following surgery. The patients attend to the clinic with the complaint of gradual dimness in the vision of the operated eye which had a good vision after surgery. He may also complain of increase in glare day by day. On slit examination there is opacification of the posterior capsule. The choicest treatment is a capsulotomy with Neodymium: YAG laser. It

is safe painless and can be performed as an outdoor procedure.

The incidence of posterior capsule opacification has marked reduced due to advances in surgical techniques, IOL designs and biomaterials.

TRAUMATIC CATARACT

Trauma is one of the most common etiological factors for a unilateral cataract in an individual. Trauma can occur at any age. It is common in children, industrial workers and people engaged in agriculture fields, forests, and construction sites.

Penetrating injury of the eye may directly injure the lens resulting in cataract.

Concussion injury may rupture the lens capsule or cause sub-capsular cataract which is star shaped in appearance. A patient with concussion injury may show a **'Vossius ring'** due to imprinting of iris pigment on to the anterior lens capsule.

Infrared irradiation results in exfoliation of anterior lens capsule. It is typically seen in the patients who are working in a glass factory as "glass-blowers".

Electric shock of high voltage can cause cataract.

Ionizing irradiation given for intraocular tumors such as retinoblastoma may produce lens opacities as complication.

TOXIC CATARACT

Corticosteroid Cataract

A corticosteroid cataract develops as a posterior sub-capsular cataract. Once the cataract develops, it may regress on early withdrawal of the coricosteroids or it may progress in spite of withdrawal of steroids. The association of corticosteroid therapy with formation of a cataract is beyond doubt or dispute. The dose and the period of therapy have no relation with the formation of cataract. It is the individual susceptibility (genetics) which has been stressed recently by some authors who noticed lens opacity after a short-term therapy and no lens changes even after a prolonged course. On the basis of these findings it seems that an alternate day therapy should be the choice as the lens changes occurs less frequently in the patients who are on intermittent therapy. Childern are more susceptible than adults.

Chlorpromazine

Chlorpromazine given for a long period may cause deposition of fine yellowish brown granules under the anterior lens capsule in the pupillary area. It may also cause retinal damage.

Other Drugs

Other drugs are busulphan, gold, and amiodarone.

COMPLICATED CATARACT
(Secondary Cataract)

The complicated cataract occurs following inflammatory or degenerative diseases of the eye. The most common cause is chronic uveitis. The other causes are degenerative myopia, retinitis pigmentosa, retinal detachment, proliferative retinopathy and following surgery for glaucoma and retinal detachment. Complicated cataract develops in the posterior sub-capsular region and thereafter gradually progresses slowly in years to evolve as mature cataract. In early stage of sub-capsular cataract a polychromatic luster is seen by the specular reflex of the slit lamp. It is diagnostic of a secondary or a complicated cataract. The patient should be thoroughly examined and investigated to control the primary disease of the eye.

METABOLIC CATARACT
Diabetic Cataract

A true diabetic cataract is rare. A diabetic cataract is due to osmotic over-hydration of the lens. It induces myopia. The cataract appears as bilateral white punctate or snowflake opacities in the anterior and posterior capsules. In some cases it matures early may be in few days. In a diabetic the senile cataract appears early and also progresses early to maturation than in a non-diabetic.

Galactosemia

This is due to severe impairment of galactose utilization due to the absence of Galactose-1-phosphate uridyltransferase (GPUT). The malady is fatal unless galactose in the form of milk and milk products is removed from the diet. Infant develops bilateral cataract "oil droplet" central lens opacities in first few days or weeks of life. The lens changes are reversible if diagnosed early and milk is withdrawn from the diet.

Galactokinase Deficiency

This is due to deficiency of galactokinase (GK) which is the first enzyme in the metabolic pathway of galactose utilization. The children are at risk to develop lens opacity early in life. It is presumed that some presenile cataracts are due to mild deficiency of galactokinase.

Mannosidosis

This is due to deficiency of the enzyme 'α-mannosidase'. The patient develops 'spoke-like' or 'wheel-like' opacities in the posterior capsule. The absence of corneal changes helps in differentiating it from Hurler's disease.

Fabry's Disease

This is due to deficiency in the enzyme-α-galactosidase A. The ocular manifestations include cornea verticillate-and spoke like lens opacities.

Lowe's Syndrome
(Oculo-cerebro-renal Syndrome)

It is a rare disease with inborn error of ammo acid metabolism which predominantly affects boys. The lens is small and thin with lens opacities which may be capsular, lamellar, nuclear or total. Glaucoma is associated in 50% cases. Mother of the child may show multiple punctate lens opacities.

Wilson's Disease (Hepato-lenticular Degeneration)

It is due to deficiency of the alpha-2 globulin, ceruloplasmin which leads to widespread deposition of copper in the tissues. Ocular features include Kayser-Fleischer ring in the peripheral part of Descemet's membrane and sunflower cataract. It can be treated with D-penicillamine.

Hypocalcemia

Both hypoparathyroidism and pseudo-hypoparathyroidism may be associated with small discrete white flecks in the lens.

Homocystinuria

It is an inborn error of metabolism due to deficiency in the enzyme cystathione synthetase. It can be confused with Marfan's syndrome. Ocular features include lens sub-luxation and glaucoma due to sub-luxation or dislocation.

Hyperlysinemia

It is a rare inborn error of metabolism due to a deficiency in the enzyme lysine dehydrogenase. The main ocular feature is the microspherophakia. Other features are motor, mental and growth retardation.

MATERNAL INFECTION CAUSING CATARACT

Rubella

The risk of fetal infection is closely related to the stage of gestation at the time of maternal infection with rubella. The risk is 50% during the first eight weeks, 33% during ninth and twelve weeks, and about 10% during 13 to 24th week. Cataract is present in about 50% of cases. There may be lens opacities at birth but may develop several weeks or months later. The opacity may involve nucleus or may be diffuse involving entire lens. Other associated defects may be micro-ophthalmos, retinopathy, glaucoma, corneal haze, squint, nystagmus and optic atrophy. Other systemic defects include deafness, congenital heart lesions, mental retardation, hepato-spleno-megaly, thrombocytopenic purpura and pneumonitis.

Other Infections

Other infections which may cause cataract are toxoplasmosis cytomegalic inclusion disease, Variola, herpes simplex and onchocerciasis.

DERMATOGENIC CATARACT

Both the skin and lens originate from ectoderm thus both the tissues may be affected simultaneously by a disease process. The lens opacity associated with skin disease is known as "Syndermatotic cataract". These occur as bilateral cataracts and can occur at any age.

Atopic Dermatitis

It is a common cutaneous disease associated with cataract. It is an allergic disorder with familial tendency. The ocular features include cataract, chronic keratoconjunctivitis, and keratoconus. Cataract occurs as bilateral posterior or anterior stellate opacities usually in the third decade of life.

Other

The other common conditions are atopic dermatitis, Rothmund's syndrome, Werner's syndrome, congenital ichthyosis, psoriasis, incontinentia pigmenti, anhidrotic ectodermal dysplasia, and congential dyskeratosis.

CONGENITAL CATARACT

About one-third of all congenital cataracts are hereditary. These cases have no association with any systemic disease or metabolic disorder. The mode of inheritance is usually dominant. The morphology of the cataract is similar in parent and child.

Capsular Cataract

Anterior capsular cataract may be associated with persistent pupillary membrane, corneal opacity and anterior lenticonus. Posterior capsular cataract occurs due to persistent hyloid artery. These have dominant inheritance and may be sporadic also.

Embryonal Nuclear Cataract

The opacity is confined to embryonic nucleus. The opacity has a powdery appearance. It is frequently bilateral with dominant inheritance.

Lamellar Cataract

The lamellar cataract is of the prenatal size, 5 mm, with riders. These are bilateral and have dominant inheritance. The effect on the vision depends on the size of lens opacity and the density of opaque lens. As the nucleus becomes compressed with age the size of the opacity appears smaller. These are usually stationary.

Sutural Cataract

These are often familyal and may have dominant inheritance. In X-linked inheritance young males are severely affected and female carriers have minor form. They may regress or develop in posterior sub-capsular opacities.

DEVELOPMENTAL CATARACT

Punctate Cataract (Blue Dot Cataract)

These appear as small round discrete opacities blue in color mostly in periphery of the cortex. No effect on vision. It is seen in many cases on routine examination when pupil is dilated.

Coronary Cataract

These occur in periphery of lens and may have brown to blue color. There is dominant inheritance. Vision is not affected. It is diagnosed on routine examination.

24

A Case with Glaucoma

CLINICAL EXAMINATION

Ocular Examination

- Look for the size and shape of the cornea. It is larger in buphthalmos and megalo-cornea. Cornea plana can be associated factor.
- Location of iris-lens diaphragm. It is placed anteriorly in cases of primary angle closure glaucoma.
- Look for the pupillary reaction. The pupil reacts sluggishly or may be dilated in cases with open angle glaucoma of long duration.
- Look for the position of lens. Its subluxation may be the cause of glaucoma. Its dislocation in the anterior chamber causes glaucoma.
- Eclipse sign: It can be elicited by throwing a penlight across the anterior chamber

from the temporal side and noting a shadow on the nasal side. It shall be positive in cases with decreased axial anterior chamber depth.

Slit Lamp Biomicroscopy

Examine the anterior segment for the following:
- Epithelial edema.
- Krukenberg's spindle (pigmentation on endothelium).
- Cells in the aqueous humor.
- Axial chamber depth.
- Iris lens daiphragm.
- Angle depth in periphery.
- Keratic precipitates.
- Rubeosis iridis.
- Pseudo-exfoliation.
- Iris atrophy.

Any of the above finding may help you clinch the etiological factor for glaucoma.

GLAUCOMATOUS OPTIC DISK CHANGES

Optic disk changes provide early and important clue for suspecting primary open-angle glaucoma.

Ophthalmoscopy

Direct ophthalmoscopy is the most common and convenient method for fundus examination. On observing any clue the fundus examination should be carried out more elaborately with slit lamp biomicroscopy using Hruby lens or Goldmann contact lens and Indirect binocular ophthalmoscopy to have a magnified and stereoscopic view for better evaluation of the optic disk changes.

Documentation Techniques

The documentation is essential for follow up to assess the progress of the malady. The documentation can be made by serial drawings, photography and photogrammetry;

- Confocal scanning laser topography (CSLT), i.e. Heidelberg retinal tomography (HRT). It is an accurate and sensitive technique.
- Optical coherence tomography (OCT).
- Scanning laser polarimetry, i.e. nerve fiber layer analyzer (NFA). It is a device that detects the glaucomatous damage to the retinal nerve fibers before the appearance of the field defects and optic disk changes.

Cup-disk Ratio

The cup-disk ratio can be recorded by numeric value or draw a picture or photograph the disk. Usually it is the horizontal cup-disk ratio which is measured. A graticule has been provided in few models of direct ophthalmoscope to record the cup-disk ratio.

- Most normal eyes have a horizontal cup-disk ratio of 0.3 or less. Cup-disk ratio of greater than 0.3 should be regarded with suspicion.
- Most cases of Primary Open Angle Glaucoma have a cup-disk ratio greater than 0.3 and also show an unequal ratio between the two eyes. Any case showing an unequal cup-disk ratio on routine fundus examination should be further investigated to exclude glaucoma.
- An estimation of only cup size has a limited value.
- Any increase in the cup-disk ratio on follow up examination has a value.

A record of cup-disk ratio must be maintained for comparison on follow up visits of the patient.

Pallor and Cupping of the Disk

The area of the disk lacking blood supply appears as a pale area. A clear color contrast is visible between the pink and pale area. The area of pallor of the disk remains same throughout the life of a normal eye. In glaucoma both the cupping and the pallor increases. In some cases of glaucoma the area of pallor and cupping correspond while in other cases the area of cupping is greater than the area of pallor. The bending of the small blood vessels as they cross the optic disk indicates the area or extent of cupping. The excavation of the disk and sharp bending of blood vessels occur late in the disease process.

Notching of the Cup Rim

There may be a notching of the physiological cup rim affecting inferior or superior or both the rim leading to a **vertically oval cup**. The notching may reach up to the disk margin. Later the cup enlarges on the temporal side. The nasal side is the last to be affected resulting in an atrophic glaucomatous cupping.

Concentric Enlargement of the Cup

A concentric enlargement of the cup is difficult to distinguish from a physiological cup if the cup-disk ratio is within normal limits.

A comparison with previous record shall help. A further increase in cup size on follow up visit is diagnostic.

Hemorrhage on the Disk

A splinter or flame shape hemorrhage on the margin of the disk is a sign of imminent damage.

Striations and Slit like Defects

Detection of striations and slit like defects are signs of glaucomatous retinal nerve fiber damage. These can be seen prior to development of cupping of the disk and loss of visual field. These defects are usually seen one disk diameter above or below the disk with bright light, clear media and well dilated pupil.

Looping Retinal Veins

The retinal veins are full and may show looping near the disk. It indicates stasis and in such cases the central retinal vein block is common.

Pulsation of the Retinal Arterioles

It may be seen at the disk margin. It is a pathognomic sign of glaucoma if intraocular pressure is high.

Glaucomatous Optic Atrophy

The optic disk appears white and deeply excavated-cupping.

TONOMETRY (Indentation tonometry/ Schiötz tonometry)

This is based on the principle of indentation of the eye by the plunger of the Schiötz tonometer. The amount of indentation is measured on a scale. The reading of the scale is converted into millimeters of mercury (mmHg) by referring to the chart available with the tonometer. Schiötz tonometer (Fig. 24.1) is the most commonly used tonometer for measuring the intraocular pressure. It is cheap, portable and easy to use. As it is an indentation tonometry the scleral rigidity plays an important factor. A patient with low scleral rigidity will show false low readings and a patient with high scleral rigidity will give false higher readings of intraocular pressure when compared with an applanation tonometer. An abnormal scleral rigidity can be detected by Schiötz tonometer by taking two readings with two different weights. If two readings are same then the scleral rigidity is normal. Different readings indicate scleral rigidity. The reading should be taken only when the tonometer lever shows the pulsation on the scale.

Method of Schiötz Tonometry

Make the patient lie down on the examination table. Instill a drop of lignocaine hydrochloride 2% and wait for a minute. Explain the patient about the method and ask for his cooperation in looking straight up and not to squeeze the lids. Ask the patient to look at a spot on the ceiling or a finger placed directly in his line of gaze so that his gaze is straight up. It is essential to apply the tonometer properly on the cornea. Separate the lids by fingers of one hand and apply the tonometer on the cornea by other hand. The tonometer must be centrally placed on the cornea. If the scale reading is 4 or less then take another reading with 7.5 gm weight. If the intraocular pressure is 20–25 mm Hg or more then repeat tonometry in morning, afternoon and evening before a patient is labeled as a case of glaucoma. Note the reading on the scale of tonometer only when the lever of the tonometer shows pulsation. The intraocular pressure varies with the cardiac pulse pressure that is why the lever shows pulsation if properly and centrally placed on the cornea. The normal reading varies from 12 to 22 mmHg.

Sources of Error in Schiötz Tonometry

- Scleral rigidity.
  The scleral rigidity is low in high myopia, dysthyroid exophthalmos and following glaucoma surgery.
- Improper calibration of tonometer.
  Each time the tonometer is used test it on the testing plate to confirm its proper calibration. The lever must move freely and easily.

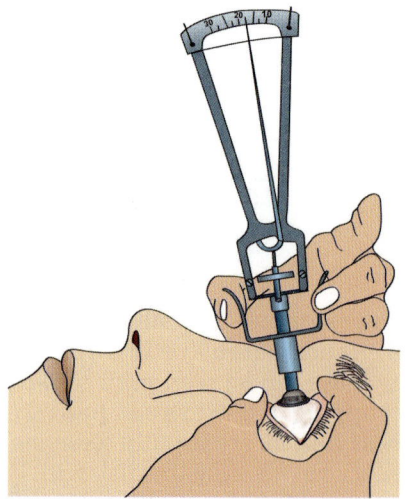

Fig. 24.1: Schiötz tonometer

- Improper application.

  The tonometer must be placed centrally on the cornea. Even slight misplacement can give a false reading. Take reading when the lever shows pulsatioan. The pulsation seen on the lever itself confirms its proper application.
- Un-cooperative patient.

Patient is un-cooperative because of apprehension and improper local anesthesia. Squeezing of the lids causes rise in pressure. Patient must be advised not to squeeze. Even separation of lids more than necessary especially in a case with prominent big eyes also causes rise in pressure. While separating the lids keep a watch on the eye. If the eye shows slight bulging on separation of lids then relieve the hold a bit.

Precautions for Schiötz Tonometry

- Sterilize the tonometer at least once a day. It can be easily sterilized by formalin vaporizer. A non-sterile tonometer can spread infection from one patient to other.
- Clean the foot plate with moist sterile cotton swab before using it on each patient.
- Occasionally a corneal abrasion may be caused by improper handling of the tonometer or due to sudden unexpected movement by the patient.
- Perform tonometry carefully.

Applanation Tonometry

In Applanation tonometry the tonometer measures the force required to flatten a small area of central cornea thus reading is not affected by the factor of scleral rigidity.

Goldmann Applanation Tonometer

It consists of a double prism that has a diameter of 3.06 mm. For tonometry instill lignocaine hydrochloride 2% as drop and wait for a minute. Stain the tear film by fluorescein strip. Make the patient sit at slit lamp and adjust the tonometer and view through the cobalt filter. When the prism touches the apex of the cornea then the viewer can see two semicircles of yellow color. These semi-circles represent the stained tear film touching the upper and lower halves of the prism. When the cornea is perfectly flattened then the inner edges of two semicircles will just touch. These circles never stay still but are constantly pulsating with the cardiac pulse. Note the reading at midpoint. Note the reading on the dial of tonometer and multiply by ten to get the intraocular pressure in mm Hg. It is the most widely used tonometer giving most accurate readings. For accurate readings it is necessary to center the semicircles on center of cornea with right thickness of the semicircles. Gentle and quick handling of the appliance is important.

Perkins Hand Held Tonometer

In this a Goldmann prism has been used with a light source and a spring. It does not require a slit lamp. It can be used with the patient in the supine position.

Pneuma Tonometer

It measures intraocular pressure by a graded flow of gas against a flexible diaphragm and gives a recorded pressure.

Air-puff Tonometer

In this method the central part of the cornea is flattened by a jet of air. Light reflected from the flattened cornea received by photoreceptor turns off the air. It gives a record of intraocular pressure.

Mackay Marg Tonometer

It is an electric applanation device. It records the intraocular pressure as a tracing on a graph paper. It measures the force required to flatten a small area of cornea against 1.5 mm plunger protruding 5 um beyond the surface footplate.

Microelectronic Tonopen

In this a microscopic strain-gauge transducer has been used to applanate the cornea converting intraocular pressure into electrical waves. A single chip computer analyses the waveforms obtained from several corneal touches and gives a digital readout.

DIURNAL VARIATION TEST

It is useful in detecting early cases of glaucoma. In the initial stage of glaucoma the patients show an exaggeration of the normal diurnal variation. Biphasic variation has been noticed in about 55% of cases. A variation in the intraocular pressure over 8 mm Hg is diagnostic. Such a case needs further investigations and early treatment with regular follow up.

PROVOCATIVE TESTS

The purpose of the provocative test is to assess the possibility of the angle to get blocked due to iris when the pupil dilates. If the angle gets blocked then there shall be a rise of intraocular pressure and the gonioscopy shall demonstrate the grade of the block of the angle.

Darkroom Rest

The patient is asked to sit in a dark room for an hour awake with the eyes open.

Prone Test

The patient is asked to lie down in a prone position for an hour.

Prone-Dark Room Test

The patient lies down in a prone position in a dark room for an hour awake with the eyes open. This test is most popular and also physiological in proper sense.

Intraocular pressure is measured and gonioscopy performed before the test and one hour after the test. An increase of 8–10 mm Hg or more in the intraocular pressure is taken as positive test in the presence of closed angle. A closure of angle is mandatory if the result is to be interpreted as positive.

A positive provocative test indicates that the angle can close spontaneously. A patient with negative test must be advised to come for follow up as angle may show closure in due course of time that may be years.

Keeping the above fact in view that there is a tendency to rise in the intraocular pressure in darkness and in a prone position the patient of latent or an intermittent glaucoma should be advised to instill an extra drop of pilocarpine when visiting a theater or engaged in a job requiring semi prone position of the head as sewing, reading, etc.

A mydriatic provocative test is unphysiological and may cause a rise in intraocular pressure even in open angle glaucoma with open angle on gonioscopy.

CORNEAL INDENTATION

Indent the central part of the cornea by a squint hook or a cotton applicator, for 30 seconds repeating 4–6 times. It may be effective in forcing the aqueous into the peripheral part of the anterior chamber and therefore opening the angle of the chamber provided there are no synechia. It helps to reduce the intraocular pressure in a short time helping the miotics to act on the pupil which is otherwise un-functional in a condition of raised intraocular pressure in a case of primary angle closure glaucoma. If the corneal indentation fails to lower the pressure then use hyperosmotic agents to lower the pressure. Mannitol is the most commonly used hyperosmotic agent. It is given intravenously. The dose is 1–2 g/kg body weight. A 20% solution is better given at the speed of about 60 drops per minute finishing the infusion in 30–40 minutes. It causes marked diuresis.

GONIOSCOPY

The purpose of gonioscopy is to visualise the angle of the anterior chamber and assess the width of the angle. A goniolens replaces the cornea and have a refractive index greater than that of cornea and tears. It eliminates total internal reflection (Fig. 24.2).

INDIRECT GONIOLENS

Goldmann Goniolens

Goldmann goniolens has a greater curvature than that of cornea therefore a viscous coupling fluid is necessary during gonioscopy. It has only one mirror for gonioscopy thus it has to be rotated 360° to inspect the entire angle. It provides a mirror image of opposite angle. It can only be used with a slit lamp.

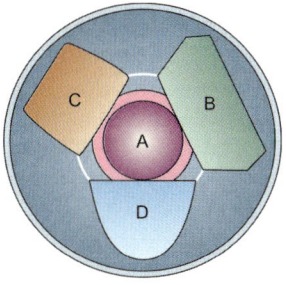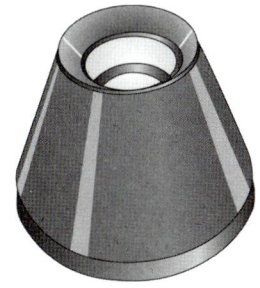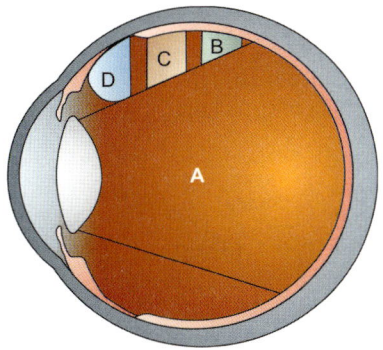

Fig. 24.2: Goldmann three mirror lens

Zeiss Goniolens

Its curvature is flatter than that of cornea so no coupling fluid is required. It has four mirrors so entire angle can be visualized simultaneously.

Avoid putting more pressure on the cornea while conducting gonioscopy. Otherwise the angle structures get distorted.

DIRECT GONIOLENS

These lenses give a direct view of the angle and are used with the patient in supine position for diagnostic or during operation for goniotomy. These lenses are used in conjunction with hand-held microscope (Fig. 24.3)

Koeppe goniolens is the most popular direct diagnostic goniolens.

Thorpe goniolens is popular surgical lens.

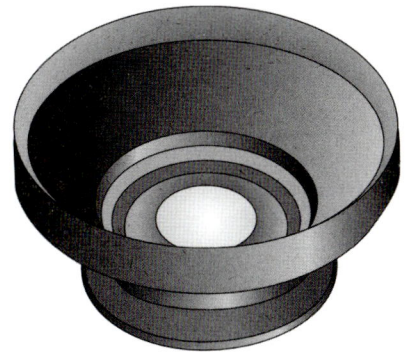

Fig. 24.3: Posterior fundus contact lens

GONIOSCOPIC STRUCTURES AT THE ANGLE

Schwalbe's Line

This is the most anterior structure in the angle. It appears as an opaque glistening white line.

Trabeculum

The trabeculum (trabecular meshwork) extends from Schwalbe's line to the scleral spur. The part adjacent to the Schwalbe's line is white in color while the remaining meshwork appears as greyish blue. Pigment can deposit in the trabecular meshwork in old age following trauma, acute glaucoma, uveitis, pseudo-exfoliation and in pigment dispersion syndrome.

Scleralspur

It is next to trabeculum and appears as narrow white band.

Ciliary Body

It appears as a band which may be brown or grey in color.

Angle Recess

Here the iris dips and gets inserted into the ciliary body.

SHAFFER'S GRADING OF ANGLE

During gonioscopy it is advisable to look and make a note about the curvature of the peripheral iris and the insertion of iris. It shall have a bearing on causing closure of the angle. Look for any abnormality at the angle, pigmentation, and peripheral anterior synechia (Fig. 24.4).

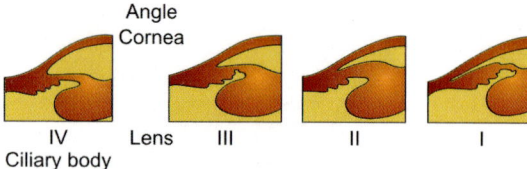

Fig. 24.4: Grades of anterior chamber angle width

Grade 0

The angle gets completely closed by the adhesion of cornea and iris in uveitis.

Grade I

Only Schwalbe's line is visible on gonioscopy. There is high risk of block of the angle.

Grade II

Schwalbe's line and trabeculum is visible on gonioscopy. There is a moderate risk of block of the angle.

Grade III

Schwalbe's line, trabeculum and the scleral spur is visible. It is open angle and not capable of closure.

Grade IV

All the structures of angle-the Schwalbe's line, the trabeculum, the scleral spur and the ciliary body is visible. It is an open angle.

PERIMETRY

Perimetry is important for the diagnosis and management of a case of glaucoma. By perimetry the visual fields are assessed thereby giving information about the damage to nerve fibers.

Confrontation Test

It is good for quick screening test for large field defects like hemianopia.

Lister Perimeter

It is useful to chart out the peripheral field defects thus having a documentation of the course of peripheral field defects in a case on examination and follow up.

Tangent Screen

With this only central fields up to 30° can be examined and charted out for record. The field defects occur in the following sequence:
- Isopter contraction.
- Baring of the blind spot.
- Small para-central scotoma.
- Seidel's scotoma.
- Arcuate or Bjerrum's scotoma.
- Ring or double arcuate scotoma.
- Roenne's central nasal step.
- Peripheral field defects.
- Tubular field defect is an indication of advanced glaucomatous field defect leaving a small island of central and temporal vision. Eventually these small islands of vision are also lost.

Goldmann Perimeter

In this appliance the target and the background illumination has a constant contrast. The test can be repeated in the patient with the same conditions and luminosity. Thus the results are more constant for comparison on follow up of a case.

Automated Perimeters

The computer performs the perimetry and records the results.

Clinical Features and Management

1. Primary open-angle glaucoma.
2. Primary angle-closure glaucoma.
3. Congenital glaucoma.
4. Low tension glaucoma.
5. Ocular hypertension glaucoma.
6. Phacogenic glaucoma.
   - Phacolytic glaucoma.
   - Phacoanaphylactic uveitis.
   - Intumescence of lens.
   - Glaucoma capsulare (exfoliative syndrome).
   - Dislocation or subluxation of lens.
   - Spherophakia-microphakia.

7. Hemogenic glaucoma.
   - Glaucoma due to hyphema.
   - Hemolytic glaucoma.
   - Ghost cell glaucoma.
8. Secondary glaucoma.
   - Hypertensive uveitis (glaucoma due to uveitis).
   - Glaucomatocyclitic crisis.
   - Angle recession glaucoma.
   - Steroid glaucoma.
   - Pigmentary glaucoma.
   - Malignant glaucoma.
   - Neovascular glaucoma.

PRIMARY OPEN-ANGLE GLAUCOMA

Primary open angle glaucoma covers majority about 80% of all forms of glaucoma. It is one of the most common cause for bilateral blindness.

Diurnal Variation of Intraocular Pressure

All the eyes have a normal diurnal variation in pressure. In normal individuals this variation is 3 to 4 mmHg. In patients with glaucoma this diurnal swing may be 20 mmHg or more. Therefore, it is essential to record intraocular pressure at different times of the day or at periodic intervals during the day to diagnose a case or to assure the patient that there is no glaucoma.

An intraocular pressure of 21 mm Hg or above should be viewed with suspicion.

Why?

High intraocular pressure is one of the most important risk factor for manifesting as primary open angle glaucoma. Therefore, the cases who show intraocular pressure of 21 mm Hg or above must be termed as ocular hypertensive cases. At this stage, there is neither loss of visual acuity nor visual fields. These cases must be followed up for changes in vision, fields and fundus. The most important risk factors are age, race and family history.

Aqueous humor outflow occurs through two routes:

Conventional route is trabecular and unconventional route is uveo-scleral. More than 80% outflow is through the conventional route. Prostaglandin analogues that improves unconventional uveo-scleral outflow are under trial.

Ophthalmoscopy

- Cupping of the optic nerve is one of the most important sign of glaucoma.
- Ophthalmoscopy may show cupping, change in the cup-disk ratio, notching of the cup rim, concentric enlargement of the cup, hemorrhage on the disk, striations and slit like defects and looping of retinal veins.
- The presence of any one or more of the above sign indicates glaucoma and case must be further subjected to investigations.

Visual Field Defects

- Documentation of the visual field defect is essential for further follow up and to assess the malady.
- Visual field should be charted in the same test conditions, using same target size, intensity, pupil and recorded by same surgeon preferably.
- Visual field charting can be done every three months.

Gonioscopy

In a case of primary open angle glaucoma the angle must be open for diagnosing primary open angle glaucoma. There are no other pathognomonic findings.

Other Factors

- Family history of glaucoma.
- High myopia.
- Retinal vein occlusion.
- Diabetes mellitus.

Differential Diagnosis

Low-tension Glaucoma

In these cases the intraocular pressure is 21 mm Hg or even less on the initial test. In these cases if there is a progressive loss of visual field then intraocular pressure should be maintained at less than 12 mm Hg.

Ocular Hypertension

Most cases show the upper end of the intra-ocular pressure. There is no cupping of the disk or any visual field loss. These require a long term follow up and should be seen as cases of glaucoma suspect.

Mimicking Conditions

- Physiological cupping.
- Coloboma of the optic disk.
- Anterior ischemic optic neuropathy.
- Chiasmal lesions.

Management

All patients with primary open angle glaucoma need regular follow up with effective treatment and control of the malady. The treatment may be medical therapy, argon laser trabeculoplasty and filtration surgery.

Medical Therapy

The aim of medical therapy is to bring down the intraocular pressure below 16 to 18 mm Hg in mild to moderate glaucoma and 12 to 14 mm Hg in severe glaucoma.

Topical Beta-blocker

Timolol maleate-0.25, 0.5% : 1–2 times daily

Topical beta-blockers are the first drug of choice.

Beta-blocker lowers the intraocular pressure by reducing the aqueous secretion due to its effect on the beta-receptors in the ciliary processes.

Its effect is reached within 1–2 hours and the action lasts for 24 hours. Superficial punctate keratopathy can occur as a local side effect. Bradicardia occurs as a systemic side effect therefore it should not be used in patients with slow pulse or heart block. Other side effects are fatigue, disorientation, confusion and depression.

Betaxolol-0.25%: 0.5%: twice a day.

Levobunolol-0.25%, 0.5%: once or twice a day.

Carteolol-1%: once or twice a day.

Topical Parasympathomimetic

Topical Pilocarpine-1, 2, 3, 4%: 3–4 times daily

Topical pilocarpine is very effective drug.

Pilocarpine acts on the ciliary muscle and thereby opens spaces in the trabecular meshwork. Thus it lowers the intraocular pressure by increasing aqueous outflow.

It is a parasympathomimetic drug that acts directly on receptors. Its pressure lowering effect begins within 20 minutes of instillation into the eye and the action lasts for 4 to 6 hours. It causes miosis and spasm of accommodation. Thus it affects vision in cases with lenticular opacities. It is very good in low concentration.

Topical Carbonic Anhydrase Inhibitor

Topical Dorzolamide-2%: 2–3 times daily

It is a topical carbonic anhydrase inhibitor.

It lowers the intraocular pressure by reducing aqueous secretion.

Topical Prostaglandin

Latanoprost-0.005% once a day.
Latanoprost is a prostaglandin in its nature.

It decreases the intraocular pressure by increasing the uveo-scleral outflow of the aqueous.

In this present era this is the first drug of choice if the patient can afford it. It is a costly drug. Therefore, for most of the patients this drug is very good adjunctive drug to beta-blocker and pilocarpine if these fail to control the intraocular pressure to desired level.

Travaprost 0.004%: once a day—It is self preserved.

Topical Adrenergic Drugs

Epinephrine hydrochloride 0.5%, 1% or 2% and dipivefrine hydrochloride 0.1% once or twice a day.

It lowers the intraocular pressure by increasing aqueous outflow by stimulating beta receptors.

Brimonidine 0.2% twice a day.

It lowers intraocular pressure by decreasing aqueous secretion.

Orally-Carbonic Anhydrase Inhibitors

Acetazolamide is given orally 250 mg every 6 hourly. It lowers the intraocular pressure within 1 hour reaching its peak at 4 hours and action lasts for about 6–12 hours. Its side effects include paraesthesia, malaise, gastrointestinal disturbance, renal stone formation, Stevens-Johnson syndrome, blood dyscrasia and transient myopia.

Start the topical medical therapy with Timolol maleate-0.25% instilled twice a day. If this is ineffective then increase the strength to 0.5%. If the tension is still not controlled then add Pilocarpine in its low concentration and instillation and increase the concentration and instillation as per need of the individual case. If the tension is still not controlled then add dorzolamide drops. Even this fails to control then add latanoprost.

Oral carbonic anhydrase inhibitors can be added only as a short-term treatment in few cases.

Monitor the effect of medical therapy by Tonometry.

In primary open angle glaucoma the medical therapy is the first choice and the surgery is the last choice.

Surgical Therapy

Argon or Diode Laser Trabeculoplasty

The regime of argon laser trabeculoplasty consists of 50 spots on the anterior half of the trabecular meshwork covering 180°.

Argon laser trabeculoplasty increases aqueous outflow facility, possibly due to shrinkage of the collagen on the inner surface of the trabecular meshwork thereby opening the inter-trabecular spaces.

It can be performed in all cases of open angle glaucoma which do not respond to medical therapy and have a clear cornea to view the trabecular meshwork. It lowers the intraocular pressure between 8 and 10 mm Hg in about 75% of cases who are on medical therapy.

Most cases need continuation of medical therapy.

Filtration Surgery

Filtration surgery is indicated in cases who do not respond to medical therapy and argon laser trabeculoplasty. In filtration surgery a fistula is created to act as a new channel for aqueous to flow out under the conjunctiva.

1. *Trabeculectomy:* It is a partial thickness fistula surgery. Trabeculectomy is the most common operation performed by surgeons. There is good control of intra-ocular pressure. It is associated with endophthalmitis, shallow anterior chamber and hypotony due to over filtration. **Sutureless trabeculectomy** is done through a valvular sclera-corneal tunnel incision. Outflow is inferior to trabeculectomy.

2. *Deep sclerectomy*

3. *Viscocanalostomy*: Deep sclerectomy and viscocanalostomy are non-penetrating filtration surgery in which anterior chamber is not exposed or entered. This technique reduces the incidence of post-operative endophthalmitis, overfiltration and hypotony.

4. *Artificial drainage shunt operations:* Artificial drainage shunts or glaucoma valve implants are plastic devices that allow aqueous outflow by creating a communication between the anterior chamber and sub-Tenon space.

Indications
- Neovascular glaucoma.
- Aniridia glaucoma.
- Intractable cases of glaucoma wherein trabeculectomy has failed even with topical antimetabolite therapy.

PRIMARY ANGLE-CLOSURE GLAUCOMA

Primary angle closure glaucoma occurs due to obstruction to aqueous outflow mainly by the closure of the angle by the peripheral iris. It can be divided into six overlapping types of angle-closure glaucoma. Each type has different clinical signs and management.

Latent Primary Angle-Closure Glaucoma

Diagnosis

Latent stage of primary angle closure glaucoma is symptomless entity. Ocular examination shows a shallow anterior chamber with convex iris-lens diaphragm. There is normal intraocular pressure. Gonioscopy shows a narrow angle. Provocative test is usually positive.

Management

A patient in a latent stage of angle closure glaucoma is most likely to pass into an intermittent stage or will develop an acute attack. It is advisable that a prophylactic peripheral iridectomy or a laser iridotomy should be performed. The patient should be advised to come regularly for follow up. If the patient has suffered an acute attack in the other eye then it is essential that either an iridectomy or iridotomy is performed or the patient uses pilocarpine 1% drops four times a day regularly and comes for follow up. Advise him to instill extra drop whenever he is exposed to dark and emotional and intellectual stress anywhere in cinema hall or even at home.

Subacute or Intermittent Primary Angle-Closure Glaucoma

Diagnosis

The attack of subacute primary angle closure glaucoma may be precipitated by any condition which results in:

Physiological mydriasis like watching television or a film in a theater especially if it is an emotional picture.

Physiological shallowing of the anterior chamber when patient is in a semi-prone position like reading, sewing and gardening.

The characteristic symptom is a rainbow colors or halos around the lights due to corneal edema. The patient may complain of dull ache or throbbing around the eye. Exposure to bright light and sleep gives relief due to constriction of pupil. Gonioscopy shows a narrow angle. Tonometry gives high reading.

Management

A peripheral iridectomy or a lesar iridotomy provides a permanent cure. Until the patient is ready for surgery keep him on miotic therapy with advise to avoid the conditions which results in physiological mydriasis and physiological shallowing of the anterior chamber. Pilocarpine 1% drops four times a day shall take care. Advise to instill an extra drop of pilocarpine if going for an emotional picture or expects situation of emotional disturbance and working long hours with head bend forwards.

Acute Primary Angle-Closure Glaucoma

Diagnosis

The patient presents with severe pain in and around the eye with marked ciliary and conjunctival congestion associated with nausea and vomiting. The patient is in an agony, crying with pain, covering the eyes with hanky and may be having a tight head band in an effort to control the pain. Once having seen a case the next case can be diagnosed form a distance as the picture and posture is so typical of a case of acute primary angle closure glaucoma. On examination there is corneal haze due to edema, anterior chamber is shallow, iris lens diaphragm is moved forward, pupil is vertically oval and fixed with no reaction to light or accommodation, aqueous flare but no keratic precipitates. Tonometry shows very high intraocular pressure. Gonioscopy shall show a closed angle. Gonioscopy can be done only after intraocular pressure has been lowered making cornea clear. Vision may be reduced to hand movements or even perception of light. Vision is recovered soon on reduction of intraocular pressure.

Since angle-closure glaucoma is usually a bilateral disease, the examination of the fellow eye should show a shallow anterior chamber and narrow angle on the gonioscopy. Presence of a wide angel in the fellow eye goes against the diagnosis of angle-closure glaucoma in the affected eye and so the diagnosis must be reviewed.

Differential Diagnosis

Acute anterior uveitis, glaucomato-cyclitic crisis, phacolytic glaucoma, neovascular glaucoma and acute conjunctivitis.

Management

A case of acute angle-closure glaucoma is an emergency case. The patient is in agony, with nausea, vomiting, dehydration, low vision and raised intraocular pressure. Therefore the following regime shall be very helpful in alleviating the symptoms and control of high pressure.

- Start intravenous mannitol 20% with about 50 drops per minute finishing in 30–40 minutes.
- Inject fortwin and phenergen through the drip.
- After mannitol start glaucose saline by drip.
- Topical pilocarpine 2% drops, one drop every ten minutes for four times and thereafter four times a day. With reduction in the intraocular pressure due to mannitol drip the pilocarpine shall be efective causing miosis and relieving the block of the angle by the iris. Pilocarpine shall be ineffective with raised intraocular pressure as the iris sphincter becomes nonfunctional probably due to ischemia of iris.
- Inject 8 mg of dexamethasone through drip set. It helps to control the uveal reaction. Follow by steroids orally.
- Topical antibiotic and steroid eye drops to prepare the case for surgery. Antibiotic drops to clear any infection and steroid eye drops to reduce the reaction so that the surgeon gets a comparatively quiet eye.
- Daimox tablets 250 mg six hourly until patient is taken for surgery in 2–3 days.
- Peripheral iridectomy or a laser iridotomy soon the patient is comfortable with reduced intraocular pressure and clear cornea permitting examination of the angle to assess the blockage. Iridectomy or iridotomy shall suffice if the angle is open 50% or more.

- Prophylactic surgery in the fellow eye or a weak miotic 1% pilocarpine four times a day and regular follow up of a case.
- Filtration surgery-trabeculectomy is the first choice if the angle is blocked more than 50%.

Post Congestive Angle-Closure Glaucoma

Daignosis

Few cases may resolve even if they do not get any medical help in time. These cases on examination show peripheral anterior synechia, glaukomflecken and patchy iris atrophy and dilated non-reacting pupil which are pathognomonic of an episode of an acute angle-closure glaucoma having occurred in past.

Management

- Topical timolol maleate and steroids drops
- Laser iridotomy if tension is not high.
- Trabeculectomy if tension is high.

Chronic Primary Angle-Closure Glaucoma

Diagnosis

Chronic primary angle-closure glaucoma results from gradual closure of the angle by synechia or subacute angle-closure glaucoma ends up in chronic primary angle-closure glaucoma.

The symptoms are similar to a case of primary open angle glaucoma. The intraocular pressure is elevated with angle closed usually in the superior quadrant and associated with cupping of the optic disk and visual field loss. Tonometry, gonioscopy, ophthalmoscopy, perimetry and symptoms help to diagnose.

Management

Initially medical therapy with laser iridotomy is the choice of management. If the pressure remains uncontrolled with increase in cupping and field loss then a filtration operation-Trebeculectomy is the choice.

Many surgeons prefer filtration surgery-Trabeculectomy as the first choice.

Absolute Primary Angle-Closure Glaucoma

Diagnosis

The eye is blind with raised intraocular pressure. It may be associated with pain, congestion, corneal haze, dilated and fixed pupil, iris atrophy, lens opacity. The eyeball is stony hard. It is an end-stage of primary acute angle-closure glaucoma which could not get medical help in time when the treatment could have saved the eye with full restoration of vision.

Management

No kind and amount of medical therapy shall be helpful. The only treatment is the destruction of secretory ciliary epithelium by cyclocryopexy, Nd: Yag laser cyclodestruction or diode laser cyclophotocoagulation. Cyclocryopexy is the favored choice.

CONGENITAL GLAUCOMA

It is a rare disease. It is inherited as an autosomal recessive trait. It is caused by the developmental defect of the anterior chamber angle.

Diagnosis

Diagnosis depends upon the observation of signs and symptoms as the patient is an infant. Parents usually seek the advice of an eye surgeon on observation of a big eye, lacrimation, photophobia and haze of cornea.
- Cornea is hazy in appearance.
- Stromal edema occurs due to corneal enlargement.
- Lacrimation.
- Photophobia.
- Enlarged eye (Buphthalmos).

Management

In each case of congenital glaucoma the following investigation must be done.
- Tonometry.
- Gonioscopy.
- Ophthalmoscopy.
- Measurement of corneal diameter.

Once the diagnosis is established the treatment is only surgical;

Goniotomy, trabeculotomy or trabeculectomy.

LOW TENSION GLAUCOMA

A case of low tension glaucoma presents with all the characteristic findings of open angle glaucoma, viz. open anagle on goniscopy, cupping of the disk and visual field loss with a normal intraocular pressure. One group of patients never show an elevated pressure even though the pressure has been documented at different times of a day over long period. Such cases do not require any treatment except a regular checkup for any further loss of field. The second group of patient shows a gradual deterioration of the visual field. Such patients must be further investigated to exclude other conditions like optik nerve or optic chiasmal tumors, any occlusion in carotid arterial system, temporal arteritis, any evidence or history of hemodynamic crisis, viz. bleeding ulcer, myocardial infarction, and vascular collapse. The conditions which mimic glaucoma such as ischemic optic neuropathy, juxtapapillary choroiditis and high myopia must be kept in mind. If there is a visual field loss and no other cause could be ascertained then lower the intraocular pressure below 12 mmHg by medical therapy or the filtering surgery.

OCULAR HYPERTENSION GLAUCOMA

Ocular hypertension glaucoma denotes clinical features with intraocular pressure above 21 mmHg yet absence of optic nerve damage, visual field loss on standard automated perimetry, normal or open angle on gonioscopy.

It is a precursor to primary open angle glaucoma. It is rather difficult to differentiate between ocular hypertension and primary open-angle glaucoma. Estimation of diurnal variation of intraocular pressure to assess peak and fluctuation in intraocular pressure is helpful.

All the eyes have a normal diurnal variation in pressure. In normal individuals this variation is 3 to 4 mm Hg. In patients with glaucoma this diurnal swing may be 20 mm Hg or more. Therefore it is essential to record intraocular pressure at different times of the day or at periodic intervals during the day to diagnose a case or to assure the patient that there is no glaucoma.

An intraocular pressure of 21 mm Hg or above should be viewed with suspicion.

Why?

High intraocular pressure is one of the most important risk factor for manifesting as primary open angle glaucoma. Therefore, the cases with intraocular pressure of 21 mm Hg or above must be termed as ocular hypertensive cases. At this stage, there is neither loss of visual acuity nor visual fields. These cases must be followed up for changes in vision, fields and fundus. The most important risk factors are age, race and family history.

Management

Topical medication by beta blockers is first choice. Lowering the intraocular pressure to 20% less than baseline or 24 mmHg can reduce the risk of manifestation of primary open-angle glaucoma in more than half the cases. The aim should be to achieve the targeted intraocular pressure. A regular follow up with all the clinical investigation is mandatory.

PHACOGENIC GLAUCOMA (Lens Induced Glaucoma, Glaucoma Secondary to Lens)

Phacolytic Glaucoma

It occurs in cases with hypermature morgagnian cataract. There is a leak of protein from the intact thin capsule of lens. The large mononuclear phagocytes laden with lens protein plug the pores in the trabecular meshwork causing rise in the intraocular pressure. There are no keratic precipitates (Fig. 24.5). There may be acute pain with congestion of the eye. The only treatment is to lower the intraocular pressure by medical therapy along with osmotic agents and remove the lens early.

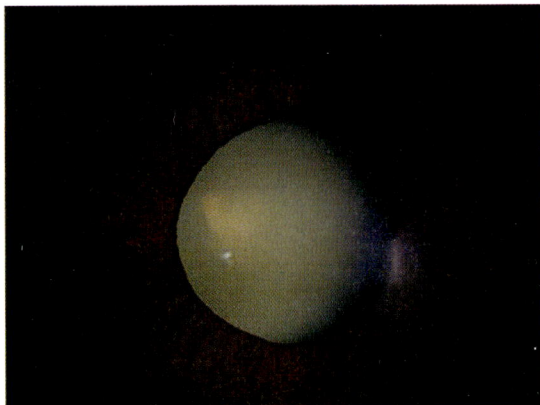

Fig. 24.5: Phacolytic glaucoma

Phacoanaphylactic Uveitis

It follows usually after the rupture of lens due to trauma or following an extracapsular cataract surgery. In this there appears an element of delayed sensitivity which manifests as an allergic type response usually seen in the second eye of a patient who has had bilateral extracapsular cataract operation. There is a marked reaction which is granulomatous type. There is a severe reaction to lens proteins showing keratic precipitates, cellular reaction in aqueous and all other signs of allergic reaction of lens protein. Treat by steroids to control the acute reaction followed by removal of lens capsule and lens material left after first surgery or trauma.

Intumescence of Lens

The rise in intraocular pressure is due to swollen lens that pushes the iris forward thereby blocking the angle and the pupil. It can occur during the maturation of senile cataract. It can occur following trauma resulting in rupture of lens capsule which allows the lens to imbibe aqueous and thus swelling of lens. Lower the intraocular pressure by medical therapy and treat by removal of lens with intraocular lens implant.

Glaucoma Capsulare

This condition is due to secretion of grey-white flake like material which gets deposited on the anterior lens capsule at the pupillary margin, zonule, ciliary processes and at the angle in the trabecular meshwork. It causes rise of intraocular pressure. It responds poorly to medical therapy and lens extraction had no benefit. Response to argon laser trabe-culoplasty is usually good. A filtration operation may be necessary.

Anterior Dislocation or Subluxation of Lens

It can be traumatic or spontaneous. Spon-taneous dislocation or a subluxation is commonly seen in conditions such as Marfan's syndrome, homocystinuria and syphilis: A trauma can cause hyphema and angle recession along with dislocation or subluxation. It causes papillary and angle block resulting in the rise of intraocular pressure. Lower the intraocular pressure by medical therapy and plan for cataract surgery with implantation.

Spherophakia (Microphakia)

It is seen commonly in *Marchesani's syndrome* and in association with other ocular congenital anomalies and inborn errors of metabolism. The lens is small and spherical, thereby causes pupillary block producing secondary angle closure glaucoma. Miotics cause further constriction of pupil and so increases the pupillary block. Mydriatics cause dilation of pupil and relieve the pupillary block. The peripheral iridectomy is the treatment of choice.

HEMOGENIC GLAUCOMA

Presence of blood in the anterior chamber or the vitreous can give rise to increase in the intraocular pressure.

Red Cell Glaucoma
(Glaucoma due to Hyphema)

There is a rise of intraocular pressure if the anterior chamber is entirely filled with blood. In such a condition the trabecular meshwork is plugged with red blood cells and there is a block of pupil with clotted blood. As the intraocular pressure is very high the initial treatment is to lower the pressure by use of carbonic-anhydrase inhibitors, osmotic agents and topical timolol. If the pressure can be lowered below 40 mmHg then one can continue medical therapy otherwise surgery to evacuate the blood is necessary to prevent blood staining of the cornea. It is advisable to nurse the patient in bed with semi-sitting position so that the blood gravitates and clear some portion of the superior angle for outflow of aqueous.

Hemolytic Glaucoma

In a condition of hyphema in the anterior chamber the large mononuclear phagocytes laden with breakdown products of hemorrhage fills the anterior chamber and plugs the pores of the trabecular meshwork causing rise in the intraocular pressure. The hemosiderin released by the lysed blood cells may cause direct damage to the trabecular meshwork causing sclerosis as occurs in a case of siderosis. Treat by lavage of the anterior chamber. Glaucoma is likely to persist if the trabecular meshwork has become sclerosed due to hemosiderin.

Ghost Cell Glaucoma

Ghost cell glaucoma occurs following vitreous hemorrhage before or during or after cataract extraction. The red blood cells after two weeks in the vitreous degenerate into ghost cells when the hemoglobin leaks out. These old red blood cells are not normal cells but are hollow (ghost) cells with rigid walls which do not allow them to pass through the pores in the trabeculae. These cells pass into the anterior chamber in aphakic eye with disturbed anterior vitreous face and gets trapped in the pores of the trabeculum thereby obstruct the aqueous outflow. These cells can be visualized in the anterior chamber by slit lamp appearing as reddish-brown cells and may lead to a diagnosis of uveitis or endophthalmitis. If medical therapy fails to keep the pressure under control then surgery to irrigate the anterior chamber to wash out the ghost cells is necessary.

SECONDARY GLAUCOMA

Hypertensive Uveitis

In case of iridocyclitis the rise in the intraocular pressure can be attributed to several factors.

- Increased viscosity of the aqueous due to formation of plasmoid aqueous.
- Posterior synechia leading to seclusio-pupil (Fig. 24.6).
- Peripheral anterior synechia.
- Trabecular meshwork is blocked by inflammatory cells and macrophages.

An energetic treatment of iridicyclitis may prevent all the factors which lead to rise in the intraocular pressure. Treat iridocyclitis and rise of intraocular pressure by medical therapy.

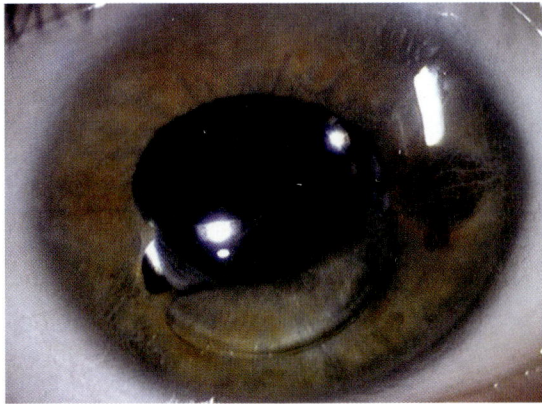

Fig. 24.6: Pupillary block glaucoma

Glaucomatocyclitic Crisis
(Posner-Schlossman Syndrome)

It is characterized by sudden and rapid rise of intraocular pressure with mild anterior uveitis. There is no pain. The patient complains of halos around the lights. Anterior chamber is not shallow. Slit lamp examination shows few fine non-pigmented keratic precipitates but no posterior synechia. It affects young adults. About 40% cases are positive for HLA-BW54. The attacks are self-limiting and resolve. During attack reduce intraocular pressure by medical therapy. A short course of topical steroids is helpful. The cases with chronic rise of intraocular pressure need surgery.

Angle Recession Glaucoma

This glaucoma is due to contusion of the eyeball. The trauma results in the tear of the ciliary body causing angle recession. The glaucoma develops after several years therefore it is essential to examine the patient with angle recession periodically for years. Treat it like any case of open angle glaucoma.

Steroid Glaucoma

Steroid induced glaucoma is a type of secondary open-angle glaucoma that develops following topical and sometimes systemic steroid therapy. The precise mechanism for the obstruction of the aqueous outflow is unknown. Glycosaminoglycans theory, endothelial cell theory and prostaglandin theory have been postulated. Treat it by withdrawing the steroids and giving medical therapy for glaucoma. It is advisable to monitor the intraocular pressure in all cases with steroid therapy for more than a month.

Instillation of topical steroid has become very common in many ophthalmic disorders because of quick relief provided by it. Some of these patients will show a marked rise of intraocular pressure within 4–8 weeks especially if the instillation is too frequent, i.e. 4–6 times a day. It resembles primary open angle glaucoma. The intraocular pressure returns to normal within 4–8 weeks on withdrawing the instillation of steroids. It is helpful to treat the case with medical therapy to keep the pressure under control during withdrawal of the drug. Monitor the pressure every 15 days until it has touched normal and maintain normalcy even after withdrawing timolol eye drops. It is necessary to monitor the pressure periodically in every case with steroid therapy-topical or systemic.

Pigmentary Glaucoma

It is characterized by presence of *Krukenberg's spindle* by deposition of the pigment on the corneal endothelium in a vertical spindle shape. There is pigment deposition in the trabecular meshwork also. It is usually bilateral and affects young myopes and seen in diabetics. Slit lamp examination shall show Krukenberg's spindle and gonioscopy shall show the pigmentation in angle. The angle is wide open. Treat like an open angle glaucoma case. The response is usually good.

Malignant Glaucoma

Malignant glaucoma occurs in cases of angle closure glaucoma who have undergone a filtering procedure surgery. The chamber is flat or fails to reform and there is a rise of intraocular pressure. It seems that the aqueous is unable to enter the anterior chamber and is forced to enter posteriorly behind the vitreous. Due to this the entire lens-iris diaphragm and the vitreous is pushed forward. Miotics aggravate the condition. First treat by aggressive cycloplegic therapy which may help in pulling back the lens. One can plan to aspirate the trapped aqueous through the pars plana. If no response then only treatment left is the removal of the lens and slashing of the anterior hyloid face to allow the aqueous to move forward. Delay hampers the prognosis and visual outcome.

Neovascular Glaucoma (Glaucoma Due to Rubeosis Iridis)

Rubeosis iridis is seen in cases with diabetic retinopathy and retinal vein occlusion. In this condition new vessels appear on the surface of the iris. These new vessels spread and bridge the angle of the anterior chamber and grow on to the corneal endothelium. It results in the block of the angle and rise of the intraocular pressure. Hypoxia of the eye is thought to be the stimulus for the growth of new vessels (Rubeois iridis). Usual therapy of glaucoma is ineffective.

Pan-retinal photocoagulation in early stage has shown regression of rubeosis due to destroying ischemic retina, minimizing oxygen demand of the eye and reducing the amount of VEGF release.

In later stage when view of posterior segment is poor, then trans-conjunctival anterior retinal cryopexy yields comparable results by retinal ablation.

Topical instillation of atropine and steroids to control the pain and reaction.

The fellow eye should be periodically examined for rise in the intraocular pressure and treated early to help avoid occurrence of central retinal vein block and neovascular glaucoma.

25

A Case with Vitreous Lesion

History

Record the history with reference to the following:
- Age on onset.
- Duration of seeing floaters or flashes.
- Ask about the shape of floaters which may be described by the patient as spots, soot, particles, spider like, a fly or a mosquito flying before the eye, cobweb, threads, earthworm like, ring, a bunch of ladies hair, cotton wool puffs, etc.
- The appearance of a flash may be described as glow, an arc of light, streak of light like an electric flash in the sky.
- Vision: It may be reduced suddenly due to floaters or gradually in due course of time.
- An intelligent patient with fresh hemorrhage may complain of seeing a dense black streak which broke into numerous minute streaks, channels, or dots causing dim vision.
- Ask about seeing any veil or a curtain coming from a side.
- Any associated systemic disease like diabetes, hypertension, anemia or leukemia.
- Any recent history of trauma may be minor and of no significance to the patient at all or body strain to lift or move something very heavy.
- Any past disease of the eye especially iridocyclitis.
- Any abnormal reflex from the pupil.

CLINICAL EXAMINATION

Visual Acuity

The symptoms in a case of vitreous opacities are floaters or flashes. There may be normal vision or it may reduce to the light perception.

Record of visual acuity is essential to assess the progress on follow up.

Ophthalmoscopy

The normal vitreous is not visible by direct or indirect ophthalmoscopy. Ophthalmoscopy helps to see the vitreous anomalies attributable either to structural change in the vitreous or invasive elements like blood and proliferative bands.

Slit Lamp Biomicroscopy with Three Mirror Fundus Contact Lens

The normal vitreous and its anomalies of retraction, condensation, liquefaction, and shrinkage can be seen by the slit lamp bio-microscopy with fundus contact lens. Slit lamp allows examination of anterior vitreous. Examine the posterior and peripheral vitreous with contact lens with mirrors.

Technique

To visualize the vitreous, set the slit lamp to the brightest level of light and adjust the beam to a narrow slit. Focus the slit beam from the greatest angle possible without missing the slit image. In this way there is a black background against which the delicate vitreous fibrils and posterior vitreous face is visible. Move the slit lamp in and out to examine the vitreous at different depths. The posterior vitreous face is visible only if the vitreous is detached. During visualization ask the patient to move the eye up and down and back to the primary position. This will make the posterior vitreous face to move a little and then it is easily visible. This movement of the eye shall help to know about the vitreous whether it is gel or liquid. With the three mirror contact lens the vitreous can be examined in different meridian and the surgeon can draw the diagram for future reference about the prognosis (Figs 25.1 and 25.2).

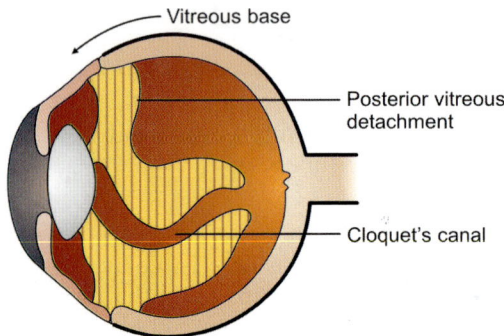

Fig. 25.1: Vertical section of detached vitreous

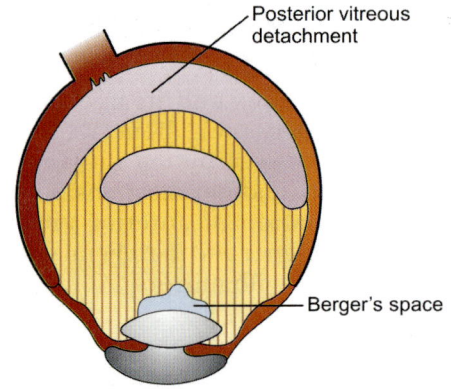

Fig. 25.2: Horizontal section of detached vitreous

Ultrasonography

B-scan ultrasonography can give much information about the vitreous and adjacent structures particularly when there is a gross vitreous opacification or other ocular media like cornea and lens are opaque. It helps to locate vitreous membranes, retinal

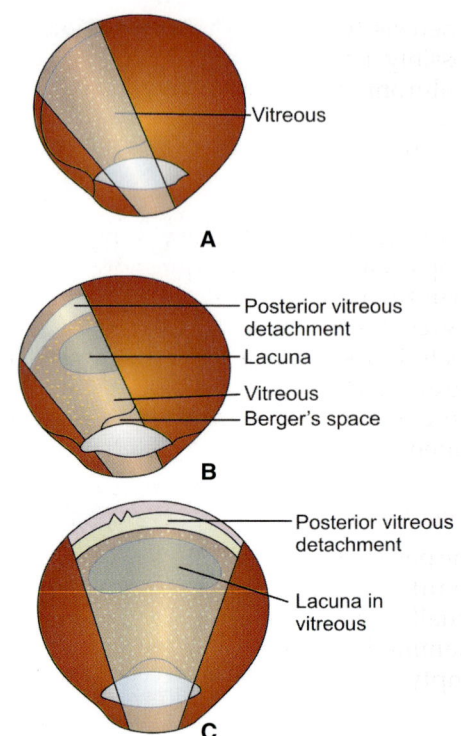

Figs 25.3A to C: Slit lamp biomicroscopy with three mirror fundus contact lens of vitreous: (A and B) Vitreous as seen through mirror of lens, (C) Vitreous seen through center of lens

detachments greater than one millimeter in depth, scleral ruptures, foreign bodies and any other lesions in the vitreous.

Clinical Features and Management
1. Synchysis and syneresis.
2. Asteroid hyalosis.
3. Synchysis scintillans.
4. Muscae volitantes.
5. Amyloidosis.
6. Posterior vitreous detachment.
7. Persistent hyperplastic primary vitreous.
8. Hereditary hyaloidoretinopathies.
9. Vitreous hemorrhage.
10. Vitreous abscess.

SYNCHYSIS AND SYNERESIS

The most common degenerative changes in the vitreous are synchysis (liquefaction) and syneresis (collapse) of the vitreous gel. It is possibly a result of breakdown of collagen or hyaluronic acid of vitreous gel.

Slit lamp Examination

Total Synchysis (Liquefaction)

In total liquefaction of the vitreous gel, the slit lamp examination does not show fine fibrillar structure of the gel. There are coarse aggregates of vitreous which are seen floating freely in the vitreous with the movement of the eye. These aggregates due to synchysis are the common cause of floaters seen by the patient.

Partial Synchysis (Liquefaction)

The partial liquefaction of the vitreous gel may result in formation of cavity or a lacuna usually seen in posterior vitreous. On slit lamp examination these lacuna appear as optically empty spaces.

Etiology

Degenerative Conditions

Senile changes, myopia and retinitis pigmentosa.

Contusion

A contusion causes an abrupt brief change in the shape of the eye. This may result in injury to vitreous where it is adherent sometimes resulting in the disinsertion of vitreous base. This is enough to result in the degeneration of vitreous.

Penetrating Injury

In penetrating injury the part of the vitreous traversed by the foreign body is damaged and show vitreous condensation, shrinkage or fibrous bands.

Thermal Trauma

Clinical use of diathermy, photocoagulation and cryo-coagulation results in the vitreous degeneration.

Systemic Connective Tissue Disorders

Marfan's syndrome, Ehlers-Danlos syndrome and homocystinuria may be associated with degeneration of vitreous.

Hemorrhage in Vitreous

Small or extensive hemorrhage in the vitreous due to any cause ultimately results in degeneration of the vitreous.

Inflammatory Processes

Invasion of the vitreous with white blood cells due to inflammation of the uveal tissue usually pars planitis or choroiditis results in the degeneration of vitreous.

Symptoms

Floaters

The floaters are opacities in the vitreous. These can stimulate the retina by casting a shadow upon it. The mind projects the corresponding dark form onto the appropriate area of visual field. These dark spots seen by the patients are unusual and annoying to him so he complains of seeing the spots in his field of vision. The relatively less mobile and central floaters are annoying and causes loss of vision. The mobile and peripheral floaters are intermittent and visible on quick movement of the eye. There are appreciated better by the patient against a bright light or a uniform light background. The onset of floaters may be acute or insidious and unilateral or bilateral. The floaters have many shapes and patient classifies them as spots, spiderlike, a fly or a mosquito flying in front up the eye, a bunch of hair, particles, cobweb, threads, worms, rings, streaks, etc. As these objects are moving therefore they are called floaters. Any case presenting with complain of seeing floaters must be thoroughly examined for any vitreous or retinal pathology. Treat if there is any disease responsible for floaters. In the absence of any pathology the patient may be assured that these floaters are harmless and due to aging.

Flashing Lights

A flashing light seen by the patient represents a cerebral awareness of stimulation of the retina by the abnormal vitreous. It is commonly associated with recent liquefaction, collapse and detachment of the vitreous due to syneresis. There is traction of the vitreous on the vitreo-retinal lesions and vitreo-retinal adhesions. Each time there is a movement of the eye which can initiate traction results in seeing a flash. To begin with this phenomenon is unilateral but another eye can get involved sooner or later. The flash is seen only for a fraction of a second. It may be seen at short interval for few minutes and then may disappear for days. The flash is better appreciated by the patient in dim illumination and on moving the eye. The flash light has been described by the patient in many forms as-a glow, a streak, an arc of light like a flash in sky, twinkle like a bright star, a flash like a flash of a camera but of much low intensity, etc. Any case presenting with complain of seeing a flash must be subjected to a thorough examination of the vitreous and retina with binocular indirect ophthalmoscope and slit lamp biomicroscopy with and without a three mirror contact lens.

Treat the case if there is positive finding responsible for flashes. If no pathology is detected advise him to a come for check up again if the flashes persist. Advice the patients to avoid strain, jerk and fast life. Examine the case thoroughly to exclude any pathological lesion in the retina and vitreous. A regular check-up every six months is advisable. Treat the lesions if needed. Assure the patient that these can occur in any person past sixth decade as a normal process of degeneration of vitreous.

ASTEROID HYALOSIS

It is an uncommon condition of vitreous that affects elderly and unilateral in 75% of cases. These are visible even by a torch and loupe if anterior and central. On slit lamp examination these appear as small reflective whitish yellow dot like opacities in hundreds attached to interlacing vitreous fibrils. Vitreous is healthy in the form of gel. These are composed of calcium containing lipids. On movement of the eye there is a little movement maintaining their original position. These do not affect the vision. These do not produce any symptoms and require no treatment.

SYNCHYSIS SCINTILLANS

Synchysis scintillans is an uncommon condition of vitreous characterized by presence of hundreds of glistening opacities, floating freely in a liquified vitreous. These opacities are composed of cholesterol crystals. These are usually settled at the bottom of the vitreous. These crystals get stirred up by the movement of the eye and again settle down. There is no predisposing factor but can follow uveitis, trauma or hemorrhage in vitreous. There are no symptoms of any kind. The patient is unaware of it. The eye surgeon happens to see these on routine examination. Require no treatment.

MUSCAE VOLITANTES

These are physiological opacities as residues of primitive hyaloids vasculature. Patient perceives these as fine dots and filaments which drift in and out of the visual field against a bright background.

AMYLOIDOSIS

Vitreous opacities may be seen in a case of systemic heredo-familial amyloidsis. Amyloid gets deposited in the virteous as fibrillar "glass-wool" deposits. Amyloid is an extracellular, amorphous, eosiophilic material that probably respresents aggregated kappa and lambda light chain derived from immunoglobins. The other ocular features may be proptosis, ophthalmoplegia, anisocoria, perivasculitis and retinal hemorrhage. The amyloid deposits in the vitreous may cause visual impairment.

POSTERIOR VITREOUS DETACHMENT

Posterior vitreous detachment is a condition of separation of the cortical vitreous from the retina anywhere posterior to the vitreous base.

It occurs due to sudden transfer of liquified vitreous from a large synchytic cavity or lacuna into the potential space between the cortical vitreous and the internal limiting membrane of the retina (sub-vitreal space). This collapse of vitreous may be accompanied by the symptoms of floaters and flashes.

A slit lamp examination will show:

- Condensed vitreous behind the lens.
- Optically empty space behind a detached posterior hyloid membrane.
- A ring like opacity (Fuch's ring) may be visible on the detached hyloid membrane anterior to the optic disk. This ring corresponds to the attachment of membrane to the optic disk. The posterior vitreous detachment may be found in many people beyond sixth decade but any case with acute posterior vitreous detachment must be subjected to thorough examination for retinal pathology, a tear or a traction site.

PERSISTENT HYPERPLASTIC PRIMARY VITREOUS

This condition is the result of failure of regression of the embryonic hyaloid vascular system. Clinically, it presents with a white reflex from the pupil. On examination, there is whitish pinkish mass behind the lens.

Clinical Features

- It is unilateral in about 90% of cases.
- There is no history of premature birth, low birth weight or having received any prenatal oxygen.
- A white reflex from the pupil is the most common presenting sign.
- Patient may be brought for squint or nystagmus.
- It is characterized by the presence of:
  - A retrolental funnel-shaped mass of fibrovascular tissue which gives rise to white reflex. It may vary in size from a small plaque just nasal to center (**Mittendorf's dot**) to a complete plaque covering the posterior lens surface. The mass is usually grey or pink.

- Identification of hyaloid artery confirms the diagnosis. The hyaloid artery may be patent or occluded. Usually it is represented by vascular remnant that extends from the mass into the vitreous cavity.
- The mass is vascular and repeated hemorrhages within the mass, vitreous and perilenticular space is common.
- The lens is clear to begin with but becomes cataractous due to rupture of posterior capsule. It may lead to swelling of the lens and secondary glaucoma of angle closure type.
- Vitreous organization may be seen at various stages of fibrosis.

Management

Closed intraocular microsurgical technique as lensectomy and vitrectomy is useful to restore some useful vision.

HEREDITARY VITREO-RETINOPATHIES

There are three types of vitreo-retinopathies in which there is degeneration of vitreous and retina.

i. *Wagner's vitreoretinal degeneration:* There is dim vision with floaters. Slit lamp examination of vitreous shows empty spaces. Ophthalmoscopy shows peripheral pigmentary degeneration and choroidal sclerosis with atrophy. Refraction is usually myopic. Electroretinogram is abnormal. It is frequently complicated by cataract and retinal detachment. There is autosomal dominant inheritance.

ii. *Favre-Goldmann disease:* There is autosomal recessive inheritance. Its manifestations include vitreous degeneration, retinoschisis, peripheral pigmentary degeneration and choroidal sclerosis with atrophy. There is nightblindness with abnormal electroretinogram. Cataract and retinal detachment may occur.

iii. *Hereditary juvenile retinoschisis:* It is transmitted as an X-linked recessive trait. There is vitreous degeneration with retinoschisis. The foveal retinoschisis may resemble cystoid macular edema

VITREOUS HEMORRHAGE

Etiology

- Proliferative retinopathy accompanying diabetes mellitus, retinal vein occlusion, Eale's disease and sickle cell anemia.
- Retinal tear with hemorrhage.
- Leukemia or anemia.
- Dysproteinemia.
- Trauma.

Preretinal Hemorrhage (Sub-hyaloid Hemorrhage)

Preretinal hemorrhage, Sub-hyaloid hemorrhage or retro-vitreous hemorrhage is located between the retina and the detached posterior hyaloid membrane. It is usually seen in the para-macular area. The blood remains unclotted and shows a change in its position with change in the position of the head. In the upright position the preretinal hemorrhage adopts a boat-shape, a semi-circular inferior border with a horizontal superior border. The blood in the lower part appears thick red and in the upper part appears yellow due to settling of red blood cells at the bottom and plasma in upper layers. The visual loss depends on the amount of hemorrhage, position of the patient and location of the hemorrhage. The blood from the sub-hyaloid region absorbs and resolves early. The retinal circulation helps in the process of fibrinolysis, phagocytosis and hemolysis which help in early resolution of blood and improvement in the vision.

Intravitreal Hemorrhage

- The effect of intravitreal hemorrhage depends on the amount of bleeding and condition of the vitreous whether in a gel form or there is liquifaction with lacuna.
- *The blood in the vitreous gel* promotes vitreous degeneration and liquefaction with formation of lacuna. The hemorrhage in the vitreous gel tends to diffuse anteriorly and centrally thus obscuring the vision and visualization of fundus. Slit lamp examination show hemorrhagic debris in the anterior vitreous and on the posterior lens capsule.

The blood in the vitreous gel readily clots along the vitreous fibers and forms finger like projections from the site of bleeding into the vitreous cavity. On slit lamp examination there is a tyndall effect (red cells and plasma proteins) within the vitreous gel between the finger like projections of blood clot. Later there are fluffy yellowish opacities and dense white yellow membranes in the vitreous. There is incomplete and slow resolution of blood from a formed vitreous gel therefore there is visual loss for a long time.

- *The bleeding in a liquified vitreous* with lacuna tends to resolve early. The blood remains unclotted and shifts with the gravity. The stirred up blood in the cavity is responsible for fluctuating visual acuity. The vision is good when the blood is settled inferiorly. The vision is blurred when blood gets stirred up due to movement of the eye.

Massive Hemorrhage in Vitreous

In this condition there may be hemorrhage simultaneously in the preretinal space, vitreous gel and lacuna of the vitreous. There is no red reflex from the eye. There is sudden painless severe loss of vision with only perception of light. In a case of repeated hemorrhage it is advisable to perform a Bright-flash electroretinography to know the condition of the retina before planning for vitrectomy.

Complications

In young people the blood may absorb within 4–8 weeks.

It leads to liquefaction of vitreous gel.

It may lead to ghost cell glaucoma.

It may become organized in fibrous bands and membranes.

It may evolve in retinitis proliferans resulting in tractional retinal detachment.

Management

Complete bed rest with 30° elevation of head and bilateral patch on the eyes.

Evaluation of case with slit lamp biomicroscopy, ophthalmoscopy, gonioscopy, ultrasonography.

Treat the causative factor.

Laser photocoagulation.

Vitrectomy is the last choice if there are bands and membranes obstructing the vision.

VITREOUS ABSCESS

The most common occurrence of vitreous abscess is following an intraocular operation, usually an intracapsular cataract surgery. The most common organisms involved are *Staphylococcus aureus*, *Pseudomonas aeruginosa* and *Proteus* and coliform species. The primary source of infection is from theater air, theater staff, contaminated solutions, infected eyelids, infected conjunctiva, instruments and drapes. It is advisable to take all the precaution to prevent the infection. Clinically, the patient complains of pain and increasing gradual loss of vision, followed soon by marked congestion and hypopyon. There is no reflex from the pupil. Treat by intensive antibiotics, steroids and plan for vitrectomy to save the eye and some useful vision.

26

A Case with Endophthalmitis

Endophthalmitis denotes inflammation of the inner structures of the eyeball—the uveal and retinal tissue associated with exudation in the vitreous.

History

Record the history with reference to the following

- Any history of recent cataract or any other intraocular operation.
- The operation was performed in a hospital or in a camp.
- Any past history of eye operation especially dacryocystitis.
- Any history of penetrating eye injury.
- Any recent history of septic fever.

CLINICAL EXAMINATION

Visual Acuity

The vision is markedly reduced, to perception of light. The projection of light may be defective.

Slit Lamp Biomicroscopy

- Corneal edema.
- Keratic precipitates and hypopyon.
- Iris muddy.
- Whitish reflex from the pupil.
- Vitreous appears hazy with inflammatory cells in the anterior chamber and anterior vitreous.

Ophthalmoscopy

There is either no reflex or a very faint reflex. Fundus is not visible.

Retinoscopy

There is a whitish grey reflex from the pupil.

Laboratory Investigations

Smear Examination of Exudates

- Giemsa stain.
- Gram's stain.
- Potassium hydroxide preparation.
- Smear examination of anterior chamber paracentesis and vitreous aspirations.

Culture and Sensitivity

- From lid margin and the conjunctiva.
- From the conjunctival flap and corneal wound or incision.
- From anterior chamber paracentesis.
- From vitreous aspiration.

Clinical Features and Management

1. Bacterial endophthalmitis.
2. Phacoanaphylactic endophthalmitis.
3. Fungal endophthalmitis.
4. Parasitic endophthalmitis.
   - Toxocariasis.
   - Cystecercois.
5. Metastatic endophthalmitis.
   - Bacterial metastatic endophthalmitis.
   - Fungal metastatic endophthalmitis.
6. Vitrectomy.

BACTERIAL ENDOPHTHALMITIS

Etiology

Exogenous Infections

Airborne from theatre air and staff, contaminated solutions used during surgery, infected eyelids and conjunctiva of patient, infected hands of the surgeon if not using the gloves, infection from instruments, drapes and sutures and any material used during surgery which is not properly sterile.

Endogenous or Metastatic Infections

It occurs due to some infected focus in the body.

- The most common organisms causing a bacterial endophthalmitis are *Staphylococcus aureus*, *Streptococci*, *Pseudomonas*, pneumococci and *Corynebacterium*.
- Postoperative endophthalmitis following intraocular operation is rare. The present estimated incidence of postoperative bacterial endophthalmitis is about 0.1 per cent.

Signs and Symptoms

- The signs and symptoms usually appear within seventy-two hours of an intraocular operation for cataract or any other surgery.
- Pain in the eye and the brow which gradually increases in intensity making patient very uncomfortable and restless.
- Gradual dim vision. Patient complains that the vision he gained after surgery is getting dim and blurred every day. The vision may reduce to just perception of light with defective projection of light.
- Edema of the upper eyelid may be the first sign.
- Conjunctiva is congested with chemosis with circumciliary congestion.
- Cornea appears hazy due to edema. Anterior chamber shows hypopyon.
- Slit lamp examination shows vitreous hazy with aggregates, debris and bands.
- The pupil shows yellow-white or no reflex (Fig. 26.1).

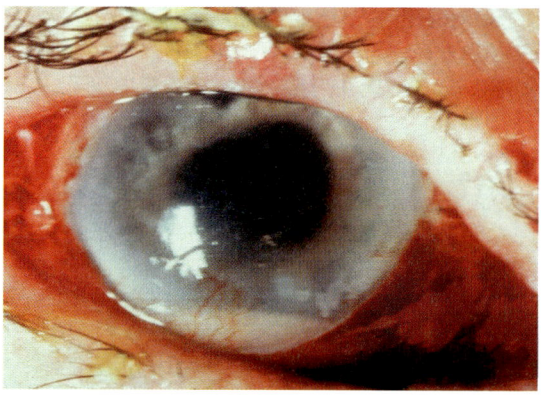

Fig. 26.1: Endophthalmitis with hypopyon

Diagnosis

- History of a cataract operation or any other intraocular surgery.
- Typical signs and symptoms.
- Leukocoria or no reflex at all.

Differential Diagnosis

- Phacoantigenic uveitis.
- Fungal endophthalmitis.
  The bacterial endophthalmitis progresses rapidly. The fungal and phaco-antigenic endophthalmitis are slow in progress.

Management

- Intensive therapy with antibiotics and steroids-topical, sub-conjunctival and systemic.
- Intracameral or intravitreal injection of Moxifloxacin can save the eye and vision.
- Topical cycloplegics.
- Topical and systemic anti-glaucoma drugs if tension is high.
- Analgesics to provide relief from pain and vitamins, minerals and nourishing diet as supportive therapy.
- Vitrectomy.

PHACO-ANAPHYLACTIC ENDOPHTHALMITIS

Phaco-anaphylactic endophthalmitis is probably an autoimmune reaction to lens protein similar to sympathetic ophthalmitis. It is difficult to differentiate it from sympathetic ophthalmia if both the eyes are involved. The phaco-anaphylactic endophthalmitis always occurs after injury to lens capsule or after an extracapsular cataract surgery. It may develop after weeks to months of lens trauma. A patient with a previous sensitization to lens protein shows a violent reaction if followed by an extracapsular cataract surgery in the other eye. The best plan is to remove the lens matter left behind. Corticosteroid therapy is effective to control the reaction.

FUNGAL ENDOPHTHALMITIS

Fungal endophthalmitis can occur following an intraocular surgery or a penetrating injury of the eye. Any case of delayed relentless uveitis following an injury or operation must be suspected for fungal endophthalmitis. Laboratory investigation of smear examination with potassium hydroxide preparation and culture sensitivity shall help to arrive at a diagnosis. Once the diagnosis is confirmed then treat by topical and systemic use of antifungal drugs. An endogenous candidal endophthalmitis can occur in association with complicated abdominal surgery, debilitating diseases and heroin addiction. Amphotericin B and flucytosine are synergistic. In a case of confirmed diagnosis an intravitreal injection of Amphotericin B 5 ug can be given. Vitrectomy is needed in all the cases to save the eye and vision.

PARASITIC ENDOPHTHALMITIS
TOXOCARIASIS (Nematode Endophthalmitis)

Toxocariasis is caused by ingestion of eggs from the faeces of dog (*Toxocara canis*) and cat (*Toxocara cati*). The infection is due to habbit of dirt eating or close contact with infected dog and cat. The infected intraocular tissues show a central focus of necrosis usually surrounding the worm with eosinophils. There is infiltration with neutrophils, plasma cells, epitheloid cells and other non-specfic chronic inflammatory cells. There is white reflex from the pupil. Presence of eosinophils and plasma cells in the retinal or vitreous abscess in a child

with white reflex from the pupil is confirmatory. If vitrectomy is not performed early then there is fibrosis and organization of the involved tissue. An early vitrectomy may save some vision.

Cysticercosis (Cestode Endophthalmitis)

Cysticercus cellulosae the larval stage of the pork tapworm *"Taenia solium"* may occasionally induce retinal or intravitreal masses that give rise to a white reflex from the pupil. The reaction is severe if the worm is dead.

METASTATIC ENDOPHTHALMITIS
Metastatic Bacterial Endophthalmitis

Metastatic bacterial endophthalmitis can occur due to infectious emboli from infection like meningitis, abdominal abscess, endocarditis, paronychia, and infected teeth. The predisposing factors include diabetes, prolonged antibiotic-steroid therapy and rheumatic heart diseases. Once the vitreous gets infected the disease process progresses rapidly with blurred vision and white reflex from the pupil. Blood culture is helpful. Vitreous culture by aspiration is a need. Start treatment with local and systemic antibiotic-steroid therapy. Intravitreal antibiotic (moxifloxacin) injections are encouraging. Consider vitrectomy.

Metastatic Fungal Endophthalmitis

Candida albicans a yeast like fungus is frequently found in human mouth, gastrointestinal tract and vagina. A metastatic endophthalmitis can occur in association with abdominal surgery, patients with immune deficiencies, leukemia, diabetes and narcotic addicts. It may present as non-granulomatous uveitis then progress to pan-uveitis and eventually in vitreous abscess. There is white reflex from the pupil. Blood culture, vitreous biopsy and culture with KOH stains are helpful. Treat with antifungal drugs systemically as antifungals have good intraocular penetration. Intravitreal anitifungal (amphotericin B-5–10 ug/0.1 ml) injections with vitrectomy may help save the eye and some vision.

VITRECTOMY

Vitreous surgery has been beneficial in the treatment of many conditions of the eye causing blindness. It shall be beneficial to both surgeon and the patient if there is a proper preoperative evaluation of a case for vitrectomy.

Preoperative Evaluation

Ocular

- Ascertain the cause of blindness by ocular examination and laboratory test.
- Visual acuity—If the patient has no perception of light or perception of light with defective projection then there are less chances for any visual recovery.
- A patient with positive macular and retinal function test has a good visual prognosis. The entopic phenomenon or Purkinje effect may be useful to evaluate the macular function. Other tests for macular function are color perception, two point discrimination and Maddox rod orientation. These are not dependable. Laser interferometry test helps to evaluate the visual potential in the presence of opaque media.
- Presence of any iris or lens pathology shall have a bearing on the outcome of vitrectomy.
- Electroretinography may be helpful.
- Intraocular pressure must be measured to have a baseline record of the pressure.
- Binocular indirect ophthalmoscopy even with opaque media may help to know about the retina.
- Slit lamp biomicroscopy with three mirror contact lens may allow visualization of fundus and posterior vitreous.
- Ultrasonography should be done to assess the posterior segment lesions. It may help to locate a detachment of retina, foreign body, and a mass behind the opaque media.
- Electroretinography and visually evoked response may help to differentiate a lesion of retina from optic nerve.
- X-ray orbit for a foreign body.

- CT scan may be helpful in certain cases where the diagnosis is not established even after all the efforts and ocular examination.

Systemic Examination

- A good history to evaluate the cause of the malady.
- A thorough systemic examination to assess the physical status for undergoing surgery.
- Routine and special laboratory test must be done.
  Electrocardiogram.
  X-ray chest.
  Complete blood picture.
  Blood sugar.
  Complete urine examination.

Indications for Vitrectomy

Vitreous hemorrhage: A patient with vitreous hemorrhage which has not cleared for the last six months and there is loss of vision so that he is not able to even move freely on covering the other eye then vitrectomy should be done.

Vitreous opacities: Any kind of vitreous opacities which obstruct the vision is an indication for vitrectomy. The most common opacities needing vitrectomy are bands, membranes, neovascular stalks, and thick floaters.

Pupillary membrane: Any membrane in the pupil which is the cause for reduced vision can be removed easily and safely with vitrectomy. The common causes for pupillary membrane are trauma, after cataract, exudates covering the pupil.

Ocular trauma: A penetrating injury usually results in many complications like cataract, vitreous escape, blood in the vitreous, iridocyclitis, hypotony, pupillary membrane, etc. due to initial incomplete management of the eye. Vitrectomy helps to reconstruct the anterior segment. A case of old trauma may also need reconstruction of anterior segment and removal of vitreous debris which is a mixture of blood, lens, and organized tissue.

Vitreous loss during intraocular surgery : Anterior vitrectomy shall help to avoid many complications which are associated with vitreous loss during surgery and during postoperative period. A vitreous loss may cause updrawn pupil, incarceration of vitreous in the wound, vitreous touch syndrome, glaucoma, hypotony, cystoid macular edema, etc.

Lensectomy: With vitrectomy instruments, the lensectomy can be performed in congenital cataract and traumatic cataract. This will avoid the complication of after cataract, pupillary membrane formation and vitreous loss and vitreous escape in the anterior chamber.

Traction detachment of retina: Vitrectomy is helpful as an adjunctive measure in a case of retinal detachment with bands and membranes causing traction.

Endophthalmitis: An early vitrectomy in a case of acute endophthalmitis may help to save the useful vision. It is also helpful in a case of treated endophthalmitis with residual vitreous opacities responsible for dim vision.

PARS PLANA VITRECTOMY

Three-port pars plana vitrectomy is the most popular surgical technique. One port is for cutting and aspiration probe. Second port is used for fiberoptic probe for illumination. Third port is used for infusion. This surgical technique provides bimanual easy handling with excellent visualization.

27

A Case with Retinal Detachment

History

Record the history with reference to the following

- Photopsia.
- Floaters thick and fine.
- Cobwebs or bunch of hairs in front of eyes.
- Small spots varying in size and number.
- Appearance of a curtain from any side of visual field.
- Visual loss.
- Any history of trauma direct or indirect.
- Any history of physical strain and stress like jumping, lifting heavy articles and pushing something heavy.
- Any history of ocular surgery like cataract, squint, removal of any growth.
- Any family history.
- Ask about using glasses for vision.

CLINICAL EXAMINATION

Visual Acuity

The visual acuity in the affected eye shall give a fair idea about the malady, the time interval and prognosis. The visual acuity in the fellow eye shall help assess about the refractive state of the patient.

Retinoscopy

There shall be a grey or white reflex from the pupil if there is a total detachment. Presence of grey or white reflex from any side indicates the area of detachment.

Direct Ophthalmoscopy

Direct ophthalmoscopy will give a fair idea about the detachment, vitreous, lens and sometimes even the hole may be located.

Binocular Indirect Ophthalmoscopy

Binocular indirect ophthalmoscopy is essential for most lesions of the retina and especially for the detachment of retina. It is a mandatory to examine both the eyes.

Advantage of Binocular Indirect Ophthalmoscopy

Low magnification

In the direct ophthalmoscopy: In an emmetropic eye the magnification is 15 and this allows only a small area of about 10° in diameter to be seen at a time The magnification in direct ophthalmoscopy depends on the refraction of the eye. In a myopic eye the magnification is greater.

In the indirect ophthalmoscopy: The magnification is independent of the patient's refractive state of the eye but depends on the power of the condensing lens used. The most commonly used condensing lens of plus 20 D gives magnification X 3.5 and the field of view is about 40°. The condensing lens of plus 30 D gives magnification of X2 and the field of view is about 60°. The main advantages of the low magnification are to visualize larger area and elimination of optical distortion.

- Stereoscopic view and better depth of focus helps to assess the elevated and solid lesions more accurately.

- It gives better illumination and resolution which helps to examine the fundus even with hazy media.
- It allows visualization of the peripheral retina which is very important to locate predisposing lesions.
- The long working distance and teaching mirror is helpful to the surgeon and students.

Slit Lamp Biomicroscopy with Fundus Contact Lens

Examination with fundus contact lens in association with slit lamp gives better magnification and therefore is helpful as follows:
- It helps in locating small breaks and holes in thin area of peripheral retina.
- It helps to examine the vitreous pathology.
- It is helpful in examination of the lesions at posterior pole especially macula.

Ultrasonography

In A scan echogram, with the sound beam at tissue sensitivity and perpendicular to the retinal surface, a retinal detachment is characterized by a single steeply rising and extremely high (100%) moderately thick retinal spike. Any change in direction causes a change in the pattern.

Electroretinogram

In a case with an attached retina, if there is a flat electroretinogram, then it indicates mass destruction of the retina with no function. In a case of total retinal detachment—the ERG is flat yet when the retina gets attached the ERG may return. Thus a flat ERG is of no prognostic significance in a case with detachment. Even though *a* and *b* waves may be absent, the early receptor potential (ERP) may still exist. The presence of ERP suggests that retinal function may return upon reattachment of the retina. The detection of ERP is not part of the usual ERG and requires special technique.

Where to look for Retinal Breaks (Holes)

- Patient's history of location of the photopsia has no value in locating the hole.
- Patient's history of seeing the shadow has a considerable value in locating the retinal hole. Look for the retinal break in the quadrant opposite to the quadrant in which the patient first noticed the shadow (Fig. 27.1).
- As 60% of all the retinal breaks occur in the upper temporal quadrant therefore look carefully and repeatedly the upper quadrant if the retinal breaks have not been detected initially.
- About 50% cases with retinal detachment have more than one break. Thus look for other break which is usually located within 90° of each other.
- The shape of the retinal detachment depends on the anatomical limits and the primary location of the retinal break. Thus a study of the shape of retinal detachment shall give a fair idea about the site of retinal hole.
- In the inferior retinal detachment wherein the sub-retinal fluid is slightly higher on the temporal side. Look for the hole in the upper temporal quadrant.
- A detachment with equal fluid level indicates a hole in the lower quadrant.
- In a bullous detachment the break is usually above the horizontal meridian.
- The presence of pigment cells in the anterior vitreous in a patient complaining of sudden photopsia and floaters strongly favors presence of a retinal tear.

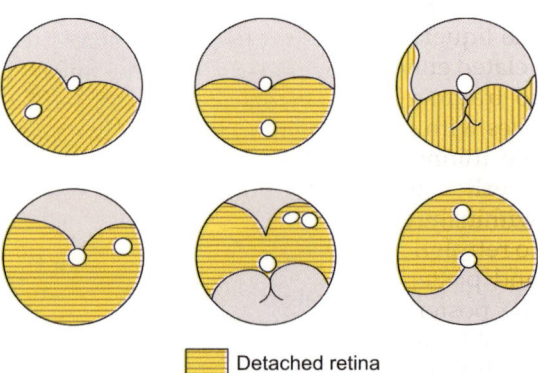

☐ Detached retina

Fig. 27.1: Shape of retinal detachment in relation to position of primary retinal break

RETINAL DETACHMENT

In the primary retinal detachment there is separation of the neurosensory retina from the retinal pigment epithelium with accumulation of sub-retinal fluid and presence of one or more retinal breaks (Fig. 27.2). The retinal detachment follows the occurrence of a retinal break. The retinal breaks are caused by two factors:

- Vitreoretinal traction.
- Peripheral retinal degeneration.

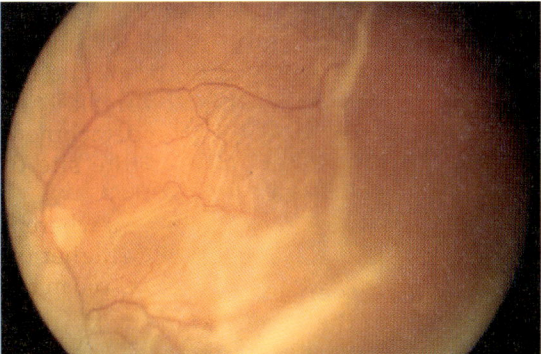

Fig. 27.2: Retinal detachment

VITREORETINAL TRACTION

The sensory retina is protected by the stable vitreous cortex gel. Any alteration in the micro-molecular structure of the vitreous gel results in its liquefaction. In most of the eyes the liquefaction of the vitreous gel is an age-related entity. Liquefaction can also occur due to trauma or occurs early in myopic. Some eyes with liquified vitreous develop a hole in the thinned posterior vitreous cortex which overlies the fovea. The liquified vitreous within the center of the vitreous cavity escapes to retrohyloid space (space between the retina and posterior vitreous) through this hole in the posterior vitreous. This passage of fluid forcibly detaches the posterior vitreous from the **internal limiting membrane (ILM)** of the sensory retina. This detachment of the posterior vitreous from the retina is called as *Posterior Vitreous Detachment (PVD)*. The remaining vitreous gel collapses and retrohyloid space is entirely filled by liquid vitreous. In majority of the eyes vitreoretinal adhesions are weak thereby the posterior vitreous detachment occurs without sequelae. The cases having strong pre-existing vitreoretinal adhesions develop breaks in the retina at the time of posterior vitreous detachment that may be occasionally delayed by months. Unless the break in the retina is treated by the photocoagulation or cryo-therapy the retinal detachment occurs sooner or later.

Tractional retinal detachment (Figs 27.3 and 27.4) is commonly associated with proliferative diabetic retinopathy, proliferative sickle cell retinopathy, retinopathy of prematurity, penetrating ocular trauma and Eales' disease.

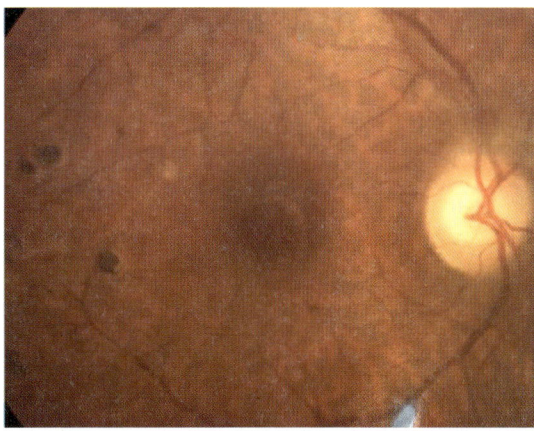

Fig. 27.3: Vitreoretinal traction syndrome

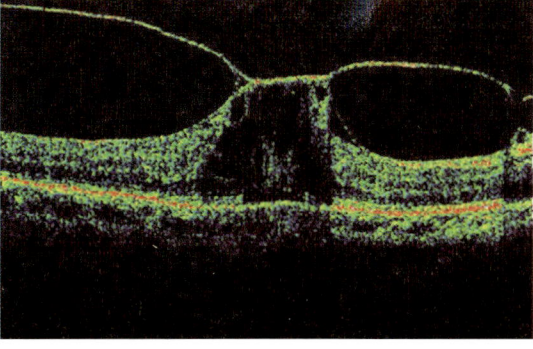

Fig. 27.4: Vitreoretinal traction syndrome-OCT

Peripheral retinal degeneration

- Lattice (palisade) degeneration
- Snail-track degeneration
- White-with pressure and white-without pressure.
- Focal pigment clumps
- Diffuse chorioretinal atrophy

Lattice Degeneration

Lattice degeneration looks like spindle-shaped areas in a group of three or four either circumferentially or radially and para-vascularly oriented islands of thin retina. It is usually bilateral commonly seen in the temporal and superior quadrant of the retina. It may be associated with snowflakes, hyperplasia of retinal pigment epithilium, white with pressure and network of white lines. The vitreous over the lattice is liquefied but have strong attachment at the margins. The lattice may show round holes within the island without any complications. Retinal break occurs following a posterior vitreous detachment at the posterior edge-of an island of lattice degeneration.

Snail-track Degeneration

Snail track degeneration appears as sharply demarcated bands with snowflakes and is associated with white with pressure. It is a variant of lattice degeneration.

White-with Pressure and White-without Pressure

The phenomenon of white-with pressure is a translucent grey appearance of the retina due to scleral pressure induced by scleral depressor during indirect ophthalmoscopy. When the retina appears translucent grey without pressure then it is called as white-without pressure. An area of retina which appears white without pressure needs a prophylactic cryotherapy.

Focal Pigment Clumps

These appear as small localized irregular patches of pigmentation often associated with vitreoretinal traction.

Diffuse Chorioretinal Atrophy

A myope may show diffuse choroidal de-pigmentation and thinning of the overlying retina in the equatorial region. It is prone to hole formation with posterior vitreous detachment.

CLINICAL FEATURES AND MANAGEMENT

Symptoms

Photopsia

Photopsia is a sensation perceived by the patient as a flash of light. It is caused by traction at vitreoretinal adhesions. In the eyes with posterior vitreous detachment the photopsia occurs due to eye movement and is more noticeable in dim illumination. It ceases after separation of adhesion or complete tearing of the piece of retina around the adhesion. It has no localizing value.

Floaters

Floaters are seen by the patient due to movement of the opacities in the liquified vitreous. The opacities may be small spots, cob-web form, bunch of hairs, linear, thick or fine.

Seeing a Shadow or a Curtain in Field

As there is spread of the retinal detachment from posterior to equator it produces field defect which is perceived by the patient as a shadow or a curtain from the side or up or below depending on the location of detachment.

Loss of Vision

If the detachment involves the fovea then there is complete loss of vision.

Signs

Marcus Gunn pupil: There is defective afferent conduction of pupillary reaction.

Intraocular pressure: It is comparatively low in the affected eye in relation to the normal eye.
- Grey-white reflex from pupil
- Opaque retina

The detached retina appears opaque with loss of the underlying choroidal pattern. The retinal vessels appear darker than the vessels on the normal retina.

Undulations: The detached retina shows undulation on the eye movement.

Posterior vitreous detachment: A retinal detachment of the long duration will show the following;
- Secondary intraretinal cysts
- Subretinal demarcation lines
- Subretinal fibrosis.

Differential diagnosis
- Acquired retinoschisis
- Choroidal detachment
- Solid detachment due to choroidal tumor
- Vitreous hemorrhage
- Retinal artery occlusion.

Investigations

Preoperative B-scan ultrasound is mandatory to planning surgery and prognosis.

MANAGEMENT

Prophylaxis

The following criteria to be kept in mind to give a prophylactic treatment with photo-coagulation or cryotherapy.
- A large break with acute posterior vitreous detachment located in the superior temporal quadrant or equatorial region.
- A retinal break in an aphakic eye.
- A retinal break associated with high myopia.
- A retinal break with a history of detachment in the fellow eye.
- A retinal break in a case with a family history of retinal detachment.
- A retinal break associated with systemic diseases like Marfan's syndrome, Stickler syndrome and Ehlers-Danlos syndrome.

Most of the lesions can be either treated with photocoagulation or cryotherapy. Equatorial or post equatorial lesions are amenable to photocoagulation. In treating a case with photocoagulation surround the break or an island of degeneration by two rows of confluent burns of moderate intensity.

The eyes with peripheral lesions and even with hazy media are amenable to cryo-therapy. In treating a case with cryotherapy, surround the lesion with a single row of cryo-application terminating the freezing soon the retina appears white.

Surgical Treatment

Scleral Buckling

Scleral buckling is a surgical procedure in which an inward indentation of the sclera is produced. This procedure helps to close the retinal break and relieve the vitreoretinal traction. The scleral buckle can be

Radial

In this the material is placed at right angle to the limbus. It is indicated in cases having large U-shaped posterior breaks.

Segmental Circumferential

In this the material is placed circumferentially with the limbus to create a segmental buckle. It is indicated in a case with multiple breaks, anterior breaks and giant tears.

Encircling Buckle

In this the material is placed around the entire circumference of the eyeball to create a buckle all around. It is indicated in the following conditions
- Breaks in three or more quadrants
- Extensive lattice degeneration
- Detachment in which the holes could not be detected
- Detachment with hazy media
- Cases in which the radial or segmental implant has failed to settle the detached retina.

Material used for Explant Buckle
- Soft silicon sponges are used both for radial and segmental circumferential buckling. The sponges may be round or oval with varying diameters usually 3 mm, 4 mm, and 5 mm round sponges and oval sponges are 5.5 × 7.5 mm.

- Hard silicon straps are used for encircling the entire globe, i.e. a 360 buckling.
- Hard silicon tyres

This is used to supplement the encircling band to achieve more indent.

Drainage of Subretinal Fluid

The drainage of the subretinal fluid is indicated in the following cases

- The hole has not been localized usually due to bullous detachment of retina.
- The retina is immobile due to proliferative vitreoretinopathy
- Eyes with detachment of retina of long duration.
- Eyes with tears in the inferior quadrant as there is tendency of the residual fluid to gravitate inferiorly when the patient is in upright position.

Drainage of the subretinal fluid provides immediate contact between the sensory retina and pigment epithelium and firm adhesion between the two though associated with complication of hemorrhage. The non-drainage of subretinal fluid can cause rise in the intraocular pressure which is temporary. Each case is to be assessed on its own merit and decide keeping in mind the advantage and disadvantage of drainage. Other surgical methods

- Intravitreal injection of air, balanced salt solution and silicon oil.
- Pars plana vitrectomy.

28

A Case with Maculopathy

History

Record the history with reference to the following:
- Ask especially about blurring of vision. The patient is able to read even 6/12. Only on asking he may say that the vision is markedly blurred, specially when the examiner ask him to compare the visual acuity by covering and uncovering the eyes alternately while looking at distance vision chart.
- Ask about alteration in the shape and size of the objects observed most of the patients are not able to appreciate this change. He is able to appreciate it on looking at the Snellen's chart when he may say that the letters are not in proper shape or small or large, in comparison to the fellow eye.

CLINICAL EXAMINATION

Visual Acuity

The patient sees blurred. His vision may improve by a line or two by putting minus lens indicating a shallow elevation of the macula.

Pupillary Reactions

The pupillary reactions are normal.

Color Vision

It is not impaired in macular disease.

Ophthalmoscopy

It is advisable to perform direct and indirect ophthalmoscopy in any case with macular pathology to have a better appreciation of the lesion in the fundus.

Slit Lamp Biomicroscopy with Fundus Contact Lens

It is helpful in detecting early macular lesions as edema, subretinal neovascular membrane, elevation of macula and pigmentary changes. It helps to differentiate lesions like hemorrhage, hole and cyst at macula.

Fluorescein Angiography

It is helpful to locate window defect at macula. It helps to plan laser therapy.

Amsler Grid Test

Amsler grid chart consists of a 10 cm square divided into smaller 5 mm squares. On keeping this chart at about 33 cm each square subtends an angle of 1°. Ask the patient to keep the chart at 33 cm and look at the central dot on the chart with right eye covering his left eye and observe and report about any distortion, wavy lines, blurred areas, or blank spots anywhere on the chart (Figs 28.1 and 28.2). Repeat the test with opposite eye. Presbyopic is advised to use his glasses. The surgeon or the patient himself can draw what he reports or sees. It is useful for follow up.

Photo-stress Test

In this test the visual pigment is bleached by light. This causes temporary retinal insen-

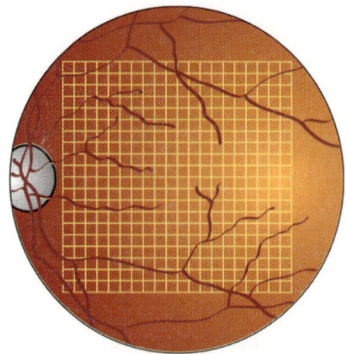

Fig. 28.1: Amsler grid superimposed on posterior pole

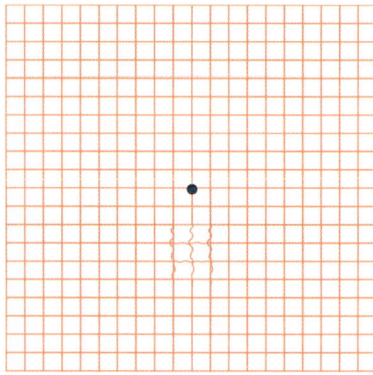

Fig. 28.2: Amsler grid showing slight distortion

sitivity which is perceived by the patient as a scotoma. The recovery of the vision depends on the ability of the photoreceptors to re-synthesize visual pigment.

This test is useful in differentiating whether visual loss is due to macular disease or optic nerve lesion.

Record the visual acuity for distance. Expose the eye to be put to test to a bright light of a pen torch for about 10 seconds. Ask the patient to read the pre test acuity line soon he recovers from scotoma. Repeat the test on the opposite eye. The patient with macular disease will take more than 50 seconds and sometimes few minutes to recover.

Optical Coherence Tomography (OCT)

It is a photographic assessment of the maculopathy for its severity prognosis and resolution.

Clinical Features and Management

1. Drusen.
2. Central serous retinopathy (CSR).
3. Cystoid macular edema (CME).
4. Macular hole.
5. Bull's-eye macula syndrome.
6. Cherry-red spot at macula.
7. Age-related macular degeneration (AMD).
8. Chloroquine maculopathy.
9. Vitreo-macular traction syndrome (VMTS).
10. Epiretinal membrane (ERM).

DRUSEN

- It is a type of macular degeneration which is related to the age. It is frequent after the age of 60.
- The lesions are usually symmetrical in both the eyes.
- Ophthalmoscopy (Fig. 28.3)
  Hard drusen appear as small discrete, yellowish white and slightly raised spots. Soft drusen have indistinct margins and become confluent.
  Diffuse drusen is indicative of wide spread abnormality of retinal pigment epithelium.
  Calcified drusen have a glistening appearance.
- Fluorescein angiography shows window defect in pigment epithelium and staining of the drusen.
- Patient may maintain good vision for a long time. The visual loss is profound and

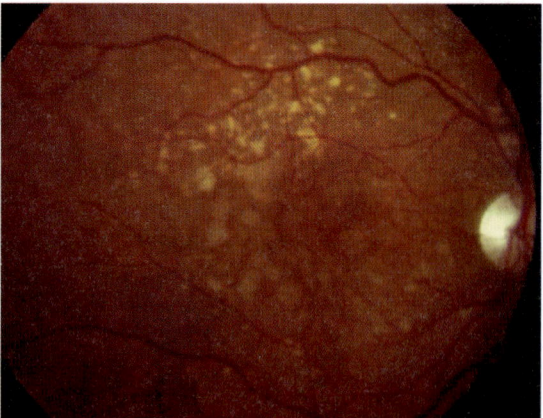

Fig. 28.3: Drusen at macula

early if associated with detachment of pigment epithelium and choroidal neo-vascularization and exudation.

- No effective treatment is available except low visual aids.

CENTRAL SEROUS RETINOPATHY (CSR)

- It is a common disorder of macula of unknown etiology.
- It affects males between the ages of 20 and 45.
- Sudden onset of blurred vision.
- Positive scotoma.
- Micropsia.
- Metamorphopsia.
- Ophthalmoscopy shows a shallow round elevation at the macula, surrounded by a reflex. Foveal reflex is absent or distorted.
- Fundus contact lens shows detachment of retina with fluid at macula.
- Fluorescein angiography shows leak and pooling at the macula.
- Most of the cases 80 to 90% undergo resolution with normal vision.
- The micropsia or metamorphopsia may persist for long time.
- There is recurrence in 40% cases.
- Some cases may develop cystoid maculo-pathy.
- As there is a tendency for spontaneous resolution so it is advisable to wait.
- Steroids for long time with maintenance dose is effective in resolution.
- Laser photocoagulation to the site of leak can be given if the site of leak is away from the fovea.

CYSTOID MACULAR EDEMA (CME)

Etiological Factors

- The exact causative factor for cystoid macular edema is unknown.
- Inflammation, vitreous traction and generalized vascular diseases like hyper-tension, diabetes and central retinal vein occlusion have been thought of.
- Prostaglandins have been implicated.
- It is seen more after an intracapsular cataract surgery.

- Implant of intraocular lens has no signi-ficant effect.
- Incidence increases with loss of vitreous.
- Incidence increases with secondary implant.

Clinical Features

i. *Angiographic cystoid macular edema*: Angiographic cystoid macular edema develops soon after cataract extraction. The incidence is more with intra-capsular cataract extraction. Fluorescein angiography shows a "flower petal" pattern. It is symptomless and resolves itself.

ii. *Clinical cystoid macular edema*: Clinical cystoid macular edema presents after few months to years of surgery. There is anterior uveitis with vitritis. Patient complains of mild irritation, redness, photophobia and dim vision. Fluorescein angiography shows "flower petal" pattern with pooling of the dye. Ophthalmoscopy shows dull foveal reflex with cystoid spaces "**Honeycomb appearance**" (Fig. 28.4). Most cases resolve spontaneously. A course of steroids or non-steroidal anti-inflammatory drugs may help.

MACULAR HOLE

- A macular hole may develop in a healthy eye in elderly people.
- It develops in myopia following trauma and solar retinopathy.

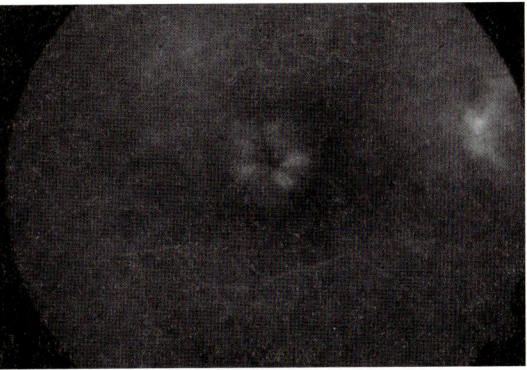

Fig. 28.4: Cystoid macular edema

- Vision is markedly reduced.
- Ophthalmoscopy shows a clear cut punched out area round or oval with few yellow spots in the base of the hole and grey halo of marginal retinal elevation (Fig. 28.5).

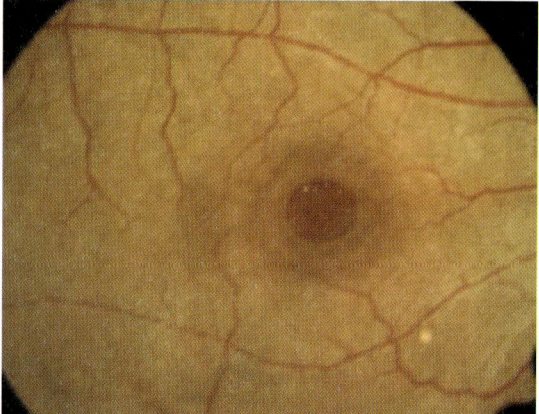

Fig. 28.5: Macular hole

- Fluorescein angiography shows an area of hyperfluorescence due to window defect in the pigment epithelium.
- Slit lamp biomicroscopy with fundus contact lens helps to differentiate the macular hole from a macular cyst.
- A lamellar hole shows a granular appearance in the base and fluorescein angiography will not show a window defect as seen in a case of macular hole (Fig. 28.6).
- Macular hole does not cause retinal detachment, therefore, no treatment is required.

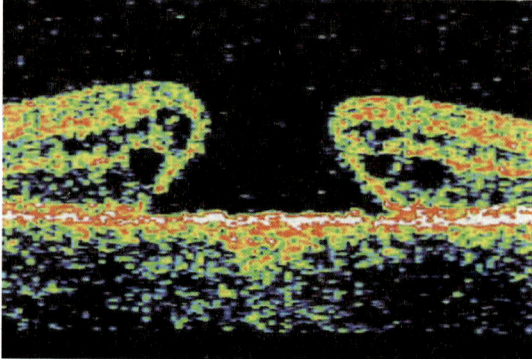

Fig. 28.6: Macular hole—OCT

BULL'S-EYE MACULA SYNDROME

The Bull's-eye macula syndrome is due to selected atrophy of retinal pigment epithelial cells.

- Inheritance is autosomal dominant.
- Dim vision in good illumination.
- Day-blindness due to dystrophy of cones.
- Defective color vision.
- Nystagmus.
- Fundus shows-typical macular pigmentary changes (bull's-eye appearance). Retinal arteries are narrowed and pigmentary changes are visible in periphery. The changes are irreversible.
- Photopic electroretinogram is subnormal or flat while scotopic response is normal. This is due to dystrophy of cones.

CHERRY-RED SPOT AT MACULA

The cherry-red spot is the most important presentation at the macula in a group of inherited metabolic diseases which comprises the sphingolipidoses.

Cherry red spot is seen in following maladies

Sphingolipidoses includes

- Tay-Sachs disease
- Niemann-Pick disease
- Sandhoff's disease
- Sialidosis types 1 and 2
- Generalized gangliosidosis

The lipids are stored in the ganglion cell layer of the retina giving the retina a white appearance. As the ganglion cells are absent at the fovea this area appears red in contrast with white surrounding retina hence it is named cherry-red spot. Later the patient develops optic atrophy.

Commotio Retinae (Berlins edema)

A commotio retinae is a condition of edema of the retina due to simple concussion, the changes are reversible and transient, though frequently it may involve permanent visual loss to a marked degree. Ophthalmoscopically the fovea stands out as a red spot against the background of milky white appearance of surrounding retina due to edema. The clinical picture resembles the appearance seen after occlusion of the central retinal artery. The picture varies considerably depending on the force impinging the posterior pole and therefore the eventual outcome which may be a normal fundus with normal vision or reduced vision with changes at the macula in the form of macular cyst, macular hole or macular degeneration.

Quinine Amblyopia

Fundus shows markedly attenuated retinal arteries, edema in the macular area with fovea shining as red spot "Cherry red spot".

Central Retinal Artery Occlusion

Central retinal artery occlusion results in irreversible loss of vision. Its frequency is 1 in 10000 out-patients cases. It is a branch of ophthalmic artery and supplies the inner retina. Its sudden occlusion results in edema of inner layers of retina. The edema gives an opaque or yellow-white appearance of the retina. The fovea appears red as the retina is thin allowing visualization of normal retinal pigment epithelium and choroid in presence of surrounding white or opaque retina. This typical appearance has been labeled as "Cherry red spot" at macula.

AGE-RELATED MACULAR DEGENERATION

Age-related macular degeneration (AMD) also known as *Senile macular degeneration* is a bilateral degeneration in aged past 60 years of age. This is a leading cause of blindness in developed countries. Risk factors are heredity, poor nutrition, smoking and high blood pressure. Prognosis of age-related macular degeneration is poor therefore it needs an early diagnosis and aggressive treatment strategy. Any permanent structural damage to the eye by other lesions should be ruled out before any treatment is commenced (Fig. 28.7).

Dry AMD (Non-exudative or atrophic or non-neovascular)

- It affects 90% of cases.

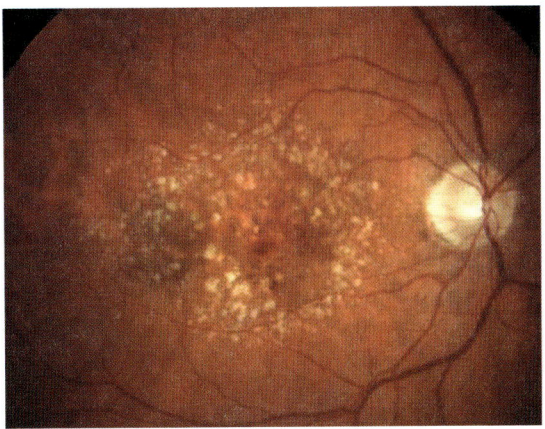

Fig. 28.7: Age-related macular degeneration

- It causes mild to moderate gradual loss of vision.
- Patient complains of difficulty in near work due to central shadowing.
- Ophthalmoscopy shows drusens.
- Dictary supplements and antioxidants are helpful in preventing or delaying the progression.

Wet AMD-(Exudative or Neovascular)

- It progresses rapidly with marked loss of vision.
- It passes through many stages and ends as disciform macular degeneration.
- Ophthalmoscopy helps in diagnosis and progress.
- Fluorescein angiography for complete categorization and sub-typing of the Wet AMD.
- Assess location of sub-foveal hemorrhage by OCT.
- Argon green laser photocoagulation for extra-foveal choroidal neovascular membrane.
- Low fluence photodynamic therapy.
- VEGF inhibitors.

CHLOROQUINE MACULOPATHY

Incidence of Chloroquine retinopathy or Maculopathy is low in well monitored and dosed patients. Incidence is low when using a dose of less than 4 mg/kg per day of chloroquine or 6.5 mg/kg per day of hydroxyl-chloroquine. Chloroquine toxicity is unlikely event if the daily dose does not exceed 250 mg daily. Chloroquine is used as a long-term therapy in rheumatic arthritis and lupus erythematosus. It is common drug as anti-malarial. Yet chloroquine does show toxicity in cases with long duration administration of controlled doses. Thus, every patient who is on long-term therapy with chloroquine should consult ophthalmologist at least twice a year to catch the malady at its pre-maculopathy stage.

Ophthalmoscopic Findings

Pre-maculopathy or Mild form of Retinopathy

Patient is asymptomatic as visual acuity and visual fields are normal. Fundus shows-light pigmentary stippling or granular appearance of the macula with loss of foveal reflex. These changes are almost similar to changes in age-related macular degeneration. These changes are reversible if drug is withdrawn.

Advanced Maculopathy or Severe form of Retinopathy

Visual acuity is affected. There is bilateral para-central field defect. Fundus shows-typical macular pigmentary changes (Bull's-eye appearance). Retinal arteries are narrowed and pigmentary changes are visible in periphery. The changes are irreversible.

It is advisable to have fundus photography as a base line within 6 months intake of chloroquine. Then it may be helpful to further assess the fundus changes later, on follow up.

VITREO-MACULAR TRACTION SYNDROME (VMTS)

In vitreo-macular traction syndrome, the vitreous is separated from the retina through-out the peripheral fundus yet remains adherent posteriorly resulting in antero-posterior traction covering macular area and optic nerve. It is usually associated with epiretinal membrane. Tractions results in retinal distortion and cystoids macular edema resulting in symptom of metamorphopsia and loss of central vision.

Fluorescein angiography demonstrates leakage, macular edema with macular puck-ering and tractional macular detachment. It may progress to macula hole.

Vitrectomy is the only choice.

EPIRETINAL MEMBRANES (ERM)

Epiretinal membranes are composed of fibroglial tissue sheets. These are non-vascularized sheets that grow over the macula after laser photocoagulation, cryopexy, retinal detachment surgery and as a complication of vascular occlusions, posterior uveitis, trauma and tumors. Epiretinal membranes may be associated with tortuosity of vessels, retinal striae, loss of foveal reflex and retinal edema (Figs 28.8 and 28.9).

It causes loss of vision and meta-morphopsia.

Most of the epiretinal membranes are idiopathic.

Vitrectomy is the only treatment.

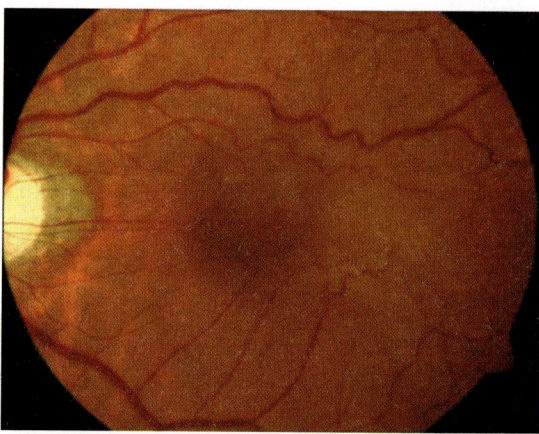

Fig. 28.8: Epiretinal membrane

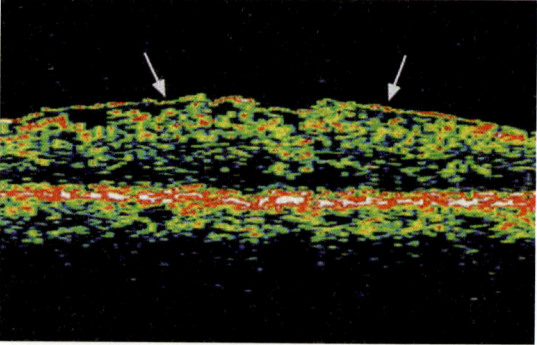

Fig. 28.9: Epiretinal membrane-OCT

29

A Case with Diabetic Retinopathy

History

Record the history with reference to the following:
- Duration of diabetes.
  Incidence of diabetic retinopathy is related to the duration of diabetes.
- Family history: The diabetes has a strong genetic component. It is transmitted as recessive trait without sex linkage. Heredity affects proliferative retinopathy.
- Insulin or non-insulin dependent type.
- Associated systemic disease like hypertension or urinary tract problem, obesity, hyperlipidemia and smoking accentuate the fundus changes.
- Controlled or uncontrolled diabetic.
- Incidence is more in females than males (4:3).
- Pregnancy accelerates fundus changes. Pregnant mothers must be more careful.

CLINICAL EXAMINATION

Visual Acuity

Patients maintain good visual acuity until the macula gets involved. A good visual acuity is not indication that he will not develop proliferative diabetic retinopathy.

Refraction

Assess the refractive state of the eyes. Also assess the reflex from the pupil. In a case of proliferative retinopathy the reflex shall appear white grey.

Ophthalmoscopy

Examine the fundus and media.

Slit Lamp Biomicroscopy with Fundus Contact Lens

It is very helpful in cases with maculopathy. It helps to examine the posterior fundus under high magnification. Any pathology in the vitreous is easily detected.

Fluorescein Angiography

It shows the areas of leakage and areas of non-perfusion and thus helps in application of photocoagulation.

Investigation

- Complete blood picture
- Routine and microscopic urine analysis
- Blood sugar-fasting and post-prandial
- Glycosylated hemoglobin (HBA1C)
- Mean plasma glucose
- Lipid, thyroid and renal profile.

Clinical Features and Management

1. Non-proliferative diabetic retinopathy (NPDR).
   - Mild
   - Moderate
   - Severe
   - Very severe
2. Proliferative diabetic retinopathy (PDR).
3. Diabetic maculopathy.
4. Advanced diabetic eye disease.

NON-PROLIFERATIVE DIABETIC RETINOPATHY

Fundus Shows

- *Micro-aneurysms:* These appear as small round dots usually seen temporal to macula. These are situated in inner nuclear layer of retina.

- *Dot and blot hemorrhages:* These appear as round hemorrhages arise from the venous end of the capillaries and located in middle layers of retina (Fig. 29.1).

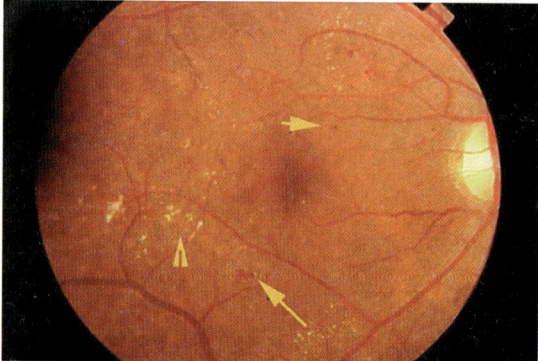

Fig. 29.1: Diabetic retinopathy

- *Flame-shaped hemorrhages:* These arise from superficial pre-capillary arterioles and follow the course of the retinal nerve fiber layer so known as flame-shaped hemorrhages.
- *Hard exudates:* These are located between the inner plexiform and inner nuclear layer of the retina. These appear as crenated yellow waxy looking spots of varying size in a circinate pattern most common at the posterior pole (Fig. 29.2).

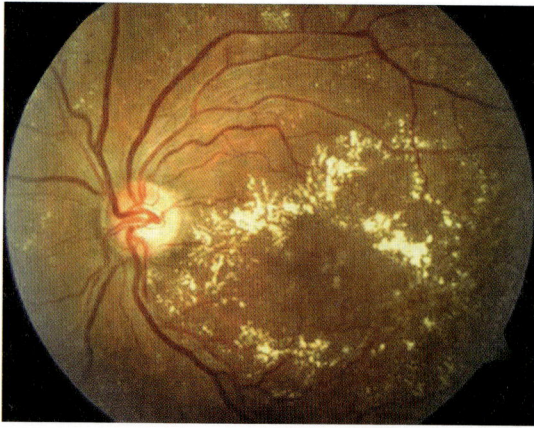

Fig. 29.2: Hard exudates

- *Cotton-wool exudates:* These are soft exudates and appear like a ball of cotton. These are due to capillary occlusion in the retinal nerve fiber layer.
- *Venous changes:* The retinal veins are dilated, tortuous and show beading, looping and sausage like dilated segments.
- *Arterial changes:* Retinal arteries are narrow and even occluded resembling retinal artery branch occlusion.

Types

- *Mild non-proliferative diabetic retinopathy* shows at least one micro-aneurysm or hemorrhage with or without any hard or cotton-wool exudates.
- *Moderate non-proliferative diabetic retinopathy* shows few micro-aneurysm, hemorrhages and exudates along with early arterial changes.
- *Severe non-proliferative diabetic retinopathy* shows micro-aneurysm and hemorrhages all over the fundus along with few venous and arteriolar changes.
- *Very severe non-proliferative diabetic retinopathy* shows large amount of micro-aneurysm, hemorrhages and exudates along with severe venous and arteriolar changes.

Management

- Strict metabolic control of diabetes.
- Control obesity and malnutrition.
- Regulate physical exercise and diet.
- Control hypertension.
- Treat anemia if present.
- Aspirin has been advised to decrease platelet stickiness.
- Regular check up of blood sugar, blood pressure and fundus at least every three months.
- Apply mild argon laser to the areas of capillary non-perfusion as shown by fluorescein angiography.
- Apply argon laser in pan retinal pattern.

PROLIFERATIVE DIABETIC RETINOPATHY

It occurs in some cases with very severe non-proliferative diabetic retinopathy. All the lesions are due to retinal ischemia.

Fundus Shows

Neovascularization: New vessels proliferate on the optic nerve head and along the major temporal retinal vessels. The neovascularization occurs when the large areas of retina is non-perfused. The vessels grow in the potential vitreoretinal space or spread into the vitreous as vascular folds. Soon, there is condensation of connective tissue around the new vessels resulting in formation of fibrovascular epiretinal membranes and fibrous bands in the vitreous.

Vitreous detachment due fibrous bands: The vitreous has a strong attachment at the areas of fibrovascular proliferation. The fibrovascular tissue continues to grow along the posterior surface of the partially detached vitreous. Later as the fibrovascular tissue is further put on traction it may cause bleeding.

Vitreous hemorrhage: Hemorrhage may occur in the vitreous gel or into the prehyaloid space. Prehyaloid hemorrhage appears as a cresent convex downwards and almost straight line at the upper end. The hemorrhage in the vitreous gel may get organized (Fig. 29.3).

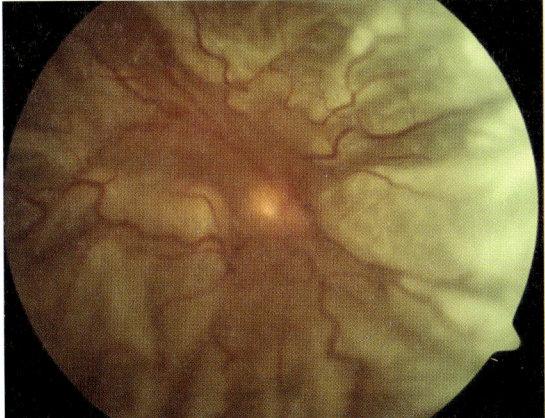

Fig. 29.3: Proliferative retinopathy

Management

- Advice the patient to avoid physical strain as it may lead to hemorrhage.
- Only treatment available is photocoagulation, by Xenon arc or argon laser.
- Pars plana vitrectomy is useful in saving some vision and prevents occurrence of detachment.
- Photocoagulation prevents occurrence of neovascular glaucoma.

DIABETIC MACULOPATHY

Diabetic maculopathy can be associated with non-proliferative or proliferative diabetic retinopathy. Diabetic maculopathy occurs due to increased permeability of retinal capillaries. It can be focal, diffuse, ischemic or circinate maculopathy.

Diabetic maculopathy is the common cause of visual loss. It is seen more in diabetics who are non-insulin dependent type. On examination-macula may show mild edema, cystic spaces and later a lamellar hole (Fig. 29.4).

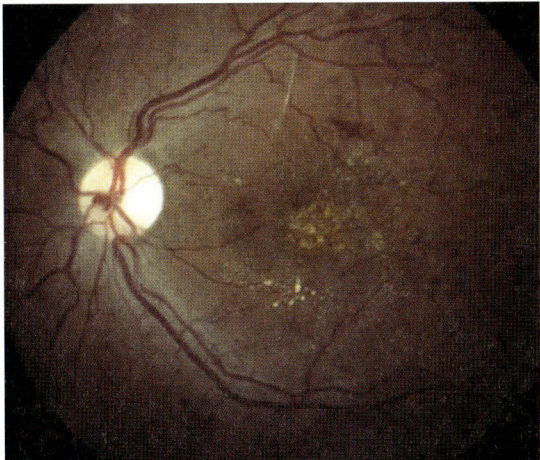

Fig. 29.4: Diabetic macular edema-1

Fluorescein angiography will show the areas of leakage (Fig. 29.5). Treat by argon laser. Treat the micro-aneurysms and apply

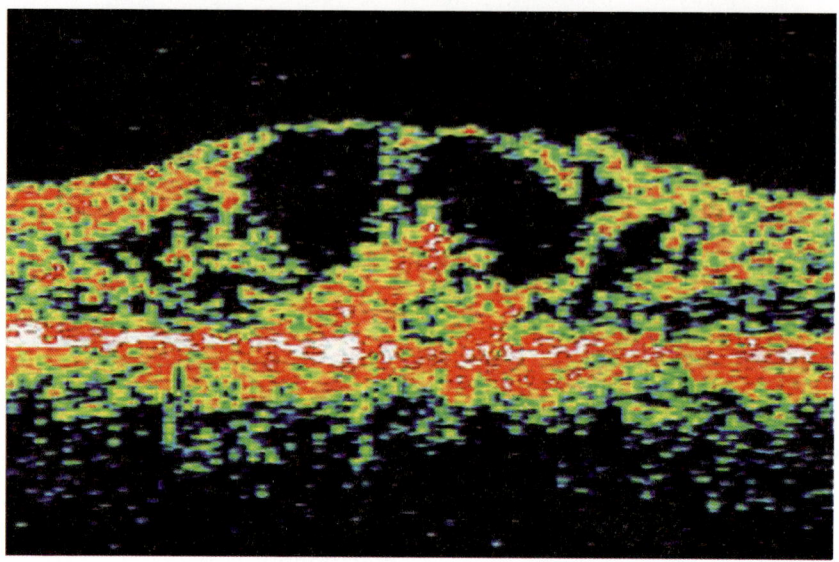

Fig. 29.5: Diabetic macular edema-1-OCT

argon laser burns to the macula area avoiding the fovea.

Management

Intravitreal steroids to reduce macular edema have been advocated to save vision.

Intravitreal injection of Vascular Endothelial Growth Factors inhibitors (VEGFs) is helpful in cases who do not respond to intravitreal steroids.

ADVANCED DIABETIC EYE DISEASE

It is the result of uncontrolled and untreated diabetic patients and diabetic retinopathy. It results in following complications:
- Persistent hemorrhage.
- Retinal detachment.
- Neovascular glaucoma.

Management as per the need of an individual case.

Management

1. Screening for diabetic retinopathy to prevent visual loss.
2. Medical therapy—Strict control of diabetes with supportive treatment; control obesity, advocate physical exercise and good controlled diet. Treat associated systemic diseases.
3. Vascular endothelial growth factors (VEGFs) inhibitors are under evaluation.
4. Intravitreal steroids are being used to save vision.
5. Photocoagulation when indicated.
6. Pars plana vitrectomy when indicated.

30

A Case with Hypertensive Retinopathy

History

Record the history with reference to the following

- Age on onset
  Hypertension in young is indicative of some underlying systemic disease. A thorough examination is essential. In an elderly it may be a normal aging phenomenon.
- Any associated systemic disease like diabetes or renal problem.
- As it is vascular disease ask for any other associated vascular problems.
- Any weight gain in recent months.
- Any emotional stress.
- Leading a sedentary or active life and lifestyle.

CLINICAL EXAMINATION

Visual Acuity

It is essential to note the vision with and without glasses to assess the progress. A reduced vision indicates involvement of macula. This case needs a thorough checkup and early control to save the vision.

Ophthalmoscopy

Usually direct ophthalmoscopy is sufficient to examine the funds in a case of a hypertensive retinopathy. Some cases may need an examination with binocular indirect ophthalmoscope to look into periphery of the fundus for any associated lesion.

Slit Lamp Biomicroscopy with Fundus Contact Lens

It is helpful to examine the macula with a stereoscopic view and high magnification.

Fluorescein Angiography

It helps to locate minute lesions which are likely to be missed by ophthalmoscopy.

Investigation

- Blood pressure thrice a day for three days.
- Complete blood picture.
- Lipid, thyroid and renal profile.
- Complete urine analysis.
- Blood sugar-fasting and post-prandial.

CLINICAL FEATURES AND MANAGEMENT

Hypertensive Retinopathy

Hypertensive retinopathy shows fundus changes in patients with systemic hypertension.

Pathogenesis

Three factors play important role in the pathogenesis of hypertensive retinopathy.

Vasoconstriction

Vasoconstriction of the retinal arterioles is the primary response to high blood pressure. This response is affected by pre-existing involutional sclerosis in elderly patients.

Arteriosclerotic Changes

It manifests as change in the arteriolar reflex and arteriovenous crossing changes due to thickening of the vessel wall.

Increased Vascular Permeability

It results due to hypoxia. It manifests as hemorrhages, exudates and focal retinal edema.

CLINICAL FUNDUS MANIFESTATION

General Attenuation

It is due to tonic contraction or due to generalized arteriolar sclerosis.

Focal Vascular Narrowing

Focal vascular narrowing should be taken as positive if the vessel involved is away from disk. It affects the vessels of first and second order usually to an extent of a disk diameter. There may be involvement of one or all the vessels. There may be one or many focal constriction. It is due to organic thickening of vessel wall.

Straightening of Arterial Tree

It is due to decrease in the length of the arteries owing to sclerotic changes behind the disk.

Gunn's Sign

There is apparent compression of vein seen as nicking on either side of crossing.

Salu's Sign

There is a deflection in the course of vein. The veins cross the artery at right angle rather than obliquely.

Both these signs may be normal in 60 per cent of cases.

Vascular Reflex

The vascular reflex is due to blood and vessels wall-the media. It is the media which changes in sclerosis.

Copper Wire Reflex

The reflex is broad and soft instead of thin and bright reflex seen in vessels of second and third order.

Silver Wire Reflex

The whole artery appears as a white reflex without any evidence of red blood column.

Sheathing of Vessels

It may be a parallel sheathing or pipe stem sheathing. It is normal near the disk.

Cotton-wool Spots

Cotton-wool spots may be seen in many other conditions such as diabetes, anemia, leukemia, and central vein occlusion. These occur at the posterior pole.

Hard Exudates

A severe hypertension can result in increased retinal vascular permeability with hard exudates accumulating particularly in outer plexiform layer in the macula (Henle's layer). This results in an ophthalmoscopic appearance of a macular star or a macular fan.

Hemorrhages

Hemorrhages in the nerve fiber layer appear as flame shaped or splinter hemorrhages which are characteristic for hypertension.

Visual Loss

The visual loss is pronounced in a case of malignant hypertension due to poor macular capillary perfusion, macular hemorrhage, retinal edema, lipid exudation, occlusion of retinal vein branch and arterioles, and sometimes due to serous detachment at macula.

Fluorescein angiography is helpful to elucidate the pathology.

Various Ophthalmoscopic Features

- Narrowing of the arterioles.
- Cotton-wool spots.
- Micro-aneurysms.

- Flame-shaped hemorrhages.
- Splinter-shaped hemorrhages.
- Hard lipid exudation.
- Arteriosclerotic changes in the form of increased light reflex, copper wire appearance and sliver wire appearance of arterioles.
- Occlusion of small branches of arterioles and venules.
- Edema of disk.
- Serous detachment of macula.

Keith-Wagener-Barker Classification of Hypertensive Retinopathy

Grade I

Retinal signs are minimal with mild narrowing or sclerosis of the arterioles.

Grade II

There is generalized or localized narrowing of arterioles. There are arteriovenous crossing changes.

Grade III

There are signs of grade II with presence of angiospastic retinopathy. There is retinal edema, flamed-shaped hemorrhages, cotton-wool spots and hard exudates (Fig. 30.1). There are marked sclerotic changes with copper wiring reflex of arterioles with Gunn, Salu and Bonnet signs of vein.

Grade IV

There are signs of grade III with silver-wiring reflex of arterioles and papilledema. There is spastic or organic narrowing of arterioles with diffuse retinopathy.

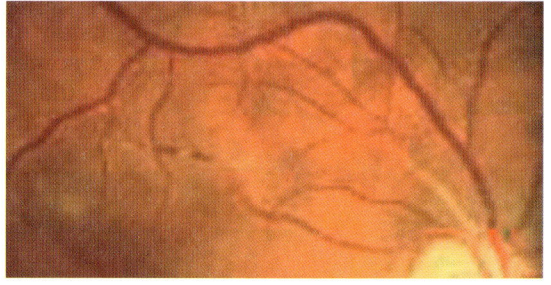

Fig. 30.1: Hypertensive retinopathy—Grade III

ARTERIOSCLEROTIC RETINOPATHY

The ophthalmoscopic findings are as follows:
- The disk appears hazy, pale and atrophic.
- Irregular lumen of vessels.
- There is copper wire or sliver wire reflex.
- There is sheathing, arteriovenous compression and tortuosity.
- Small hemorrhages scattered, superficial or deep may be seen.
- Hard exudates are seen.

Clinical Types

1. *Hypertension without sclerosis:* Seen in young patients. Good prognosis if hypertension is well controlled.
2. *Hypertension with involutionary (senile) sclerosis:* Seen in elderly patients with arteriosclerotic changes in the fundus. Good prognosis if hypertension is well controlled.
3. *Hypertension with compensatory arteriolar sclerosis:* Seen in young patients with well advanced fundus changes due to benign nephrosclerosis akin to renal or albuminuric retinopathy. Poor prognosis.
4. *Malignant hypertension:* Seen in young patients with fundus changes akin to hypertensive neuroretinopathy. Poor prognosis.

Prognosis

- Prognosis of hypertension with Keith-Wagener grade I and grade II is very good. The process is reversible if hypertension is controlled.
- Prognosis of hypertension with Keith and Wagener grade III and grade IV is poor.
- Antihypertensive drugs have helped to save the damage to brain, heart and kidneys and thus increased survival rate.
- An early diagnosis and proper and regular treatment of hypertension prevents the development of the hypertensive retinopathy.

Management

- Strict control of hypertension with regular check up by cardiologist.

- Buy a good quality of blood pressure instrument-preferably mercurial rather than automatic and learn the art to record the blood pressure by self. Except your own self, none shall be able to record Blood pressure when you would like it to be recorded. This will help you to adjust the doses as per your own need to maintain blood pressure of 140/80 mm Hg for most of 24 hours of the day.

- Regular physical exercise with guidance of physician coupled with yoga and meditation.
- Strict control of weight as per age and height by work up and diet.
- Anyone can live a long and healthy life by just keeping a watch on the Self and caring the self, if you really wish to enjoy the world created by your effort with setting Sun of age.

31

A Case with Central Retinal Vein Occlusion

History

Record the history with reference to the following:

- Age: It is common in the sixth and seventh decades of life.
- Hypertension: Hypertension increases the risk of vein occlusion. Thickened artery compresses the vein where the two share a common adventitia at the arteriovenous crossings in the retina and just behind the lamina cribrosa.
- Any history of diagnosed glaucoma. Any eye with raised intraocular pressure is at high risk for central retinal vein occlusion.
- Any systemic disease like diabetes, sarcoidosis and Behcet's disease.
- Ask about metamorphopsia.

CLINICAL EXAMINATION

Visual Acuity

- It is slightly reduced in a case of non-ischemic type of central retinal vein occlusion.
- It is markedly reduced in a case of ischemic central retinal vein occlusion.
- In a case of branch block there is some loss of field and vision along with metamorphopsia.

Direct Ophthalmoscopy

Examine the fundus and media.

Indirect Ophthalmoscopy

It is essential to examine the periphery of the fundus especially for a branch block.

Slit Lamp Biomicroscopy with Fundus Contact Lens

Examine the macula especially for any edema, cystic spaces and hemorrhage.

Intraocular Pressure

The intraocular pressure is low when the occlusion occurs. It is 20 to 30% lower than the unaffected eye due to diminished flow. In a case of branch block there is no change in the intraocular pressure. Later it tends to rise, a phenomenon particularly observed in those cases in which an initial fall in intraocular pressure is absent. Glaucoma occurs in 20% cases of central retinal vein occlusion within three months due to neovascularization in the iris and angle.

Tonometry

- If there is high intraocular pressure in both the eyes and almost equal then treat the case for glaucoma also.
- If the intraocular pressure of the affected eye is higher than the fellow eye then the affected eye is at higher risk for neovascular glaucoma.

Fluorescein Angiography

- It is essential to know the condition of macula. Wait for the retinal hemorrhage to absorb to obtain a good fluorescein angiogram. If fluorescein angiogram shows macular non perfusion then photocoagulation shall be of no value.

- If fluorescein angiogram shows macular edema then argon laser photocoagulation should be performed.

Optical Coherence Tomography (OCT)

OCT quantifies macular edema and helps to monitor the treatment.

CENTRAL RETINAL VEIN OCCLUSION
(Retinal apoplexy, Hemorrhagic retinitis)

Etiology

The occlusion of a retinal vein occurs due to changes in both the arteries and veins, the arterial changes being primary. There are many factors such as.

Incidence of Vein Occlusion

It affects both the sexes equally usually after the middle age. It affects one eye and later the other eye also gets involved. It is more common than central retinal artery occlusion.

Constriction of Flow
(Pressure on the Vein by Sclerotic Retinal Artery)

There is a constriction of central retinal vein by the chronic sclerotic process involving the central retinal artery just behind the lamina cribrosa and at arteriovenous crossings where the two share a common adventitia. This sets in irritative proliferation of endothelium which accelerates the process of obliteration of lumen.

Stagnation of Circulation
(Hyperviscosity of blood and thrombosis)

Stagnation of the flow can occur due to arterial obstructive disease either at lamina cribrosa or at the arteriovenous crossing in retina. There may be arterial spasm in hypertensive disease or in quinine poisoning. Other conditions which can cause stagnation of flow or thrombosis are cardiac insufficiency, endocarditis, fevers, leukemia, sickle cell disease, diabetes, polycythemia, hyperlipidemia and lowering of blood pressure.

Primary Venous Disease
(Periphlebitis retinae)

Periphlebitis retinae affect the central or peripheral veins.

Primary Open-angle Glaucoma

Primary open-angle glaucoma and retinal vein occlusion are associated. The association is due to venous stasis induced by raised pressure in the exit veins.

Local Inflammation

Orbital cellulitis, facial erysiplelas and cavernous sinus thrombosis and Eales' disease,

CLINICAL FEATURES AND MANAGEMENT

Visual Acuity

It is always affected to some extent or markedly reduced depending on the condition of the macula. If the macula has developed edema then it causes marked loss of vision.

Veins and Hemorrhages

Initially there is moderate dilation of veins with scattered punctate hemorrhages. Thereafter the veins are dilated with loops. The retina is splashed with gross hemorrhages of all sizes and irregular mainly in central region.

Macula

It may appear dull with no foveal reflex. There may be hemorrhage at the macula. There may be edema at the macula. Later it may show cystic spaces, pigmentary disturbances, lamellar hole and pucker.

Patient complains of metamorphopsia when there is macular edema.

Macula gets involved in central retinal vein and temporal retinal vein occlusion. Macula escapes in the block of inferior temporal vein branch.

Clinical Features of Pre-occlusion of Retinal Vein

The veins are full, tortuous and engorged with retinal edema along the course. Venous pulsation is absent. The part of the disk may show swelling. The most important fundus finding is an appearance of new formed veins at the disk with small hemorrhages. The hemorrhages are arranged around the terminal veins like *"berries on a twig"*. Few coiled venous channels may be seen. At this stage the patient may complain of a transient obscuration of vision. Manage by photocoagulation and control of intraocular pressure.

Clinical Features of Central Retinal Vein Occlusion

The central retinal vein occlusion may be:

i. **Non-ischemic occlusion or venous stasis retinopathy**: It is the most common clinical type of retinal vein occlusion affecting about 75% of cases.
   Ophthalmoscopy: The fundus changes are mild to moderate. Early cases show mild tortuosity of veins, flame-shaped hemorrhages in periphery, mild papilledema and mild or no macular edema. Late cases sheathing around the main vein, few coils at disk, partially absorbed hemorrhages, and cystoid macular edema or no edema.
   The malady resolves with no visual loss in about 50% of cases. The visual loss is due to cystoids macular edema. A short course of oral steroids for 2–3 months is effective in resolving cystoid macular edema.

ii. **Ischemic occlusion or hemorrhagic retinopathy**
   It refers to acute or sudden complete occlusion of the central retinal vein. Patient comes with complain of sudden loss of vision in the affected eye.
   Ophthalmoscopy: Early cases show marked tortuosity of veins, massive retinal hemorrhages-Splashed-red ink appearance, numerous cotton wool exudates, papilledema and edema and hemorrhages at macula. Late cases show marked sheathing around veins, collaterals at disk, neovascularization at the disk and periphery and chronic cystoid macular edema with pigmentary changes.

It is easy to differentiate two clinical types by fundus picture. Further cases with ischemic occlusion show afferent papillary defect, visual field defect and reduced amplitude of *b*-wave of electroretinogram.

Clinical Features of Retinal Vein Branch Occlusion

Superior temporal branch is commonly involved. Macula gets involved in central retinal vein and temporal retinal vein occlusion (Fig. 31.1). *Macula escapes in the block of inferior temporal vein branch.*

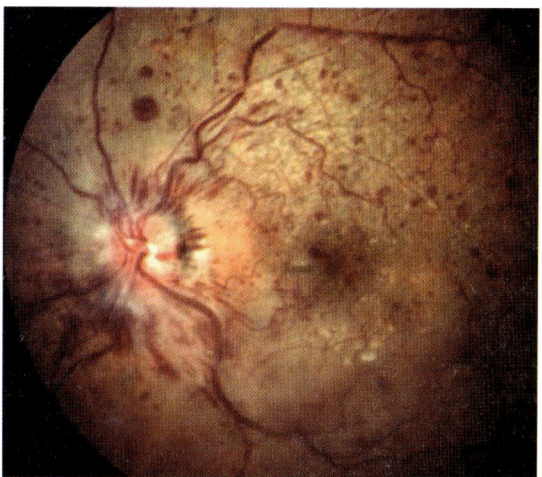

Fig. 31.1: Central retinal vein occlusion

Ophthalmoscopy: The banking of the veins distal to arteriovenous crossing (Bonnet's sign) is often seen at the site of an impeding occlusion. The vein distal to crossing is surrounded by a white halo due to transudation through its walls while the associated artery shows sheathing and small flame-shaped hemorrhage. On occlusion the fundus changes are confined to the part. As the macula is supplied by both the arteries, there may be loss of central field due to hemorrhage and exudates in central area.

A communication is established between adjoining veins through capillaries. The clot may become canalized. The new vessels are tortuous and coiling upon themselves and ending blindly without any useful purpose.

Complications

- Chronic maculopathy-edema, cyst, pigmentation, scarring, hole.
- Neovascular glaucoma.
- Rubeosis-iridis.
- Vitreous hemorrhage and proliferative retinopathy.
- Tractional retinal detachment.
- Epiretinal membrane.

Management

- Treat the cause: the inflammatory periphlebitis.
- Topical timolol maleate to control high intraocular pressure.
- There is controversy about use of anti-coagulants.

- Vasodilators are useful if the arterial spasm is the causative factor. It is useful if at all only in early stage.
- Systemic steroid therapy in some cases is helpful especially with macular involvement.
- Intravitreal injection of triamcinolone acetonide: 4 mg/0.1 ml have been used in both types to treat macular edema and neovascularization.
- Grid laser photocoagulation for macular edema in branch occlusion.
- Pan Retinal Photocoagulation is helpful to re-establish the circulation and saves vision and prevents neovascular glaucoma.
- Intravitreal anti-VEGF treatment is gaining importance to treat macular edema and neovascularization.

A Case with Retinitis Pigmentosa

History

Record the history with reference to the following:
- Age when he realized about the night blindness.
- Any family history.
- Refractive state of the eye.
- Any associated systemic illness as few syndromes are associated with night blindness.

CLINICAL EXAMINATION

Visual Acuity

About 25% patients retain good vision though the field of vision may be very narrow. Visual loss is gradual and most of them maintain 6/60 vision even after the age of 50.

Field of Vision

- There is ring scotoma in early stage
- There is progressive contraction of peripheral field leaving ultimately only a tubular central field of 2 or 3°.

Ophthalmoscopy

Examine the fundus and media.

Slit Lamp Biomicroscopy with Fundus Contact Lens

It is required if there is a lesion at macula.

Tonometry

Glaucoma may be associated with retinitis pigmentosa. A record of intraocular pressure shall be helpful to exclude or diagnose and treat.

Dark Adaptation (Adaptometry)

The test is clinically useful in the cases who complain of night blindness due to disorder of the retina as in a case of retinitis pigmentosa.

Electroretinogram (ERG)

Elctroretinogram demonstrates the responses of the retina to full-field stimulation by a flash of light.

The electroretinogram is the record of an action potential produced by the retina when it is stimulated by light of adequate intensity (Fig. 32.1).

An active electrode embedded in a contact lens is placed on the cornea. A reference electrode is placed on patient's forehead. The potential between the two electrodes is then amplified and the response is displayed on a

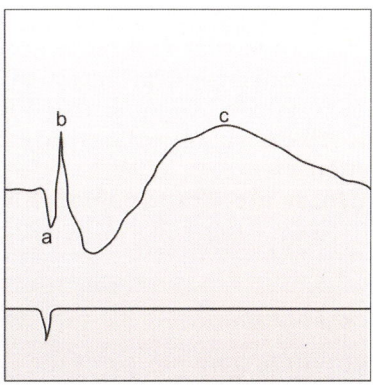

Fig. 32.1: Normal electroretinogram (ERG)

pen recorder. The electroretinogram can be obtained both in the light adapted (photopic) and dark-adapted (scotopic) states. The usual response is biphasic.

'*a* wave'

The initial negative deflection is the '*a* wave'

'*b* wave'

The second positive deflection is the '*b* wave'. The amplitude of the '*b* wave' increases with dark adaptation and decreases in the intensity of the light stimulus.

An electroretinogram shows the function of the first two neurones of the retina. It does not help in the diagnosis of the function of the ganglion cells and optic nerve.

Electroretinogram response is flat (extinguished) in retinitis pigmentosa, central retinal artery occlusion, retinal detachment, choroideremia, gyrate atrophy and siderosis.

Electroretinogram response is subnormal in cone-rod dysfunction, sector retnitis pigmentosa, or central retinitis pigmentosa and the condition of advanced retinopathy wherein large areas of retina has become atrophic or ischemia.

Electroretinogram response is negative in cases with gross disturbances of the retinal circulation such as central retinal artery occlusion and less commonly in central retinal vein occlusion, birdshot chorioretinopathy, quinine toxipathy and siderosis.

Electroretinogram is used to monitor cases with drug and chemical toxicity such as chloroquine and ethambutol.

Pattern Electroretinogram (PERG) helps to assess the function of macula and to differentiate between macular and optic nerve dysfunction as a cause for delayed visual evoked potential response. An abnormal VEP with normal PERG suggests optic nerve dysfunction.

Multifocal Electroretinogram (mfERG) helps to assess the central macular cone function.

Electrooculogram (EOG)

The electrooculogram measures the standing action potential which exists between the cornea which is electrically positive and the back of the eye which is electrically negative. It is based on the activity of the retinal pigment epithelium and the photoreceptors. This means that an eye blinded by any lesion proximal to photoreceptors will show a normal electrooculogram. An advanced disease of the retinal pigment epithelium will show a significant electrooculogram response.

EOG helps in the diagnosis of Best macular dystrophy in which the EOG light rise is abolished in the presence of normal ERG.

Visual Evoked Potential (VEP)

The visual evoked potential test assesses the functional integrity of the visual pathways. The visual evoked potential gets affected by a lesion anywhere in the visual pathway from ganglion cells to visual cortex.

Visually evoked potential is an electrical signal generated by the visual cortex in response to light stimulus of the retina (Fig. 32.2). As most of the visual cortex represents the macula therefore this test is essentially a method of testing the macular function. This is the only test which can assess the function of the visual path way beyond the retinal ganglion cells. Thus an abnormal visual evoked potential response with a normal electroretinogram and electrooculogram suggest lesion of visual pathway from the ganglion cells to the visual cortex.

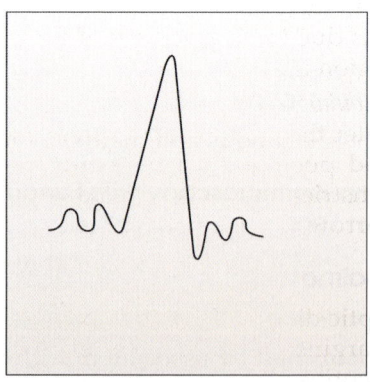

Fig. 32.2: Normal visual evoked potential response (VEP)

TYPICAL RETINITIS PIGMENTOSA

Clinical Features

Inheritance

- *Autosomal recessive:* This is the most common mode of inheritance. Sporadic cases which do not have a family history also belong to this group. In these cases there is an early and severe form of retinitis pigmentosa.
- *Autosomal dominant:* This is the next common mode of inheritance. In these cases there is a benign course of retinitis pigmentosa thereby the loss of vision and field is late.
- *X-linked recessive:* This is the least common mode of inheritance. There is a severe form of retinitis pigmentosa with early development of symptoms. Female carriers may have a normal fundus. Some cases may show involvement of a sector of fundus.

Visual Symptoms

- *Nightblindness:* Nightblindness is the characteristic feature that manifests several years before the visible fundus changes. It is due to degeneration of rods.
- Visual loss is usually gradual as many patients may maintain 6/60 vision even after 50 years of age.

Visual Field Changes

- *Ring scotoma*
  It is due to involvement of the equatorial region in early stage.
- *Tubular field of vision*
  Later the ring scotoma spreads anteriorly and posteriorly presenting peripheral constriction of visual field resulting in a narrow tubular field of vision.

Ophthalmoscopy

- Optic disk is pale and waxy with blurred margins and ultimately evolves as consecutive optic atrophy (Fig. 32.3).
- Arteries are extremely attenuated and appear thread like in later stage.

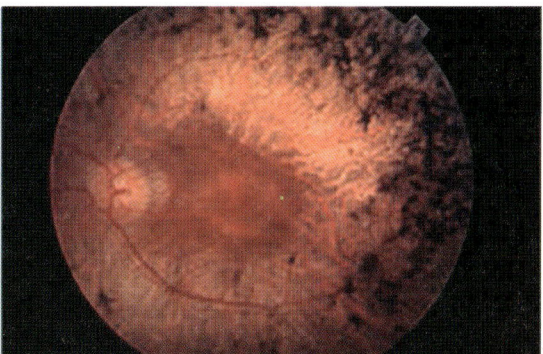

Fig. 32.3: Retinitis pigmentosa with pigments in mid-periphery

- Small irregular clumps of pigment scattered throughout the fundus mostly seen along the retinal veins or over the veins. Pigments resemble bone corpuscles in shape. Initially the pigmentary changes affect the equatorial region only projecting a ring scotoma. Later the pigmentary changes spread anteriorly and posteriorly projecting only a small tubular field of vision.
- Some cases may show cystoid macular edema which is the cause for early visual loss.

Other Features

- Posterior capsular cataract which also results in loss of vision.
- Open-angle glaucoma.
- Patients are usually myopic.
- Keratoconus.
- Posterior vitreous detachment.

Management

- There is no effective treatment for retinitis pigmentosa.
- It is treatable but not curable.
- Many measures have been adopted such as; vasodilators, placental extracts, transplantation of rectus muscles/omentum and vitamins but without any result.
- **Stem cells injection** from bone marrow is under trial and showing encouraging results. Stem cells have capacity for self

renewal and differentiation into mature cell type.

- Low vision aids are helpful.
- Rehabilitation as per his socio-economic status.
- Counseling-general, family and genetic counseling is needed.

ATYPICAL RETINITIS PIGMENTOSA

Some cases may not show typical pigmentary manifestation though fundus shows attenuation of arteries, waxy pale disk and flat ERG.

Retinitis Pigmentosa Sine Pigmento

It is characterized by all the clinical features of typical retinitis pigmentosa except the absence of pigmentary changes in the fundus.

Retinitis Punctata Albescens

It is characterized by presence of innumerable discrete white dots scattered between posterior pole and equator without pigmentary changes. There is subsequent development of pigmentary changes, waxy pale disk and attenuation of arteriols-the characteristic features.

Sectorial Retinitis Pigmentosa

There is involvement of only one quadrant of the fundus. The progress of the disease is very slow.

Pericentric Retinitis Pigmentosa

All the fundus finding are like that of a typical retinitis pigmentosa but the fundus changes are confined to central fundus sparing the periphery.

SYNDROMES WITH RETINITIS PIGMENTOSA

Laurence-Moon-Bardet-Biedl Syndrome

It is an autosomal recessive genetic disorder. Its five classical features include polydactyly or syndactyly, retinitis pigmentosa, obesity, mental retardation, and hypogonadism. Some cases may also show brachycephaly, short stature, congenital heart disease, deafness and various neurological disorders. This syndrome can be confused with Alstrom-hallgren syndrome in which there is retinitis pigmentosa, obesity, deafness and diabetes mellitus and no polydactyly, mental retardation and hypogonadism.

Friedreich's Ataxia

It is characterized by retinitis pigmentosa, posterior column disease, ataxia and nystagmus.

Kearns-Sayre Syndrome

It is characterized by retinitis pigmentosa, chronic progressive external ophthalmoplegia and heart block.

Refsum's Syndrome (Heredopathia atactica polyneuritiformis)

It is an autosomal recessive inherited syndrome. Its main features include atypical retinitis pigmentosa, peripheral neuropathy and cerebellar ataxia. Nightblindness due to pigmentary retinopathy is the presenting symptom. Ophthalmoscopy shows a salt and pepper type of changes. Sudden death can occur due to acute heart failure or respiratory paralysis.

Cockayne Syndrome

It is characterized by childhood dwarfism with a characteristic birdlike facies, deafness, nystagmus, ataxia, progressive mental retardation and atypical pigmentary retinopathy in form of a salt-pepper fundus.

Usher's Syndrome

It is characterized by congenital non progressive sensory neural deafness of varying severity with pigmentary retinopathy; thus the patient suffers from deafness and blindness. It is an autosomal recessive inherited syndrome.

Bassen-Kornzweig Syndrome (Acanthocytosis)

It manifests with atypical retinitis pigmentosa, neuromuscular disease like Friedreich's ataxia, celiac disease and malformation of erythrocytes. Disturbances of ocular motility and ptosis may also be seen.

Favre-Goldmann Syndrome

There is vitreoretinal degeneration with poor night vision. It shows an autosomal recessive inheritance pattern. Its features include atypical retinitis pigmentosa, vitreous degeneration (Liquefaction), retinoschisis, lens opacities and marked electroretinogram abnormalities.

Mucopolysaccharidoses

This group of inborn errors of metabolism is characterized by corneal stromal infiltration, retinal pigmentary retinopathy, optic atrophy, skeletal anomalies, mental retardation and facial coarseness.

33

A Case with Optic Nerve Lesion

History

Record the history with reference to the following:
- The visual loss has been gradual, sudden or in few days.
- Any associated history of non specific fevers.
- Any history of specific fevers due to measles, chickenpox and mumps.
- Any septic focus in the system as sinusitis, genitourinary tract infection and orbital infection.
- Any peri-ocular tenderness on movement of the eye or by pressure on the eyeball.
- Any headache frontal, occipital or temporal.
- Any tenderness in the scalp even on combing hairs.
- Any history of pipe smoking or intake of alcohol.
- Intake of drugs for a long period especially ethambutol, isoniazid and chloramphenicol.
- Any history of headache which becomes worse on coughing or straining.
- Any history of vomiting without feeling of nausea.
- Diplopia in any particular field of gaze.
- Any difference in the level of the two eyes.

CLINICAL EXAMINATION

Visual Acuity

Most of the patients with optic nerve lesion will have a reduced visual acuity. There is acute loss of vision in cases with optic neuritis. In other lesions the vision loss is progressive. Therefore, record the visual acuity carefully for further comparison and follow up to assess the progress of the malady.

Ocular Movements

The ocular movements may be affected in a case with optic nerve tumor. There may be a peri-ocular pain on the movement of the eye in a case of optic neuritis.

Pupillary Reactions

A normal reaction of the pupil to light does not exclude an optic nerve lesion. A change in the pupillary reaction is suggestive of optic nerve lesion. An ill-sustained reaction of the pupil beyond doubt strongly favors optic neuritis.

Ophthalmoscopy

Examine the fundus with direct and indirect ophthalmoscope and note the finding about the size, shape, color, margins and cup of the disk. Look for any pits in the disk. Make a note of cup-disk ratio. If there is a swelling of the disk then make a note about the swelling in the dioptre-the difference in focusing the retina and the disk margin. Look for any sheathing of the vessels at the disk and close to the disk.

Color Vision

An optic nerve lesion results in a defective color vision in the affected eye. An eye with a defective color vision sees the colored objects as if "washed-out". A simple and quick way to detect a uniocular color vision defect is to ask the patient to compare the color of a red color object held by him. Thereafter the color vision defect can be confirmed with Ishihara's plates.

The presence of dim vision with normal color vision in the affected eye goes against the optic nerve lesion.

Light Brightness or Contrast Sensitivity

An optic nerve lesion causes depression of the light brightness sensitivity. The patient perceives the light in a room dim with the affected eye in comparison to the normal eye. An intelligent patient usually complains that though he can see everything but dim with the affected eye, i.e. contrast sensitivity is impaired.

Visual Fields

A quick screening can be done by confrontation test. On suspicion, the patient should be subjected to proper visual field charting on perimeter and tangent screen. Optic nerve lesion may produce four types of visual field defects; central scotoma, centrocaecal scotoma, altitudinal field defect and arcuate defects. The field defects are more marked to red color than the white.

Amsler Grid Test

For central visual fields.

X-ray Skull

To detect any lesion of pituitary.

CT Scan, MRI and MRV

It is required to diagnose a lesion of pituitary and tumors of optic nerve.

Cerebrospinal Fluid Analysis

It is helpful in diagnosis of meningitis.

Fluorescein Angiography

It is helpful in the diagnosis of papilledema.

Erythrocyte Sedimentation Rate (ESR)

Erythrocyte sedimentation rate is frequently very high in cases of giant cell arteritis with

levels in excess of 100 mm/hour or more. At the same time ESR has been found to be normal in biopsy positive cases. One must interpret the erythrocyte sedimentation rate with clinical findings.

C-reactive Protein

It is invariably high in a case of giant cell arteritis.

Temporal Artery Biopsy

Temporal artery biopsy should be done on the same side of ocular involvement. It is advisable to obtain a long piece of artery at least 2.5 cm and several sections to confirm the artery involvement.

Visually Evoked Potential (VEP)

It shows reduced amplitude and delay in the transmission time.

Clinical Features and Management
1. Optic neuritis
2. Arteric anterior ischemic optic neuropathy
3. Diabetic papillopathy
4. Toxic optic neuropathy
5. Leber's optic neuropathy
6. Glioma of optic nerve.
7. Meningioma of optic nerve sheath
8. Papilledema
9. Optic atrophy

OPTIC NEURITIS

Types of Optic Neuritis

- *Papillitis* refers to involvement of the optic disk in inflammatory or demyelenating disorders. More common in children.
- *Neuroretinitis* refers to involvement of the optic disk and macular region.
- *Retrobulbar neuritis* refers to involvement of the optic nerve behind the eyeball. More common in adults and with multiple sclerosis.

Etiology

- *Idiopathic:* Most often the cause of the optic neuritis is not established.
- *Hereditary:* Leber's disease

- *Inflammatory:* Post-viral is the most common cause in the children. The attack may occur following a specific or a non-specific fever of viral origin such as measles, mumps, chickenpox, whooping cough, or glandular fever. It may be related to septic focus of meningitis, sinuses and orbit.
- *Demyelinating disease:* Optic neuritis is the most common ocular manifestation of multiple sclerosis. It is the presenting feature in 25% of cases. Recurrence in the same eye or opposite eye indicates increased risk for multiple sclerosis. A patient with optic neuritis must be watched periodically for any sign and symptoms of multiple sclerosis.

Symptoms

- *Visual loss* is sudden and progressive even to the extent of finger counting and perception of light. Patient may complain of episodic transient loss of vision during exertion which recovers on rest.
- *Veiled vision in bright light*: Patient complains of seeing through a dark grey veil which covers his entire field of vision. The light in the room appears dim in the affected eye in comparison to the normal eye.
- *Tenderness:* Patient complains of tenderness on the movement of the globe especially in upward movement commonly felt in retrobulbar neuritis.
- With loss of vision there is some loss of color appreciation.

Signs

- Reduced visual acuity.
- Decreased brightness of light.
- Ill-sustained pupillary reaction to light is diagnostic if elicited without any doubt.
- Positive central or centro-caecal scotoma.
- Impaired color vision.

Ophthalmoscopy

Ophthalmoscopy may show any of the following three features.

Papillitis: There is a swelling of the disk with blurred margins and filling of the optic cup. The retinal vessels are dilated and tortuous. The vitreous shows inflammatory cells.

Neuroretinitis: It has all the fundus findings of papillitis with a macular star.

Retrobulbar neuritis: The fundus appears normal as the lesion is behind the globe. Few cases may show a temporal pallor of the disk in late stage.

Treatment

Systemic steroid is the treatment of first choice. Most of the patients do recover the normal vision with residual defect in the color vision and light brightness. Visual prognosis is good in cases of multiple sclerosis.

ARTERIC ANTERIOR ISCHEMIC OPTIC NEUROPATHY (AAION)

Arteric anterior ischemic optic atrophy is segmental or generalized infarction of the optic nerve. It affects elderly people usually over the age of 60.

Etiology is caused by giant cell arteritis—a disease of unknown etiology.

The common vessels affected are superficial temporal artery, ophthalmic artery and posterior ciliary arteries.

It can be idiopathic.

It can be due to miscellaneous factor associated with collagen vascular disorders.

Symptoms

- There is a sudden and marked loss of visual acuity.
- Patient may have a peri-ocular pain
- Patient may point towards a tender temporal artery.
- Patient may complain of transient obscuration of vision prior to onset of the malady.
- Headache and scalp tenderness may be present in some cases.
- Jaw claudication
- Neck stiffness
- Weight loss with loss of appetite

Ophthalmoscopy

There is a swelling of the disk with blurred margins.

Peripapillary hemorrhages-splinter-shaped.

Later the optic atrophy sets in with cupping of the disk.

Other Ocular Lesions

- Attacks of amaurosis fugax.
- Central retinal artery occlusion.
- Anterior segment necrosis.
- Ocular muscle paralysis.
- Cortical blindness.

Investigation

- Erythrocyte sedimentation rate is high.
- C-reactive protein is invariably raised.
- Elevated platelets.
- Temporal artery biopsy may give a positive report.

Treatment

Systemic steroid is the choice.

In a case of multiple sclerosis-start intravenous methylprednisolone 1 gm daily for 3 days followed by oral steroid.

Start with (2 mg/kg body weight) or 120 mg of prednisone daily tapering it to 10 mg a day in about one month time. The daily does of 10 mg is maintained for about three months. Reduce further depending on the symptoms of the patient and erythrocyte sedimentation rate. Patient needs treatment for about 1–2 years. Some patient may need steroid for rest of life.

Differential Diagnosis

Non-arteric anterior ischemic optic neuropathy (NAAION): It affects elderly and healthy people who have hypertension as the only sign of systemic vascular disease. The only symptom is a sudden loss of vision not accompanied by pain in the eyes. The field defect consists of an altitudinal hemianopia commonly involving the lower half. Some patients may have an arcuate defect or a central scotoma. The color vision is diminished in proportion to the level of visual acuity. In contrast to this in a case of optic neuritis the color vision is severely impaired irrespective of the visual acuity. On ophthalmoscopy—there is a sectorial edema of the disk with splinter shaped hemorrhage. Later the optic disk becomes pale but do not show cupping of the disk. There is no effective treatment.

Chronic simple glaucoma: As the optic disk in cases of anterior ischemic optic neuropathy show cupping in later stage, therefore, it is essential to differentiate it from cupping of glaucoma. The cupping of anterior ischemic optic neuropathy is very shallow and does not reach up to the margin of disk and the intraocular pressure is normal.

DIABETIC PAPILLOPATHY

Clinical Features

- It affects diabetic in the 20–30 age group.
- About 75% of cases show malady in both the eyes.
- The initial loss of vision which is usually mild is recovered in few months.
- Ophthalmoscopy—may show mild edema of the disk with no other finding. There may be marked swelling of the disk with hemorrhages, exudates and cystoid macular edema with or without macular star.

Differential Diagnosis

- Papilledema.
- Papillitis.
- Anterior ischemic optic neuropathy.

Diagnosis

- Early age with absence of symptoms of any kind expect mild loss of vision.
- Mild loss of vision in comparison to fundus findings.
- Patient is a juvenile onset diabetic.
- Recovery of vision occurs in few months.

Treatment

Good control of diabetes.

TOXIC OPTIC NEUROPATHY

Toxic optic neuropathy embraces all the conditions of optic nerve damage due to ingestion of exogenous poisons, drugs and tobacco. The most common of these are ethyl alcohol, methyl alcohol, lead, arsenic and thallium. The common drugs are ethambutol, chloramphenicol, isoniazed and streptomycin. Intake of tobacco in the form of cigar pipe and chewing is common. Some of these affect the nerve fibers directly while others affect the ganglion cells of the retina which results in the degeneration of optic nerve fibers.

Tobacco Amblyopia

- It occurs due to excessive smoking of tobacco in form of cigars or strong tobacco mixture. An associated intake of alcohol with deficiency of protein and vitamin B complex enhances its toxic effect. It is usually labeled as "tobacco-alcohol amblyopia".
- There is gradual and progressive loss of vision with fogginess and difficulty in near work.
- Visual field charting shows bilateral centro-caecal scotoma more for red target. The peripheral field remains intact.
- The amblyopia is due to degeneration of the ganglion cells of retina at macular area affecting the papilla-macular bundle which results in loss of central vision.
- Ophthalmoscopy shows a little pallor of the disk.
- Treat by
  - Complete abstention from smoking and drinking alcohol.
  - Intake of diet rich in protein and vitamins.
  - Intramuscular injection of vitamin B_{12}, 1000 units biweekly for 10 weeks thereafter oral vitamins.
  - Visual prognosis is slow but good if treated early.

Methyl Alcohol Amblyopia

- It occurs due to drinking wood alcohol or drinking methylated spirit. Spurious liquor is the common cause for mass drinking which results in death or blindness if the patient survives.
- There are generalized symptoms of acute poisoning—headache, dizziness, nausea, vomiting, abdominal pain, delirium, stupor followed by coma that may end in death.
- If the patient survives then there is blindness due to damage of ganglion cells which results in optic atrophy.
- Ophthalmoscopy show a pale disk with blurred margins and attenuated vessels that manifests as bilateral primary optic atrophy in due course of time.

Ethambutol Amblyopia

- It affects the optic nerve if intake of the drug is more than 15 mg/kg per day. Its effect is more in diabetics and alcoholic.
- Direct effect on the nerve has been proposed by some and interference with zinc metabolism by others.
- Neuritis is reversible if the drug is discontinued or dose is reduced and kept on 15 mg/kg per day or less.
- Visual field defect may be a bitemporal hemianopia indicating the seat of affection being the chiasma.
- There is an impaired color vision for red and green.
- Ophthalmoscopy shows a swollen disk with hyperemia and splinter-shaped hemorrhages.

Treat by

Stop or reduce the intake of drug less than 15 mg/kg per day. Keep a watch on the fundus and field changes and color vision at regular intervals during treatment by ethambutol. Injection of hydroxocobalamin is helpful. Diet rich in protein and vitamins is necessary.

Quinine Amblyopia

- It occurs due to intake of quinine even in small dose in susceptible persons. Quinine is used in malaria.
- There may be a complete loss of vision. Pupils are dilated and fixed. Some cases

may recover central vision giving him a tubular vision. The peripheral fields are contracted.

- Deafness and tinnitus may be associated.
- Ophthalmoscopy shows a pale disk with markedly attenuated blood vessels. Later it manifests as optic atrophy.

Oral Contraceptives

- Oral contraceptives are usually a combination of progestrogens and oestrogens. These may play role in the production of vascular occlusive disease particularly in females who suffer from hypertension, migraine and any other vascular syndromes.
- Treat by withdrawing the use of drug and giving vitamins.

LEBER'S OPTIC NEUROPATHY

It is a rare hereditary disorder affecting healthy young males. Only 15% of the patients are females. Males cannot transmit the disease to their offsprings. It is the females who transmit the disease to the next generation.

There is a gradual progressive loss of vision to blindness in due course of time. Other eye gets involved sooner or later. There is a centro-caecal scotoma which becomes absolute. Ophthalmoscopy show mild hyperemia and swelling of the disk and dilation of pericapillaries. Later there is a clear optic atrophy. The pupillary reaction to light is normal in spite of severe loss of vision. No treatment except genetic counseling.

GLIOMA OF OPTIC NERVE

- It affects usually children between the ages of 4 and 8.
- It manifests as a gradual and painless unilateral axial proptosis.
- Vision is affected early.
- Fundus shows optic atrophy or papilledema and venous engorgement.
- CT scan shows an enlargement of the optic nerve in a fusiform shape.
- An early diagnosis and early lateral orbitotomy helps to save the vision and the eye.

MENINGIOMA OF OPTIC NERVE SHEATH

- The tumor arises from arachnoidal villi so there is compression of optic nerve which results in early loss of vision.
- Later the tumor bursts through the dura to from mass within the muscle cone giving rise to slowly progressive unilateral proptosis with limitation of ocular movements.
- The triad of symptoms
  - Visual loss for a long time.
  - Pale swollen optic nerve head.
  - Opticociiliary shunt is pathognomonic for optic nerve sheath meningiomas.
- CT scan show a diffuse enlargement of optic nerve.
- An early removal of tumor shall save the life of child though the vision is lost due to damage to optic nerve by tumor and by surgical procedure.
- Radiotherapy has been found to save vision.

PAPILLEDEMA

Papilledema is a term reserved for the passive swelling of the optic nerve head due to raised intracranial pressure which is almost always bilateral although it may be asymmetrical. The most common cause for raised intracranial pressure is space occupying lesion of brain-the tumors.

Disk edema or disk swelling is a term that includes all the causes of active or passive edematous swelling of the optic disk.

Clinical Features

Etiology of Disk Edema or Swelling

- *Congenital:* Pseudo-papilledema.
- *Inflammation*: Papillitis and neuroretinitis.
- *Ocular:* Posterior uveitis, central retinal vein occlusion and hypotony-low intra-ocular pressure.
- *Orbital*: Orbital tumors, orbital cellulitis and Graves' ophthalmopathy.
- *Vascular:* Marked anemia, uremia and Anterior ischemic optic neuropathy.
- *Intracranial*: Increased intracranial pressure.

Etiology of Papilledema

- *Congenital:* craniosynostosis.
- *Intracranial space-occupying lesions:* The brain tumors, abscess, tuberculoma, subdural hematoma and aneurysm. Space-occupying lesions in any position except medulla oblongata may induce papilledema. Papilledema is most commonly associated with tumors in posterior fossa due to obstruction to flow of cerebrospinal fluid. Papilledema is least with pituitary tumor. The tumors of cerebellum, midbrain and parieto-occipital region induces early papilledema than tumors in other regions.
- *Intracranial infection*: Meningitis and encephalitis.
- *Intracranial hemorrhage*: Cerebral and subarachnoid hemorrhages.
- *Head injury*: that results in diffuse cerebral edema may induce papilledema.

Etiopathogenesis

Stasis of axoplasm in prelaminar region of the optic disk due to alteration in the pressure gradient across the lamina cribrosa results in the development of papilledema.

General Symptoms

Patient usually consults a physician with general symptoms of headache, projectile vomiting, pulsatile tinnitus and transient obscuration of vision which is posture induced. Headache becomes worse on coughing and straining. Vomiting is without nausea.

Ocular Symptoms

- Visual acuity and papillary reactions are normal for a long time until the optic atrophy sets in.
- Patient may complain of diplopia.

Ocular Signs

- Visual acuity and pupillary reactions are normal in early stage. The vision reduces and pupillary reactions becomes sluggish in later stage with manifestation of optic atrophy.
- Color vision is normal in early stage.

Fundus Picture

In an early case
- There is blurring of the disk margin; the nasal margin is involved first followed by superior, inferior and then temporal.
- Blurring of the peri-papillary nerve fiber layer.
- Absence of the spontaneous venous pulsation at the disk.
- With increase in edema of the disk; disk becomes hyperemic and veins are full, tortuous and show bend at the margin and looping.

In later stage
- The optic cup is filled and swelling increases usually up to 1–2 mm (1 mm elevation is equivalent to 3 dioptres).
- Flame-shaped hemorrhages and cotton wool spots.
- Hard exudates appear at the macula in a star shape or fan shape.
- With time the disk shows post papilledematous optic atrophy with pale disk and sheathing of vessels.

End-stage

Ophthalmoscopy shows a picture of post neuritic optic atrophy or post papilledematous optic atrophy or secondary optic atrophy.

Visual Field

- Enlargement of blind spot is present.
- Later there is peripheral construction of visual fields due to optic atrophy.

Differential Diagnosis

- Papillitis
- Pseudoneuritis—the cause is high hypermetropia, nuclear sclerosis of lens, congenital excess of glial tissue, opaque nerve fibers and drusen of disk.

- Central retinal vein block.
- A peripillary hemangioma.

Diagnosis

- Typical fundus picture.
- Normal visual acuity in relation to findings at the disk.
- Normal fields.
- Enlargement of blind spot.
- Fluorescein angiography shows dye leaking beyond disk in surrounding tissue.
- Raised intracranial pressure.
- CT scan and MRI may show intracranial lesions.
- Presence of venous pulsation goes against the diagnosis of papilledema.

Treatment

- Treat the cause.
- Record the peripheral fields. Beginning of constriction of peripheral fields indicate that the optic atrophy is setting in. Patient requires an early decompression to save the vision.

OPTIC ATROPHY

Optic atrophy occurs due to damage to the axons between the retinal ganglion cells and the lateral geniculate body. It is the end result not only for optic nerve lesions but also for the lesions of retina, optic chiasma and optic tract. Thus the optic atrophy is characterized by loss of axons. There is no regeneration. The supporting and connective tissue elements show proliferation in a case heading for optic atrophy.

Classification of Optic Atrophy

Primary Versus Secondary Optic Atrophy

i. *Primary optic atrophy:* It results from the lesions proximal to the optic disk without papilledema or swelling of the disk. The common causes are multiple sclerosis, idiopathic retro-bulbar neuritis, intracranial space-occupying tumors such as pituitary tumors pressing directly on the anterior visual pathway, toxic amblyopias and tabes dorsalis.

ii. *Secondary optic atrophy:* It is more commonly seen than the primary optic atrophy. It is always preceded by the congestion and swelling of the optic disk. There is a marked proliferation of glial and fibrous tissue on and around the disk. On ophthalmoscopy—the disk shows a palor with blurred margins of the disk. There is loss of physiological cup. The vessels show sheathing within the peripapillary region.

Descending Versus Ascending Optic Atrophy

i. *Descending optic atrophy:* Any intracranial tumor which can cause compression of the optic nerve results in descending type of optic atrophy. It proceeds from the region of optic tract towards the optic disk. This can be either primary or secondary depending on whether the tumor caused papilledema or not.

ii. *Ascending optic atrophy:* It is the result of degeneration of ganglion cells and nerve fiber layer of retina due to any retinal disease affecting these structures. The ascending optic atrophy may occur in the conditions such as toxic retinopathy, ischemic retinopathy, following retinal photocoagulation and retinitis pigmentosa. It is usually of a secondary type of optic atrophy.

Ophthalmoscopic Classification

1. Primary optic atrophy.
2. Consecutive optic atrophy.
3. Glaucomatous optic atrophy.
4. Post-neuritic optic atrophy.
5. Ischemic optic atrophy.

Clinical Features of Optic Atrophy

Loss of Vision

It may be sudden or gradual and partial or total. Ophthalmoscopic picture has no relation to visual acuity.

Pupillary Reaction

Pupil is usually semi-dilated. The direct light reflex is sluggish. Cases with retrobulbar neuritis may show an ill-sustained papillary reaction. A case of glaucomatous optic atrophy shows dilated and fixed pupil.

Fundus Picture

Primary optic atrophy: Optic disk is white or whitish blue in hue with sharp margins. Lamina cribrosa is visible clearly in the physiological cup and retinal vessels are normal.

Consecutive optic atrophy: Optic disk is yellow and waxy in appearance. The margins are blurred and vessels are attenuated. It occurs following destruction of ganglion cells due to degenerative or inflammatory lesions of the choroid and or retina. Its common causes are diffuse chorioretinitis, retinitis pigmentosa and central artery occlusion.

Glaucomatous optic atrophy: It is characterized by deep cupping of the optic disk and nasal shifting of the vessels (Fig. 33.1). It results due to high intraocular pressure in primary open-angle glaucoma.

Post-neuritic optic atrophy: Optic disk appears dirty white in hue. Its margins are blurred. Physiological cup is shallow and lamina cribrosa not visible. Retinal vessels are attenuated. There is perivascular sheathing.

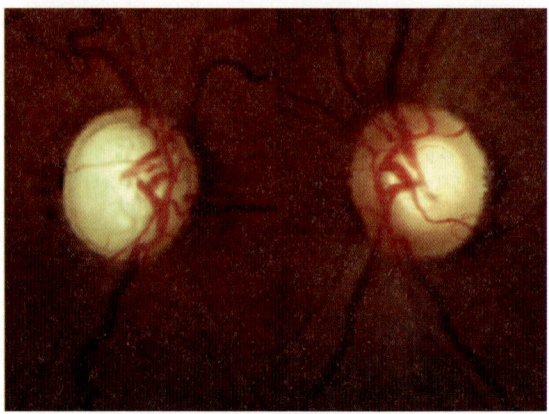

Fig. 33.1: Glaucomatous optic atrophy

It occurs as a sequelae to papilledema or papillitis.

Ischemic optic atrophy: Optic disk appears pale with blurred margins. Vessels are markedly attenuated. It occurs in giant cell arteritis and Quinine amblyopia.

Management

Treat the underlying cause. It may help to preserve some useful vision.

Early diagnosis and energetic management shall help the patient to save some vision.

A Case with Myopia

34

History

Ask specially about the following points:
- Either of the parents using minus lenses.
- Any systemic abnormality in the family.
- Any history of toxemia, rubella, toxoplasmosis in the prenatal period.
- Any history of premature delivery or low birth weight.
- Any febrile childhood illness.
- Any debilitating illness in childhood.
- Posture of the child while studying.
- Illumination in study room.
- Likes to play out door or insists for indoor games.
- Normal daily diet to know about intake of proteins and vitamins.
- Any record of visual acuity or eye checkup.
- Any attempt to narrow the palpebral aperture on seeing at a distance.
- Headache after near work.
- Seeing floaters in the field of vision.

CLINICAL EXAMINATION

Visual Acuity

A patient with myopia will have a reduced visual acuity. While recording the visual acuity on Snellen's chart the eye surgeon must keep a watch on the eyes of the patient as he can narrow his palpebral aperture to create a horizontal slit to have a better vision and show better acuity than actual.

Eyeball

A patient with physiological myopia usually shows a normal eyeball.

A patient with pathological myopia may show a prominent large eyeball.

A patient with a large or a small cornea must be further examined to find the cause and exclude micro-cornea or a macro-cornea.

Anterior Chamber

Anterior chamber is deep in a case of a pathological myopia. It usually does not show any change if myopia is less than six diopter.

Gonioscopy

The presence of anterior insertion of iris or iris processes or pigmentation in the angle indicates the greater risk of the patient to be a glaucoma suspect. The patient must be subjected to provocative tests and regular check up for intraocular pressure.

Intraocular Pressure

Intraocular pressure must be recorded on each visit and in every case of myopia especially patients with progressive myopia. A raised intraocular pressure is one of the causative factor for progressive myopia.

Ophthalmoscopy

Direct ophthalmoscopy is an essential part of examination of a case of myopia. If there are fundus changes then the patient must be examined by indirect binocular ophthalmoscope. Usually there are no fundus changes in a case of physiological myopia. A case of pathological myopia shows the following changes:

- Crescent at the disk with a large cup.
- Posterior staphyloma.
- Disk may show a crescent, tilting and supertraction.
- Macula show hyperpigmentation or Fuch's spot.
- Chorioretinal changes are seen in the form of hemorrhages, areas of focal atrophy, degenerative changes in the periphery and breaks in the retina.
- Liquified vitreous with floaters.

Visual Fields

A case of a pathological myopia may show central field defects which are enlargement of the blind spot, central, paracentral and arcuate defects. The central field defects are due to small areas of atrophy. Arcuate defects are seen if there is an association of glaucoma. Enlargement of blind spot is due to crescent at the optic disk.

Refraction

Assess the error of the refraction.

Slit Lamp Examination

It helps to examine the media and detect any lens opacity or thin scars of the cornea, changes in the iris and condition of vitreous.

Ocular Movements

In a case of myopia there is a negative angle kappa which creates an illusion of a convergent squint. In a case of uncorrected high myopia less accommodation is required for certain amount of convergence leading to development of a high AC/A ratio. This results in exophoria which may break in an exotropia.

Other Clinical Findings

- An apparent convergent squint.
- A real divergent squint.
- Proptosis-unilateral if only one eye is myopic.

- Pupil dilated with sluggish reaction.
- Lateral aspect of the globe is flat. It is seen on asking the patient to adduct the eye.
- ERG is normal. It may be subnormal in degenerative myopia.

Posterior Staphyloma

The most frequent and most important type of posterior staphyloma is that affecting the posterior pole. In this tessellation and pallor extend in a horizontal elliptical area from two disk diameter to five disk diameter nasal to the optic nerve to macular area. This can attain great degree of ectasia with its nasal wall usually having the sharpest margin and the greatest slope. On ophthalmoscopy—Posterior staphyloma gives an appearance of a vertical crescentic shadow located nasal to optic disk with a substantial difference in diopteric correction for the fundus area on either side of its dark concave arc. The shadow corresponds to the sharp nasal margin of the posterior staphyloma with its concavity towards disk.

Special Investigation Prior to Radial Keratotomy

Corneascope

A corneascope shows corneal irregularities which otherwise may pass unnoticed. A case with corneal irregularity is an unsuitable case for radial keratotomy.

Keratometry

A keratometer reading of the case to be operated for the radial keratotomy is essential. A patient with higher reading shall give better results following surgery. A patient with low reading may remain under corrected. The effect of radial keratotomy is achieved by flattening the central cornea. If the central cornea is already flat indicated by low reading of about forty-two then the operation is less likely to make it more flat. If the central cornea has more curvature indicated by higher reading of about forty-seven then there are more chances for it to become more flat thereby giving better result.

Ultrasonic Pachymeter

It is an important investigation in all the cases to be taken for radial keratotomy. It gives an idea about the corneal thickness. The surgeon can accordingly adjust the diamond knife, the depth to which he can go safely without producing a micro or a macro perforation. A thick cornea with a steeper slope from center to periphery shall give better results than a thin cornea. A thick cornea provides deeper incisions which gives more correction of myopia.

Intraocular Pressure

A patient with an intraocular pressure of 12 to 20 is a suitable case. A patient with low intraocular pressure shall have under correction of myopia. A patient with intraocular pressure on the lower side shall need more incisions and re-deepening of the incisions.

Clinical Features and Management
1. Myopia
2. Axial-physiological myopia.
3. Axial-pathological myopia.
4. Curvature myopia.
5. Index myopia.
6. Congenital myopia.

MYOPIA

Myopia or short sight is that form of refractive error wherein parallel rays of light come to focus in front of the sentient layer of retina when the eye is at rest.

AXIAL-PHYSIOLOGICAL MYOPIA

In this myopia-the eye remains healthy. The visual acuity can be corrected to normal with lens and there are no degenerative changes in the fundus. The peripheral retinal degeneration may occur later in life. The myopia does not progress after adolescence when the myopia has reached about five diopter.

AXIAL-PATHOLOGICAL MYOPIA

- It is degenerative and progressive.
- It is strongly hereditary.
- It is common in women.
- It has racial tendencies-common in Jews and Japanese.
- Many factors have been thought to play a part in its development:
  - Excessive accommodation and convergence
  - Vascular congestion due to bend head for near work.
  - Endocrinal and nutritional imbalance.
  - Debility and illness.
- Increase in length of the eye affects the posterior pole and surrounding retina.
- Visual field show contraction and ring scotoma in some cases.
- ERG is subnormal due to chorioretinal atrophy.

Symptoms

- The eyeball is large and prominent.
- The patient has dim vision for distance.
- The patient complains of seeing floaters-black spots.
- May notice flashes of light signs.

Signs

- The eyeball is prominent.
- The anterior chamber is deep.
- The pupil reacts sluggishly.
- An apparent convergent squint due to a large negative angle kappa.
- Scotoma may be present both central and peripheral.
- It may progress to minus 25 D or more.

Ophthalmoscopic Findings

- Generalized atrophy of retina and choroid (Fig. 34.1).
- Crescent near the disk on temporal side or all around.
- Supertraction crescent on the nasal side
- Patches of choroidal atrophy with pigments around.
- Foster Fuch's fleck or spot—A dark circular area in the macula may occur suddenly due to proliferation of pigmentary epithelium associated with an intrachoroidal hemorrhage.
- Posterior staphyloma.
- Vitreous is liquified with floaters.

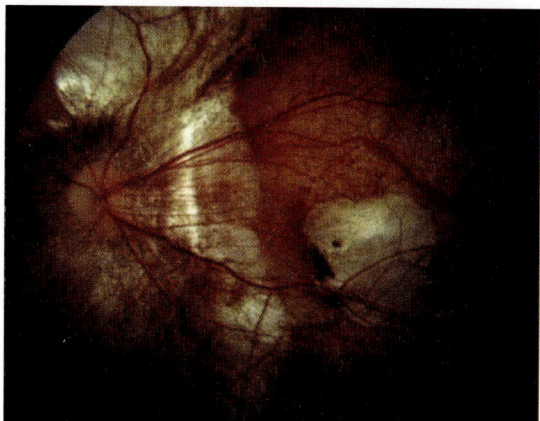

Fig. 34.1: Pathological myopic degenerative changes

Complications

- Posterior cortical opacity of lens.
- Retinal detachment.
- Hemorrhage in the vitreous.
- Foster Fuch's spot.
- Posterior vitreous detachment.

Counseling

- Two high myopes should not marry. If marry, then should not have offsprings as there is strong likelihood of passing this axial-pathological myopia.
- Explain about the visual hygiene, proper posture, height and illumination for reading and writing.
- Good diet rich in protein and vitamins.

CURVATURE MYOPIA

It can result due to increased curvature of cornea as in a condition of keratoconus. A condition of anterior and posterior lenticonus can cause marked degree of myopia. The curvature of anterior lens can increase in spasm of accommodation or in lens subluxation and dislocation.

INDEX MYOPIA

Myopia can result due to decreased refractive index of the cortex of lens in diabetes. Myopia can result due to sclerosis of lens nucleus in incipient cataract.

CONGENITAL MYOPIA

Rarely the child is born with congenital myopia of about 10 D. It is non progressive. There is convergence of both the eyes.

Myopia may be Associated with Systemic Disorders

- Albinism.
- Mongolism.
- Marian's syndrome.
- Ehlers-Danlos syndrome.
- Homocystinuria.
- Laurence-Moon-Biedl syndrome.

Myopia Associated with Ocular Disease

- Night blindness (nyctalopia).
- Achromatopsia.
- Microphthalmos.
- Keratoconus.
- Microphakia.
- Ectopia lentis.
- Coloboma.
- Choroideremia.
- Gyrate atrophy.
- Retinitis pigmentosa.
- Myelinated nerve fibers.

MANAGEMENT OF MYOPIA

Optical

Spectacles

Resilens offer safety over glass lens. Myopes are more likely to be involved in injury and many eyes are lost due to shattering of glasses, causing rupture of globe.

Contact Lens

Contact lens gives an improvement in the appearance, visual acuity and field of vision.

Low Vision Aids

Telescopic lens are helpful for the distance vision. A high myope gets adjusted to read at his far point comfortably.

REFRACTIVE SURGICAL PROCEDURES

Radial Keratotomy (RK)

This procedure involves deep radial incisions in the peripheral part of the cornea leaving the central 4 mm optical zone. On healing, these incisions flatten the central cornea thereby reducing its refractive power. It gives good correction in low to moderate myopia of 2 to 6 D.

Photorefractive Keratectomy (PRK)

In this technique, central optical zone of anterior corneal stroma is photoablated using Eximer laser to cause flattening of the central cornea. It gives good correction for –2 to –6 D of myopia.

Laser-assisted in situ Keratomileusis (LASIK)

In this technique, a flap of 130–160 micron thickness of anterior corneal tissue is raised. Then the midstromal corneal tissue is ablated directly with an *excimer laser beam* to flatten the cornea. This is the most considered choice of treatment for myopia of up to –12 D.

Femtosecond Laser Technology

This laser creates flaps with a consistent thickness. Thus minimizing flap complications. Femtosecond laser vaporizes tissue inside the cornea. Presently, the laser is used to cut a corneal flap during LASIK. Femtosecond laser technology has enhanced the safety profile of refractive laser surgery.

Phakic Intraocular Lenses (PIOLs)

Phakic intraocular lenses compete with LASIK surgery for refractive error of –8 D and –12 D. These have overtaken LASIK in cases with myopia beyond –12 D. Phakic intraocular lens implants are placed in anterior chamber with angle fixation. Angle fixation implants are better than iris fixation implants.

The advantages of phakic intraocular lens implant in comparison with LASIK are as follows:

- Preserves corneal asphericity.
- Less reduction in contrast sensitivity.
- Better than spectacle and contact lens corrected visual acuity.
- Maintains accommodation.
- Minimizes surgical complication.
- Optical zone can be varied.

- Can be easily removed or exchanged.
- All types of spherical ametropia, astigmatism and even presbyopia can be corrected.
- Colorants or filters can be included as desired or needed.
- Well tolerated.

These refractive implants placed in anterior chamber with angle fixation can induce cataract or corneal endothelial damage.

Let us hope that these too can be overcome by further improvement in the technique or material.

Implantable Collamer Lens (ICL)

The implantable collamer lens (ICL) is a phakic intraocular lens. It is permanently implanted in the eye behind the iris and in front of the natural lens. These were previously called as "Implantable contact lenses". It is out of use. More and more surgeons are using phakic intraocular lens-angle fixate.

Refractive Lens Exchange

The refractive lens exchange IOLs are available from –10 to +35 D. This wide range provides opportunity to potentially treat a fairly large range of refractive errors. Ophthalmologists are familiar with procedure of implant. The refractive lens exchange is performed on a normal eye with normal vision with spectacles or contact lens with no retinal lesion of any kind. The disadvantage is that it is an intraocular procedure and the fact that retinal complications increase with removal of the crystalline lens.

MYOPIA HYGIENE

Proper Posture

Advise myopic not to read with a stooping position. He should be advised to keep his back straight while reading or writing. For this the height of the table and chair should be adjusted to give him proper posture and height to maintain proper distance from the books. Proper posture will help avoid congestion of the eye due to stooping and proper distance shall help avoid extra effort on the accommodation and convergence.

Correction of Refraction

The patient must get himself examined every 6 months to correct his refraction so that there is no strain on the eyes and proper balance is maintained

Nutrition

Pay proper attention to the intake of animal protein and vitamins. The intake of food should be properly timed to provide a child with calories all the day.

Early Treatment for any Febrile or Systemic Illness

Any febrile or debilitating illness can cause increase in myopia. It is advisable to take an early treatment to check progress of myopia.

Illumination and Ventilation

The study room should be properly illuminated. The light should not fall directly on the book or the eyes. The room should have proper ventilation for flow of fresh air.

Avoid Hard and Jerky Exercise or Games

A patient with myopia of 10 D or above must be advised to avoid hard exercises and games which involve jerks and fast movements. It is advisable to get interested in indoor games.

Marriage Counseling

Two high myopes should avoid marriage. As it is a hereditary disease. The offsprings are likely to have myopia.

35

A Case with Heterophoria—Latent Squint

History

Record the history with reference to the following:

- Eye strain.
- Headache and a feeling of tiredness after near work even for half an hour.
- Any blurring of vision. The patient usually complains about the feeling of words running together. Feels comfort on closing one eye while reading.
- Discomfort at all distance.
- Any momentary feeling of diplopia.
- Any difficulty in judging the distance.
- Any difficulty in playing fast games, moving objects or watching television or a film in theater.
- Any appearance of squint in a child after day's work.
- Any specific symptom related to near work.

CLINICAL EXAMINATION

Visual Acuity

Record the visual acuity for distance and near both with glasses and without glasses. Usually the vision is normal. Correct refractive error.

Refraction

It is a must in every case. In a child the retinoscopy should be done under full cycloplegic effect. Assess the refractive state of the eyes and prescribe glasses accordingly. Prescribe full correction for hypermetropes and slightly under correction for myopes. Correct the astigmatism how soever minor it may be.

Cover-Uncover Test

It is the most important and easy test to perform even in children. It should be carried out for distance and near. Perform cover-uncover test and also an alternate cover test. Make a note about the type of heterophoria which may be exophoria, esophoria or hyperphoria. Note about the recovery whether quick or slow or even breaks in heterotropia.

Convergence and Accommodation Test

Convergence Test

Place the face part of the Livingston Binocular gauge on the patient's infraorbital margin and ask the patient to hold the gauge with his left hand. Move the rod in the groove at the farthest end. Ask the patient to fix his gaze at the black part of the rod and move the rod towards the patient. Note the reading on the gauge at the point where the examiner notices the divergence of one or both the eyes. This will give the convergence power. The normal reading is from 6 to 10 cm in young adult. This is the objective test for convergence.

The subjective test for convergence is more delicate. In this the box with a cross in which a black vertical line card is placed is moved from farthest end towards the patient instead of the rod in the groove. Ask the patient to look at the line in the cross and report as soon as the line becomes double or moves to right or left. Note the reading at this point. Normal reading is less than 20 cm but more than objective test for convergence.

Accommodation Test

Test the accommodation uniocularly and binocularly. Ask the patient to report when he observes the letters in the box card becoming blurred as the box is moved steadily and slowly towards the patient. The normal reading in young adult is about 10 cm or less. Make proper allowance for the presbyopia in elderly. It is advisable to repeat the test at least twice for satisfactory results.

AC/A Ratio

AC/A ratio is defined as the change in vergence induced by a unit stimulus to accommodation.

AC/A ratio—the amount of convergence measured in prism diopters per unit change in the accommodation. That is one diopter of accommodation is associated with 4 prism diopter of accommodative convergence. A high ratio results in esotropia and a low ratio causes exotropia when patient looks at near objects.

Maddox Rod Test

Maddox rod test (Fig. 35.1) measures deviation of heterophoria for distance.

The patient is made to sit comfortably in a dark room with a white spot light fixed at the distance of six meters. Put a trial frame on the patient and place Maddox rod in the right eye with grooves in the horizontal direction. The patient is able to see a red vertical line with the right eye and a spot light with his left eye.

- If the red line appears to cut across the spot light then there is orthophoria.

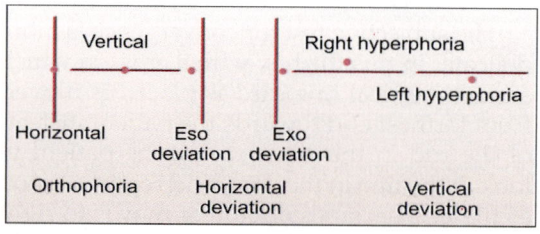

Fig. 35.1: Maddox rod test.

- If the red line appears on the side of the white spot light then there is either esophoria or exophoria. Then place the prisms in gradually increasing strength in front of the left eye until the red line appears to cut across the white spot light. The strength of the prism is the amount of heterophoria.

Repeat the test by placing the Maddox rod with grooves in vertical direction. In this case the red line appears horizontal.

- If the line cut across the spot light then there is orthophoria.
- If the line is above or below the spot light then there is either right or left hyperphoria. Then put the prisms in increasing strength so that the line cut across the spot light. The strength of prism is the amount of vertical heterophoria.

The amount of deviation can be read directly if there is a graduated tangent scale with a spot light placed six meters from the patient. A Maddox hand frame has a rotating Maddox rod on one side and rotating prisms of increasing strength on the other side. Thus by the use of a Maddox hand frame one gets direct reading.

Maddox Wing Test

Maddox wing test (Fig. 35.2) measures the amount of heterophoria for near fixation.

The patient is asked to hold the Maddox wing by its handle and look through the two site holes with both the eyes open and observe the arrow and numerical numbers. The right eye sees only a white vertical arrow and a red horizontal arrow. The left eye sees only horizontal and vertical row of numbers. Ask the patient to read the white horizontal number that coincides with the white vertical arrow. This gives the amount of exophoria or esophoria. The odd number give esophoria and even number give exophoria.

Ask the patient to read the red vertical number that coincides with the red horizontal arrow. The even number gives the amount of Left hyperphoria and odd number gives the amount of right hyperphoria.

To get the correct reading set the red horizontal arrow parallel with the horizontal

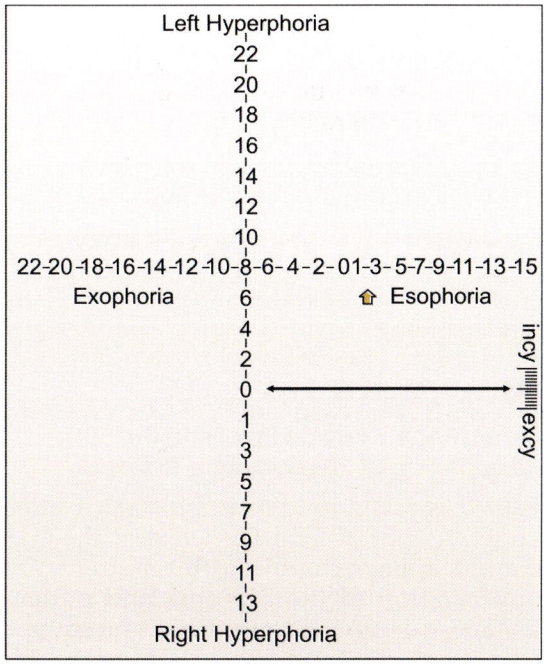

Fig. 35.2: Maddox wing test.

row in numbers. The amount of deviation is direct in prism diopters.

Measure Fusional Reserve

Fusional reserve can be assessed with synoptophore or prism bar. The normal values are as follows:
- Vertical fusional reserve: 1.5 –2.5.
- Horizontal negative fusional reserve (abduction range): 3–5.
- Horizontal positive fusional reserve: (adduction range): 20–40.

HETEROPHORIA

Heterophoria or latent squint is a condition of the eyes in which the eyes are kept in alignment due to fusion. There is deviation of the eyes soon on breaking the fusion.

Types of Heterophoria

Exophoria

In exophoria there is a tendency of the eyes to deviate outward.

Convergence weakness type: The exophoria is more for near than for distance. The Maddox wing reading is higher than the Maddox rod reading.

Divergence excess type: The exophoria is more for distance than for near. The Maddox rod reading is higher than the Maddox wing reading.

Esophoria

In esophoria there is a tendency of the eyes to deviate inwards.

Convergence excess type: The esophoria is more for near than the distance. The Maddox wing reading is higher than the Maddox rod reading.

Divergence weakness type: The esophoria is more for distance than the near. The maddox rod reading is higher than the Maddox wing reading.

Hyperphoria

In hyperphoria there is a tendency of one eye to deviate upwards. It is a relative condition in which one eye is hyperphoric and the other eye is hypophoric.

It is mandatory to use the term right or left hyperphoria depending on the eye that remains deviated up as compared to the other eye.

Cyclophoria

In cyclophoria there is a tendency for torsional deviation of the eye. It can be incyclophoria or excyclophoria. It is rare.

Orthophoria

In Orthophoria there is no deviation of eyes even after breaking the fusion. Few people are orthophoric. Some degree of heterophoria is universal.

Clinical Features and Management
1. Etiology and symptom
2. Esophoria
3. Exophoria

ETIOLOGY

- *Error of refraction:* The most important cause for heterophoria is an error of refraction.

  In hypermetropia there is more demand for accommodation and so for more convergence which results in esophoria. In myopia there is less demand for accommodation and so for less convergence which results in exophoria.
- Any occupation which requires more and constant near work demands more and constant accommodation and convergence therefore it precipitates esophoria.
- Dissociation factor predisposes for phorias. Prolonged use of one eye dissociates the fusion. It is seen in the individuals using microscope or watch makers using uniocular magnifying glass.

SYMPTOMS

Eye Strain

The eye strain is due to extra effort by the extraocular muscles to overcome the latent deviation. The occupation plays an important part. Any occupation requiring near work can precipitate esophoria and so eyes strain to overcome it.

Headache

To begin with there may be a feeling of tiredness or discomfort which may give a feeling of dull headache. Patient may complain of dull ache of the eyes or deep seated pain behind the eyes. Later there is headache which occurs even after reading for half an hour. There is headache after watching television or a film. Patient complains of headache on exposure to bright light even sunlight.

Blurring of Vision

There is blurring of vision. The letters in a book appears running in each other. The patient feels comfortable by closing one eye momentarily.

Difficulty in Changing Focus

There is difficulty in playing fast games wherein the focus has to be changed very frequently such as badminton, tennis, ping-pong, etc.

Difficulty in Judging the Distance

Patient with heterophoria finds problem in judging the distance while parking car, cricketers, tennis players, and pilots especially while landing.

MANAGEMENT OF ESOPHORIA

Divergence Exercise Involving the Recognition of Physiological Diplopia

Patient is asked to look at a distant fixation target. A spot of light flashed near the eyes should appear double to the patient. On appreciation of the diplopia and patient looking at distant target the light is substituted by a pencil and then with a stereogram. This stereogram is slowly moved away from the eye until fusion of the two pictures is achieved by the patient. At this point of fusion the accommodation is correct for the card and in excess of the convergence which is correct for the distant fixation target. In this exercise the convergence is relaxed and accommodation is used to see the picture clearly.

Divergence Exercise with Diploscope

It has been designed to improve the relative divergence of the eyes. Ask the patient to see the letters of diploscope through the holes in the septum. If he can see the letter –D O G- then the patient is orthophoric. Ask the patient to look at distant object beyond letters and see the four holes and letters in it. If he can see clearly – D O O G-then the convergence is completely relaxed and to see the letters clearly uses accommodation without convergence.

Divergence Exercise with Remy Separator

Ask the patient to look at a distant object through the transparent slides and make an attempt to superimpose and fuse the pictures in the instrument. In this exercise also the convergence is completely relaxed by fixing at a distant object and accommodation is used to see the pictures clearly.

Divergence Exercise with Prisms

Prisms in increasing strength with base-in are placed before the eyes maintaining the target as single induces relaxation of convergence. For this purpose the use of a prism bar is ideal.

Divergence Exercise with Synoptophore

The arms of the synoptophore are set in a position so that patient can achieve fusion. Then the arms are moved slowly to stimulate divergence. Fusional slides are used for this purpose. Exercise on synoptophore also helps in treating the suppression by reeducating binocularity.

Use of Relieving Prisms

The prisms are used in cases where in the esophoria is equal for distance and near. These are useful in cases which show no tendency to increase in esophoria. These are helpful in elderly people in whom surgery is not indicated.

Surgery

- *Esophoria with convergence excess-with high AC/A ratio:* Recession of one or both the medial rectus muscle is an ideal operation.
- *Esophoria with divergence weakness with low AC/A ratio:* Resection of one or both the lateral rectus muscle is an ideal choice.
- *Esophoria with equal for distant and near with normal AC/A ratio:*In these cases a limited recession of medial rectus and limited resection of lateral rectus muscles is indicated. There should be a sufficient gap between the two operations to observe and assess the results of the first surgery.

MANAGEMENT OF EXOPHORIA

Convergence Exercises Involving the Recognition of Physiological Diplopia

There is a distant fixation light. Ask the patient to see at a pencil/pen held by one hand and close to the eye at about 20 cm in line with the distant fixation light. The light should appear double. With the perception of diplopia ask the patient to hold a stereogram—a card with identical pictures at an arm's length by the other hand and holding a pencil/pen in other hand halfway between the stereogram and eyes. On fixing the gaze at the pencil, the card should appear double showing four pictures. On moving the pencil towards the stereogram the two pictures merge into one with a stereoscopic effect. When the picture is clearly seen then the accommodation is used for the card and convergence is maintained for the pencil. It gives a convergence exercise.

Convergence Exercise with Diploscope

Ask the patient to see the letter through the holes and if he can see the letters -D O G- clearly then the amount of the convergence and accommodation used is correct for the distance of the letters from the eyes. Ask the patient to look at an imaginary spot on septum between the two middle holes in the septum and read the letters. In this case the convergence is increased and a superimposed -D- and -O are seen through the one hole and superimposed-O- and -G- are seen through the other hole. If the letters are seen clearly then the accommodation is correct for the distance but the convergence has increased without increase in accommodation. This exercise improves the relative convergence of the eyes.

Exercises to Improve Convergence

This can be done at home by a patient. Ask the patient to hold a pencil, a card with picture or a word at arm's length and then gradually bring it towards the eyes maintaining fixation. Diplopia manifests if patient fails to maintain fixation. Then repeat the test. It should be carried out 4 times each day for five minutes.

Jump Convergence Exercises

In this patient is asked to change fixation repeatedly and quickly from distant to near target, e.g. from infinity to 20 cm. This near distance can later be reduced to even up to 5 cm.

Convergence Exercises with Prisms

An increasing strength of prism with base-out placed before the eye induces convergence. A prism bar is ideal for this.

Exercise with the Synoptophore

The arms of the synoptophore are slowly moved to stimulate convergence. After fusion has been achieved the single vision is further maintained by use of accommodative convergence.

Relieving Prisms

Prisms with base-out may be prescribed for near work in some cases to help them overcome the annoying symptoms.

Surgery

- *Exophoria of divergence excess type-with high AC/A ratio:* Recession of one or both lateral rectus muscle is the choicest surgery.

- *Exophoria with Convergence weakness type with low AC/A ratio:* Resection of one or both medial rectus muscle is the choice.

- *Exophoria with normal deviation for distant and near with normal AC/A ratio:* In this liberal recession of lateral rectus and limited resection of the medial rectus muscle is advised. There should be a sufficient gap between the two operations to observe and assess the results of the first surgery.

36

A Case with Heterotropia—Manifest Squint

History

Enquire emphatically with patience about the following factors:

- Age of onset.
  Squint manifesting in early age shall require a surgical correction. Squint manifesting late is likely to be accommodative and responds to glasses and orthoptic treatment.
- Medical history—birth weight, developmental and neurological.
- Family history of squint.
  Ask about the history of any family member having a squint and at what age and therapy.
- Any variation in the squint.
  The child may show squint in the evening and may be normal in the morning. The child is squinting with one eye only or alternates.
- Squint is constant or intermittent.
- Squint associated with double vision-diplopia.
- Observe for any change in head posture.
- Any association with trauma whether physical or psychic.
- Any association with febrile illness such as measles, malaria, flu.
- Using glasses. If using glasses then since what age.
- Any previous record of ocular check up and treatment—glasses, occlusion or surgery.

Clinical Examinations

1. Inspection.
2. Visual acuity.
3. Refraction.

4. Ocular movements
5. Cover test
6. Test for convergence and accommodation
7. Maddox rod test
8. Maddox wing test
9. Hirschberg's test
10. Prism and alternate cover test
11. Worth's four light test
12. After image test
13. Tests on synoptophore.

Inspection

Observe for head posture, facial asymmetry, deviation of the eye and nystagmus.

Visual Acuity

Test the visual acuity of each eye separately and with both the eyes wherein the case has a binocular single vision. Test the vision with glasses and without glasses for distance and near vision. A pin-hole test gives information that the impairment of vision is due to refractive error or due to an organic cause.

Refraction

It is essential to assess the refractive state of the eyes. In young children it is better to examine under full cycloplegic effect. Correct the error of refraction if any and prescribe the glasses. Note the visual acuity with glass. Observe for any deviation of eyes with and without glasses for distance and near vision.

Ocular Movements

Ocular movements are of three types—ductions, versions and vergences (Figs 36.1 and 36.2).

Uniocular movements are labeled as "Ductions". Ductions include the following:

- Adduction.
- Abduction.
- Elevation (supraduction).
- Depression (infraduction).
- Intorsion (incycloduction).
- Extorsion (excycloduction).

Binocular movements are label as "versions and vergences". These movements are synchronous, symmetrical and include the following.

Versions

- Dextroversion (right gaze).
- Levoversion (left gaze).
- Supraversion (up-gaze).
- Infraversion (down-gaze).
- Dextroelevation (right and up-gaze).
- Dextrodepression (right and down-gaze).
- Levoelevation (left and up-gaze).
- Levodepression (left and down-gaze).
- Dextrocycloversion (rotation of both the eyes to right).

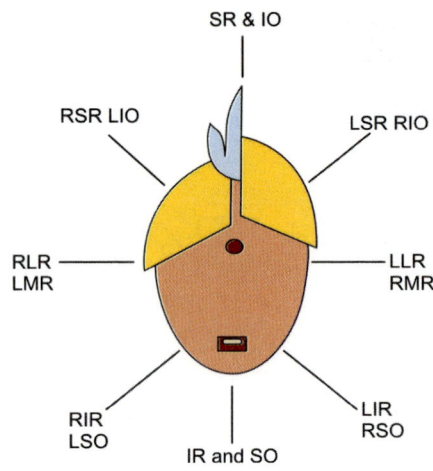

Fig. 36.2: Ocular movements

- Levocycloversion (rotation of both the eyes to left).

Vergences

Convergence: Convergence is an inward movement of both the eyes due to simultaneous contraction of the medial rectus muscles of both the eyes.

Divergence: Divergence is an outward movement of both the eyes due to

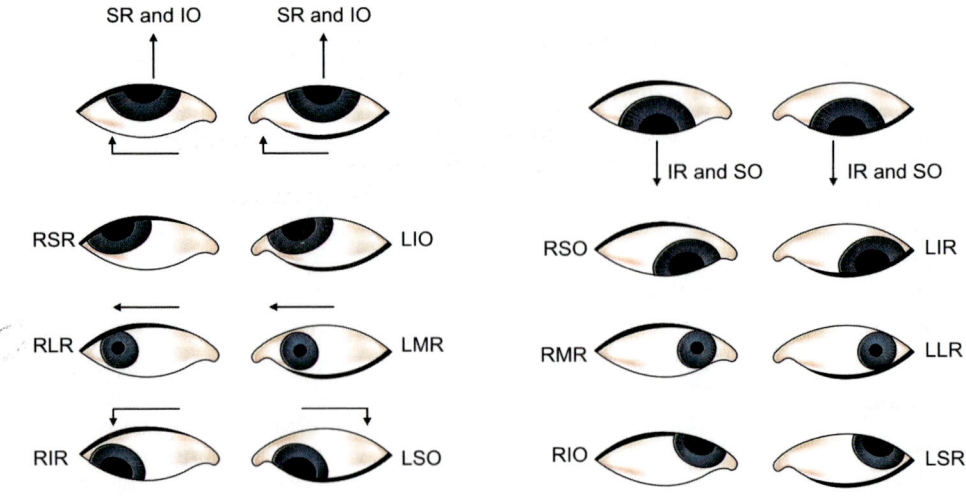

Fig. 36.1: Ocular movements

simultaneous contraction of lateral rectus muscles of both the eyes.

Cardinal Position of Gaze and Yoke Muscles

There are six cardinal positions of gaze and six pairs of yoke muscles.

Cardinal positions	Yoke muscles
• Dextroversion (right gaze)	Right lateral rectus Left medial rectus
• Levoversion (left gaze)	Left lateral rectus Right medial rectus
• Dextroelevation (right and up-gaze)	Right superior rectus Left inferior oblique
• Dextrodepression (right and down-gaze)	Right inferior rectus Left superior oblique
• Levodepression (left and down-gaze)	Left inferior rectus Right superior oblique
• Levoelevation (left and up-gaze)	Left superior rectus Right inferior oblique

Actions of Ocular Muscles

Muscles	Primary action	Secondary action
Lateral rectus	Abduction	None
Medial rectus	Adduction	None
Superior rectus	Elevation	Adduction and intorsion
Inferior rectus	Depression	Adduction and extorsion
Superior oblique	Depression	Intorsion and abduction
Inferior oblique	Elevation	Extorsion and abduction

Hering's Law of Equal Innervations

Hering's law implies that equal and simultaneous innervation flows to a pair of muscles that contract simultaneously (yoke muscles) in different binocular movements of the eye such as right lateral rectus and left medial rectus in dextroversion, both medial recti in convergence and right superior rectus and left inferior oblique in dextroelevation.

Sherrington's Law of Reciprocal Innervations

Sherrington's law of reciprocal innervation implies that increased innervation and contraction of a muscle is automatically associated with a reciprocal decrease in innervation and relaxation of its antagonist muscle. For example-in dextroversion, there is an increased innervations flow to right lateral rectus and left medial rectus muscle is accompanied with decreased innervations flow to right medial rectus and left lateral rectus muscles.

Agonist Muscle

The primary muscle moving the eye is labeled as agonist muscle. All the muscles are agonist muscles when they move the eye in any given direction.

Antagonist Muscles

The muscle which acts in the opposite direction to the agonist muscle is called as antagonist muscle to that agonist muscle. For example-medial and lateral recti, superior and inferior recti and superior and inferior oblique muscles are antagonist to each other in the same eye.

Contralateral Antagonist Muscles

These are a pair of muscles one from each eye having opposite actions. For example-the right lateral rectus and left lateral rectus are contralateral antagonist muscles.

Synergist Muscle

The muscle which acts in conjunction with the agonist muscle to produce a given movement is labeled as synergist muscle. For example-superior rectus and inferior oblique of same eye are synergistic elevators.

Contralateral Synergist or Yoke Muscles

These are a pair of muscles (one from each eye) that contract simultaneously during version movements. For example, right lateral rectus and left medial rectus are yoke muscles for dextroversion movement of the eye.

Cover-Uncover Test

The examiner sits in front of the patient at the same level and asks the patient to look at the forehead of the examiner. In young children a light is thrown in the eyes by a torch so that he is able to fix the eyes towards the light. The examiner then covers one eye of the patient with the occluder or back of the palm of his hand and observes the other eye. Each eye is tested in turn. The test is conducted for the distant fixation as well as for the near fixation in the primary position of the eyes. It should be conducted in the main positions of conjugate gaze especially if there is a suspicion of a vertical deviation. The cover test should be repeated making it a cover-uncover test and alternate cover test several times before arriving at a conclusion about the orthophoria and heterotropia.

The cover-uncover test provides the following information

- Orthophoria: if there is no movement of the eyes.
- Heterophoria: if the eyes show a movement.
- Exophoria: if the eye moves outwards.
- Esophoria: if the eye moves inwards.
- Hyper or hypophoria: if there is vertical movement of the eyes.
- The squint is a manifest or a latent.
- The squint is unilateral or alternating.
- The squinting eye is steady or unsteady, central or eccentric or wandering.
- In a concomitant or non-paralytic squint: the primary and secondary deviations are equal.
- In a paralytic squint: the secondary deviation is greater than the primary deviation.

Convergence and Accommodation Test

Convergence Test

Place the face part of the livingston gauge on the patient's infraorbital margin and ask the patient to hold the gauge with his left hand. Move the rod in the groove at the farthest end. Ask the patient to fix his gaze at the black part of the rod, and move the rod towards the patient. Note the reading on the gauge at the point where the examiner notices the divergence of one or both the eyes. This will give the convergence power. The normal reading is from 6 to 10 cm in young adult. This is the objective test for convergence.

The subjective test for convergence is more delicate. In this the box with a cross in which a black vertical line card is placed is moved from farthest end towards the patient instead of the rod in the groove. Ask the patient to look at the line in the cross and report as soon as the line becomes double or moves to right or left. Note the reading at this point. Normal reading is less than 20 cm but more than objective test for convergence.

Accommodation Test

Test the uniocular and binocular accommodation. Ask the patient to report when he observes the letters in the box card becoming blurred as the box is moved steadily and slowly towards the patient. The normal reading in young adult is about 10 cm or less. Make proper allowance for the presbyopia in elderly. It is advisable to repeat the test at least twice for satisfactory results.

Maddox Rod Test

Maddox rod test measures deviation of heterophoria for distance.

The patient is made to sit comfortably in a dark room with a white spot light fixed at the distance of six meters. Put a trial frame on the patient and place Maddox rod in the right eye. The patient is able to see a red vertical line with the right eye and a spot light with his left eye.

- If the red line appears to cut across the spot light then there is orthophoria.
- If the red line appears on the side of the white spot light then there is either esophoria or exophoria. Then place the prisms in gradually increasing strength in front of the left eye until the red line appears to cut across the white spot light. The strength of the prism is the amount of heterophoria.

Repeat the test by placing the Maddox rod with grooves in vertical direction. In this case the red line appears horizontal.

- If the line cut across the spot light then there is orthophoria.
- If the line is above or below the spot light then there is either right or left hyperphoria. Then put the prisms in increasing strength so that the line cut across the spot light. The strength of prism is the amount of vertical heterophoria.

The amount of deviation can be read directly if there is a graduated tangent scale with a spot light placed six meters from the patient. A Maddox hand frame has a rotating Maddox rod on one side and rotating prisms of increasing strength on the other side. Thus by the use of a Maddox hand frame one gets direct reading (Fig. 36.3).

Fig. 36.3: Maddox hand frame

Maddox Wing Test

Maddox wing test measures the amount of heterophoria for near fixation.

The patient is asked to hold the Maddox wing by its handle and look through the two site holes with both the eyes open and observe the arrow and numerical numbers. The right eye sees only a white vertical arrow and a red horizontal arrow. The left eye sees only horizontal and vertical row of numbers. Ask the patient to read the white horizontal number that coincides with the white vertical arrow. This gives the amount of exophoria or esophoria. The odd number give esophoria and even number give exophoria.

Ask the patient to read the red vertical number that coincides with the red horizontal arrow. The even number gives the amount of left hyperphoria and odd number gives the amount of right hyperphoria.

To get the correct reading set the red horizontal arrow parallel with the horizontal row in numbers. The amount of deviation is direct in prism diopters.

Hirschberg's Test

It is rough test to find out the angle of a manifest squint. The examiner sits in front of the patient and throws the light from a small pen-torch on the patients's face from about 33 cm and instructs him to look towards the light. The examiner then notices the position of corneal reflex (Fig. 36.4).

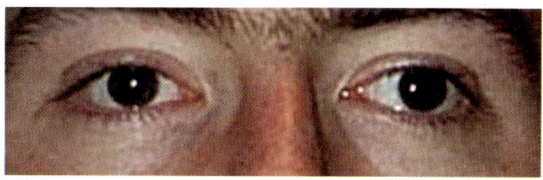

Fig. 36.4: Hirschberg's test —positive

- If the light reflex is central in both the pupils then there is no squint.
- If the cornea reflex is in the center of one eye and at the pupillary border of the other eye then the patient has an angle of about 20° of squint.
- If the corneal reflex is at the limbus then the patient has an angle of about 45° of squint.
- Some books describe it differently; 16° if the light reflex is at the pupillary border, 32° if the light reflex is midway between the pupil and limbus and 48° if the light reflex is at the limbus.

It is one of the most useful and practical method of assessing the angle of squint before and after the surgery and also on follow-up visits.

Prism and Alternate Cover Test

This test measures the total deviation latent and manifest and does not differentiate heterotropia from heterophoria.

Place the prism in front of one eye with the base of the prism placed in direction that is opposite to the deviation, e.g. in convergent squint place the prism with base-out and in divergent squint place the prism with base-in. The end point is reached when there is no ocular movement. The strength of the prism gives the angle of deviation. Perform the alternate cover test.

Worth's Four Light Test

The apparatus consists of a box with four lights arranged in a diamond formation and illuminated internally. The two lateral lights are green, the upper one is red and the lower one is white (Fig. 36.5). The patient is made to sit at six meters from the test box and wears a red-green filter goggles. Ask the patient about the number of lights visible to him and in what color.

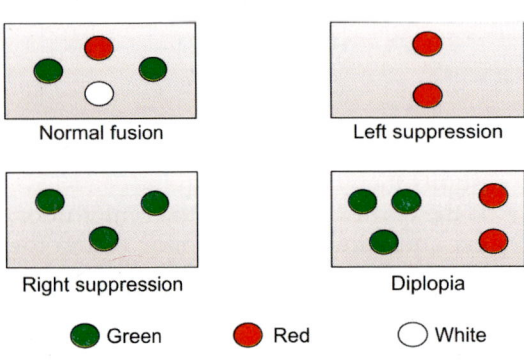

Fig. 36.5: Worth's four dot test

The test provides the following information:

- With binocular single vision and fusion the patient sees four lights two green, one red and one slight orange in color.
- If patient can see four lights in the presence of a manifest squint then he has abnormal retinal correspondence (ARC).
- If patient can see only two red lights then he has suppression in left eye.
- If patient can see only three green lights then he has suppression in right eye.
- If patient can see two red lights and three green lights then he has diplopia.
- If patient sees red and green lights alternately then he has alternate suppression.

After Image Test

This test is to find out the retinal correspondence. This test is done in a dark room. Make the patient sit and cover his right eye. Expose the left eye to a horizontal beam of light (a fluorescent tube light) for ten seconds. Now close the left eye and expose the right eye to a vertical beam of light for ten seconds. Turn off all the lights in the room.

Ask the patient to open both the eyes and draw and describe what he sees;

- If the two after images are seen as a cross then the patient has a normal retinal correspondence.
- If the patient has abnormal retinal correspondence then the two images will not cross and appear in the form of T on its side or the components of T may be separated.
- In a case of an esotropia with abnormal retinal correspondence the vertical after image (belonging to right eye) will be seen to the left of the horizontal after image (belonging to the left eye). These findings are reversed in a case of an exotropia.

Synoptophore

It is an instrument for assessing the angle of squint, grades of binocular vision, presence of suppression, amblyopia and abnormal retinal correspondence.

Three Grades of Fusion

Grade I: Simultaneous Perception

Two dissimilar test slides are presented to macula. A slide with a bird is placed in front of one eye and a slide with a cage in front of the other eye. Ask the patient to move the arms so as to put the bird in the cage.

- If the patient is not able to see the two pictures simultaneously then he has either suppression or amblyopia.
- If he can put the bird in the cage then he has a fusion of grade I.

Grade II: Fusion under Stress with Amplitude of Fusion

A pair of test slide are used which individually lack some details but when superimposed then forms a complete picture. The classic example is slides with rabbit. In one slide the rabbit lacks the tail and in another slide the rabbit lacks the bunch of flower.

- If patient is able to superimpose the slides to form a complete picture—a rabbit with tail and a bunch of flowers then he has a fusion of grade II.
- The power to fusion must also have a range. It is tested by moving the arms of the synoptophore so that eyes have to converge and diverge in order to maintain fusion. The normal amplitude of fusion is 25–30 diopters. The normal amplitude for divergence is 5 diopters.

Grade III: Stereopsis

The test slides are devised to give an impression of depth. The best example is of bucket which is appreciated in three dimension. Both the slides have a bucket but pictures have been taken from slightly different angle.

If the patient is able to superimpose the slides to one bucket then he has a fusion of grade III.

Retinal Correspondence

If the patient is able to superimpose the slides of grade II fusion then the patient has a normal retinal correspondence. The other test is an after image test.

Anomalous (Abnormal) Retinal Correspondence

In abnormal retinal correspondence the retinal elements of the squinting eye adopts an abnormal relationship with the fovea of the non-squinting eye. It can be diagnosed by the "after image test". It requires no treatment. Treatment is necessary for suppression and amblyopia.

Suppression

Suppression is a temporary active cortical inhibition of the image of an object formed on the retina of the squinting eye. Suppression is produced due to subconscious active neglect of the vision in the squinting eye by the visual cortex. It occurs during binocular vision, i.e. both the eyes open. When the normal eye is covered the squinting eye takes up the fixation. Suppression occurs when there is confusion and diplopia. It can be easily diagnosed by Worth's four dot (light) test. The patient wears red and green glasses. The target has four lights, one red, two green, and one white. If there is no suppression the patient can see four lights; one red, two green and one red-green light. If there is suppression then he will see either two red lights or three green lights or see the lights alternately. In the presence of diplopia the patient will see five lights.

Amblyopia

Amblyopia refers to a condition of partial loss of vision in one or both the eyes in absence of any organic lesion of the eye and visual pathway.

The amblyopia develops faster in the first six months of the life and usually does not evolve after six years of age.

Types of Amblyopia

- Strabismic amblyopia.
- Stimulus deprivation amblyopia (amblyopia ex anopsia).
- Anisometropic amblyopia.
- Isoametropic amblyopia.
- Meridonial amblyopia.

Management of Amblyopia

- Treat the amblyogenic causative factor during early age.
- Treat the opacities of the lens or cornea.
- Correct the refractive error.
- Occlusion therapy of the sound eye to force the use of amblyopic eye is the easy and choicest treatment.

VARIOUS CLASSIFICATION OF SQUINT

According to the Direction of Squint

- Esotropia-manifest convergent squint.
- Exotropia-manifest divergent squint.

- Hypertropia-manifest sursumvergent squint.
- Hypotropia-manifest deorsumvergent squint.
- Cyclotropia-manifest torsional squint that can be either incyclotropia or excyclotropia.

Concomitant or Incomitant Squint

Concomitant Squint (Non paralytic Squint)

In concomitant squint the eyes move in a completely coordinated manner so that the angle of deviation is equal in all the direction of gaze.

Incomitant Squint (Paralytic Squint)

In the incomitant squint the eyes move in an in-coordinated manner so that the angle of deviation varies in different directions of gaze.

According to Squint Manifestation

Constant Squint

In constant squint there is squint in all the direction of gaze at all the distance of fixation of gaze and irrespective of eye fixed.

Periodic Squint

In a periodic squint the squint manifests either for a distance fixation or for a near fixation. In a periodic convergent squint the deviation is present for near but absent for distance fixation. In a periodic divergent squint the deviation is present for distance fixation but absent for near fixation.

Intermittent Squint

Intermittent squint manifests when the child is tired after full day at school or after a mild illness. It may not manifest if the child is not put to study that is when not using accommodation.

Squint May be Uniocular or Alternating

Uniocular Squint

In a uniocular squint the squinting eye is always the same except under cover test during which the squinting eye may take up fixation but reverts back to squint soon the cover is removed from the non-squinting eye.

Alternating Uniocular Squint

In alternating squint either eye may show squint when the other takes up the fixation. In a cover test-cover the right eye and left eye takes up the fixation. On uncovering the right eye, the right eye show a squint and left eye is fixed. Now cover the left eye and right eye takes up the fixation. On uncovering the left eye, the left eye shows squint and right eye is fixed. There is no preference for any eye to take up fixation.

Squint is Accommodative or Non-accommodative

Accommodative Squint

The squint manifests on using accommodation, i.e. when the patient is fixing for near work and no squint when fixing for distance.

Non-accommodative Squint

A non-accommodative convergent squint manifests even in the absence of any accommodation effort by the patient. These cases show an increased deviation on exercising accommodation.

Apparent Squint (Pseudo-squint)

An apparent squint is the term applied to a clinical condition wherein there is a false appearance of a squint with absence of any deviation of the eyes.

Apparent Convergent Squint

It is associated with the presence of epicanthus with flat bridge of nose and a large negative angle alpha.

Apparent Divergent Squint

It is associated with the marked narrowing of the lateral canthi and presence of a large positive angle alpha.

Clinical Features and Management

1. Convergent squint
   Accommodational convergent squint
   - Fully accommodational squint.
   - Accommodational with convergence excess.
   - Accommodational with divergence weakness.
   - Partially accommodational squint.

Non-accommodational convergent squint
   - Unilateral convergent squint.
   - Alternating convergent squint.
   - Secondary convergent squint.
2. Divergent squint

Primary divergent squint
   - The divergence excess type.
   - The convergence weakness type.
   - The mixed type.

Secondary divergent squint
Apparent divergent squint
3. Vertical squint
4. Microtropia
5. A.V and X phenomenon
6. Inverted Y or Lambda phenomenon
7. Surgery for squint.
8. Guide lines for squint surgery

Convergent Squint

Accommodational Convergent Squint

The accommodational convergent squint occurs usually at the age of 3 to 5 years when the child starts playing with toys, reading and writing, eating, thereby using his accommodation. To begin with the accommodational squint is of intermittent type which gradually passes into the constant or an alternating squint. There are four types of accommodational squint.

Fully accommodational convergent squint: A case of fully accommodational squint does not show squint for distance or near with correction of refractive error and use of glasses. There is a constant convergent squint soon on removing the glasses. These cases are managed by prescription of suitable glasses.

Accommodational with convergence excess: The patient shows no squint for distance with glasses but shows a squint for near work even with distance glasses used for near work. This type of patients can be managed by additional plus glasses for near work.

Accommodational with divergence weakness: There is a manifest convergent squint for distance even with glasses but show esophoria for near work. These cases need surgical correction.

Partially accommodational squint: There is a constant convergent squint for distance and near even with glasses. The angle of squint is reduced by glasses but not fully. These cases always need surgical correction. These patients may have a normal binocular vision or may not have a binocular function.

Non-accommodational Convergent Squint

Unilateral convergent squint (Fig. 36.6)
- Early onset from birth or early infancy.
- Onset may be abrupt following a minor trauma or an insignificant illness such as flu or influenza.
- The squint is usually constant type.
- There is an early suppression and amblyopia or development of abnormal retinal correspondence and eccentric fixation.
- There may be an organic cause in the macular area.
- An early diagnosis may help to initiate free alternation by occlusion.
- An early surgery shall help to achieve parallelism of the eyes and so a chance for the development of a normal binocular single vision.

Alternating convergent squint
- Early onset of squint. Probably the infant is born with a squint although at birth the

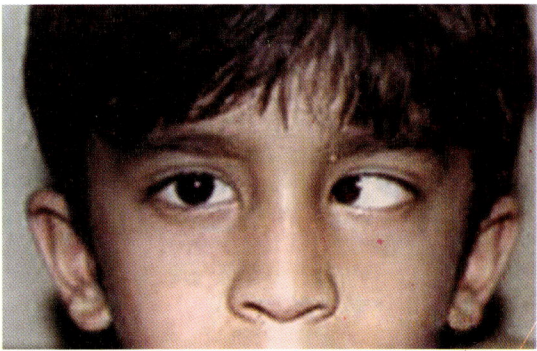

Fig. 36.6: Unilateral convergent squint

squint may not be obvious. The squint tends to increase as the child grows and uses his accommodation.

- The angle of deviation is large about 25° or more.
- Vision is equal in both the eyes due to free alternation.
- There is no error of refraction or the error is insignificant and equal in both the eyes.
- There may be some limitation of abduction of each eye. There may be some elevation of each eye on the contralatero-version.
- Operation is the choicest treatment for cosmetic purpose. Some cases may develop a binocular vision after a good corrective surgery.

Secondary convergent squint: A secondary convergent squint may result due to the following factors:

- A lesion of ocular media such as corneal or lenticular opacity and pseudoglioma.
- A lesion in the afferent pathway such as optic atrophy and chorioretinal atrophy.
- Anisometropia
- Congenital myopia involving one or both the eyes.
- A surgical over-correction of a divergent squint.
- Associated with vertical deviations of the eye.
- Operation is indicated for cosmetic purpose to correct the deviation.

Divergent Squint

Primary Divergent Squint

It is of three types:

The divergence excess type

- Patient is unaware of the squint as the divergence occurs in a position of rest that is when the patient is looking at a distance object and not fixing at anything particular.
- Cover test show a latent squint with good recovery for near but becomes manifest for the distance.
- Later the squint tends to become a constant type.

- Maddox rod reading is more than Maddox wing.
- Worth's four light test may show either a crossed diplopia or suppression.
- Surgery is helpful and provides a good binocular vision.

The convergence weakness type

- There is orthotropia for distance but exotropia for near.
- Cover test show a latent squint for distance with good recovery but becomes manifest for near fixation.
- Maddox wing reading is higher than the Maddox rod reading.
- Convergence is poor.
- Convergence exercise may help
- Surgery gives good result.

The mixed type

- There is divergence of the eye at all the distance whether near or far. This is due to divergence excess and convergence weakness. The angle of deviation is same for distance and near.
- Surgery gives good result.

Secondary Divergent Squint

A secondary divergent squint may result due to the following factors:

- A gross defect or loss of vision in one eye promotes deviation of the eye. The age of the patient plays an important part. Divergence occurs usually if the defect is congenital or the onset has occurred before the age of six months. Divergence also occurs after adolescence when the convergence becomes weak. The process of divergence accelerates with the onset of presbyopia.
- Anisometropia.
- Aniseikonia.
- Associated with vertical deviations of the eyes.
- Due to an abnormality of orbit as in oxycephaly.
- Myopia may lead to divergence due to less use of accommodation.
- A surgical over-correction of a convergent squint.

- Operation is indicated for cosmetic purpose. A slight over-correction is advisable.

Apparent Divergent Squint

It is seen in the following conditions:
- A large positive angle alpha.
- A case with wide interpupillary distance.
- In exophthalmos.
- A case with wide palpebral fissure.
- A case with marked narrowing of lateral canthi.

Vertical Squint (Hypertropia or Hypotropia)

A primary vertical squint is of a rare occurrence. Many cases of hyperphoria may manifest as hypertropia for a temporary period in a condition of fatigue. A primary vertical deviation remains constant in the absence of a horizontal deviation in any part of fixation. Such a condition is a theoretical concept. A vertical squint is almost always associated with a horizontal or torsional deviation in certain position of gaze. In the intermittent type of a vertical deviation the patient usually complains of diplopia, headache and eye strain, due to the effort to maintain fusion. In cases of constant squint there is an early occurrence of amblyopia and suppression with no complaint from the patient.

Squint with both a horizontal and a vertical deviation may be a case of primary vertical squint with secondary horizontal squint or a primary horizontal squint with a secondary vertical component. In a case with primary vertical squint there is a dissociation of the eyes breaking down the binocularity. This case with a prior heterophoria or an accommodational factor will develop a horizontal squint. This is seen in early childhood wherein the child brings about the factor of convergence and accommodation thus causing convergent squint with vertical primary deviation.

In a case with primary horizontal convergent squint there is some vertical deviation in the form of elevation in adduction.

In a case with primary horizontal divergent squint there is some vertical deviation in the form of elevation of diverging eye, the elevation increases in abduction.

In vertical heterotropia, there is a manifest vertical deviation of the eyes in the opposite direction so that one eye is hypertropic when the other eye is fixing and when the hypertropic eye is fixing the other eye is hypotropic.

A secondary vertical squint can occur in an eye with constant convergent squint. The eye when in position of convergence the inferior oblique which is a stronger muscle in adduction than its direct antagonist the superior oblique elevates the eye. Most of these cases show good prognosis after operation on horizontal muscles.

An alternating hypertropia or hypotropia may occur wherein one eye moves either upward or downward when the other is used for fixation.

The following various factors may be the cause for vertical deviation of eye
- Asymmetry of face.
- Imbalance between the elevators and depressors.
- Variations in the insertions.
- Abnormal bands and attachment.
- An incomitant deviation becomes a comitant in due course of time.

Treatment

- Treatment is surgical correction of the deviation.
- Correct the deviation which is more. If it is a primary vertical deviation correct by surgery on vertical muscles.
- If horizontal deviation is more than correct by surgery on horizontal muscles.
- A small vertical deviation may disappear after correction of horizontal deviation.

Microtropia

Microtropia is an ocular disalignment with an angle of deviation so small that it would normally be seen only on dissociation of the eyes and it manifests as phoria. A squint under 10 prism dioptres may be included in this tropia. It is an esodeviation.

- The visual acuity of the affected eye is little low due to amblyopia.
- There is a crowding phenomenon.
- In reading, single letters of a word appears fuzzy or at times disappear or become intermingled with next letter.
- Amsler chart show a relative scotoma on the right side of the central fixation point in the right eye microtropia and on the left side of the central fixation point in the left eye microtropia. Due to this, the last letters of a word are blurred in right microtropia and first letters are blurred in the left microtropia.
- The essential feature is the presence of harmonious abnormal retinal correspondence in a small angle squint associated with eccentric fixation and amblyopia.
- Cover test may not be able to demonstrate the small angle of squint because the angles of eccentricity and anomaly coincide.
- The four diopter prism test is highly sensitive test to detect even a small angle of squint up to 2°. A four diopter prism is placed base-out in front of the non-amblyopic eye (eye with normal vision) which causes a shift of the retinal image of fixation light slightly to the temporal side of the fovea, where upon, the eye adducts to get refixation. This movement of recovery by the non-amblyopic eye is also reflected in the amblyopic eye by abduction according to Hering's law. This movement is easily visible by the observer.
- Correct any error of refraction if any and prescribe glasses.
- It is advisable to leave microtropia alone.

A, V And X Phenomenon

The A, V, X, Y and inverted Y or Lambda phenomenon, are cyclovertical deviations of the eyes usually found in association with a concomitant squint whether convergent or divergent. As a general rule, there is slight relative alteration in the relative positions of the eyes when they move from primary position to upwards and downwards. If this phenomenon becomes obvious then it constitutes an important feature of a squint.

A-Phenomenon in Esophoria or Esotropia

The eyes show more convergence on looking upwards than when looking downwards.

A-Phenomenon in Exophoria or Exotropia

The eyes show more divergence on looking downwards than when looking upwards.

V-Phenomenon in Esophoria or Esotropia

The eyes show more convergence when looking downwards than when looking upwards.

V-Phenomenon in Exophoria or Exotropia

The eyes show more divergence when looking upwards than when looking downwards.

X-Phenomenon

There is some degree of divergence in the primary position which increases both on looking upwards and downwards.

Y-Phenomenon

The eyes show normal position (orthotropia) in primary gaze and down gaze, but show divergence (exotropia) in upward gaze.

Inverted Y or Lambda Phenomenon

The eyes show normal position (orthotropia) in primary gaze and upward gaze but show divergence (exotropia) in the downward gaze. From practical point of view, it is the A and V phenomenon which are important. Usually these are found on a routine examination unless there is associated squint. In some cases parents may notice that the squint becomes less obvious or disappears when the child is looking down for reading or taking meals. This can happen if the A-phenomenon is associated with esotropia. In some patient the squint becomes more obvious when he is looking upwards indicating a V-phenomenon associated with exotropia.

It has been suggested that a difference of at least 15 prism diopter on upward or downward movement is necessary to constitute the A-phenomenon and at least 25 prism diopter to constitute the V-phenomenon.

Management

- Any patient with a marked degree of A or V-phenomenon may require treatment.
- If the condition do not show improvement on correction of refractive error and prescription of glasses then surgery is the only treatment.
- There are three approaches to surgical treatment: surgery on the horizontal recti, the vertical recti or obliques.
- Each case to be decided on its merit.
- It is advisable to limit the surgery first to horizontal recti muscles.
- It is advisable to look for A and V-phenomenon in every case of squint to plan the management and surgery.

Surgery for Squint

There are three types of operation for extraocular muscle surgery for squint.

1. Weakening of the Muscle

Recession of muscle: In recession, the muscle is cut at its insertion and re-attached posterior to its insertion to decrease its pulling power. It can be performed on all the six extraocular muscles.

Marginal myotomy: Marginal myotomytomy is performed to further weaken the already recessed muscle. It increases the length of the muscle and thus reduces its pulling power.

Myectomy: It is rarely used surgical procedure wherein a contracted rectus or oblique muscle is cut at its insertion and left.

2. Strengthening of the Muscle

- *Resection of muscle:* In resection, the muscle is cut at its insertion and thereafter a desired length of piece is cut from this and the muscle is re-sutured at its original insertion. This increases its pulling power. It is suitable only for four rectus muscle.

- *Tucking of muscle:* In this operation procedure, the muscle is not incised at its insertion. The sutures applied at a desired point are sutured at the insertion. This enhances its pulling power. This is good for superior oblique muscle in cases of fourth nerve palsy.

- *Advancement:* In this procedure, the muscle is cut at its insertion and re-sutured at a point anterior to its insertion nearer to limbus.

3. Change the Direction of the Action of a muscle

The procedure to change the direction of action of muscles is used to correct A and V-phenomenon. The horizontal rectus muscle can be transposed to about two-thirds of its original insertion.

Guide Line for Squint Surgery

- There is a limit for recession of extra-ocular muscles. A recession beyond the equator shall be ineffective. The muscles reach the equator as follows:

Medial rectus	5.5 mm
Lateral rectus	8 mm
Inferior rectus	4 mm
Superior rectus	4 mm

- For resection-there is a limit of 10 mm for medial and lateral rectus muscle.
- The goal of surgery is to achieve cosmetically straight eyes with good vision preferably binocular vision.
- The deviation in the primary position helps to decide amount of surgery and number of muscles to be operated on.
- Do not perform a graded muscle surgical approach or procedure. Adjust the amount of correction desired by operating on more muscles.
- The results of recession and resection by a definite millimeters are variable as each patient has his own problem. Assess the case individually and thereafter plan the surgery.
- It is advisable to under-correct in the young patients. A residual deviation of

about 10° or so may disappear if stereoscopic vision is established.

- Roughly 1 mm of recession or resection of the medial rectus muscle corrects about 3° of squint.
- Roughly 1 mm of recession or resection of the lateral rectus muscle corrects about 2 degrees of squint.
- When recession of medial rectus muscle is combined with resection of lateral rectus muscle then there is an increased correction of about 25% over the amount of correction if two operations are done separately with interval.
- The stronger muscle in the line of action of the deviated eye is chosen for recession. Later, if there is still some deviation then resect the opposite weaker muscle.
- The recession operation gives greater amount of correction of deviation than a similar amount of resection operation on the same muscle.
- Permanent over-correction of divergent squint is relatively rare. The over-correction tends to disappear in 6–8 weeks. The exotropia should be slightly over-corrected.
- Over-correction of convergent squint always persists.
- In esotropia, a recession of medial rectus to 5 mm gives good results in accommodative esotropia.

- A combination of 5 mm recession of medial rectus and 8 mm of lateral rectus resection is next stronger procedure for esotropia. It corrects about 25° of esotropia or more.
- A bilateral lateral rectus resection is a weak procedure for esotropia.
- A bilateral medial rectus recession is a strong procedure suitable for a case of esotropia with definite V-phenomenon.
- In esotropia, attempt to correct the smallest deviation demonstrated by the patient.
- In exotropia, attempt to correct the largest deviation demonstrated by the patient.
- In constant exotropia, one can plan to operate as follows:
  - In a lesser degree of exotropia, one can plan for recession of lateral rectus muscle and resection of medial rectus muscle in same eye.
  - Recession of both the lateral rectus muscles and resection of both the medial rectus muscles is a strong procedure.
- Large recession (more than 5 mm of medial rectus muscle) and large resection (more than 10 mm of lateral rectus muscle) tends to limit the adduction.
- In alternating squint, simultaneous bilateral surgery dividing equally in both the eyes gives good results.

37

A Case with Paralytic and Restrictive Squint

History

- Age of onset.
- Duration.
- Mode of onset-sudden or gradual.
- Any systemic illness preceding squint-fever or flu.
- Any trauma even mild.
- Squint is intermittent or constant.
- Unilateral or alternating.
- Diplopia.
- Family history.
- Systemic history of diabetes.
- Hypertension, thyroid disorder and any neurological symptoms.

CLINICAL EXAMINATION

- Inspection.
- Visual acuity.
- Refraction.
- Head posture.
- Look for ptosis.

Ocular Movements

Test uniocular as well as binocular movements in all the six diagnostic directions of gaze and straight upwards and downwards. There is limitation of the movement in the direction of action of the paralyzed muscle.

Pupillary Reaction

Pupillary reaction may be abnormal in secondary deviation due to affection of the retina and optic nerve.

Ophthalmoscopy

It reveals associated lesions of media, retina and optic nerve.

Cover Test

It will show that the secondary deviation is greater than the primary deviation. When the patient is fixing with the normal eye the deviation of the affected eye is called as primary deviation. Now cover the normal eye and let the patient fix with the affected eye and observe the normal eye behind the cover. The normal eye takes up the position brought about by the contraction of overacting synergist muscle. This is secondary deviation. In a recent case of palsy the secondary deviation is always greater than the primary deviation. In course of time due to changes in the antagonist and synergist muscles, it begins to present features of concomitant (non-paralytic) squint. A measurement of the primary and secondary deviation can be done by neutralization with prisms and most readily with prism and cover test.

Hess Screen Test

The equipment consists of a Hess screen, green spot light, switch board and red-green filter goggles. The Hess screen (Fig. 37.1) is made of a wood and painted grey. There are small circular apertures which are covered by pieces of red mica. There is a light source behind each aperture with red mica. The illumination of

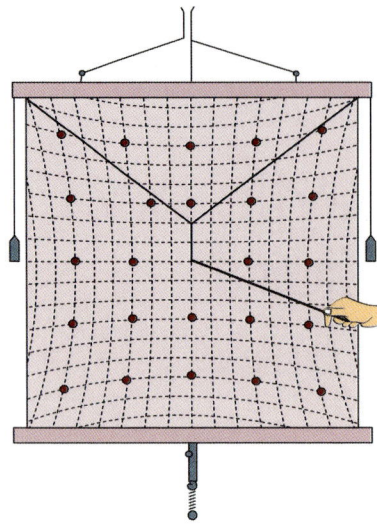

Fig. 37.1: Hess screen

each aperture is controlled by a switch board. Each of the red mica light in the screen can be switched on in turn by insertion of a plug in the corresponding switch in the switch board.

Explain the patient what he is supposed to do. He is seated in front of the screen with a spot light in his hand. Place red-green filter goggles with red filter glass in front of the right eye. The clinician then switch on the red mica light onto the screen and the patient is asked to superimpose his green spot light on to the red light. In normal case the two lights should be nearly superimposed in all nine positions of gaze. After completion of charting reverse the goggles and repeat the test and chart out the findings.

The Hess screen test gives the following information on comparing two charts:

- The smaller chart indicates the eye with paretic muscle.
- The larger chart indicates the eye with the overacting muscle.
- The smaller chart shows the restriction of field in the main direction of action of the paretic muscle.
- The larger chart shows the enlarged field in the main direction of the action of the yoke muscle.

- A record of primary and secondary deviation can be obtained which later helps in assessing the progress.
- Charting done at suitable intervals helps in judging the progress of a case.
- If paresis persists then the shape of both the charts will change. The charts will become more and more concomitant and it becomes impossible to determine the primary paretic muscle.
- Thus Hess screen test is useful in the diagnosis of the paretic muscle and very useful as a prognostic guide.

Diplopia Test

It is useful to chart the diplopia in a case of a paralytic squint. It is purely a subjective test. Mostly the patient is uncooperative. One cannot rely only on the diplopia charting. Other investigations should be performed and due weight age be given. The charting is done in a semi dark doom. Patient is asked to stand study and should move the eyes to see the bar light and not the head. The clinician stands in front with a bar light or a candle light. The red-filter goggles are placed on the patient's face with red glass in front of the right eye. The slit bar light is moved about in the field of binocular fixation in all the nine position from a distance of about four feet from the patient. The position of the images as seen by the patient are recorded upon chart with nine squares the red image with red pencil and green image with green pencil showing the tilt of the image, the distance from each other and the level between the two images.

The following information is derived from the diplopia chart:

- The diplopia is horizontal or vertical.
- The area of single vision and diplopia.
- The distance between the two images in the area of diplopia. The separation is maximal in the position of gaze of that muscle. The furthest displaced image belongs to the eye with muscle palsy.
- The images are seen on the same level or not.
- One image is tilted or both are erect.
- Diplopia is homonymous or crossed.

Forced Duction Test

Non-invasive Investigation

- Orbital ultrasonography.
- CT scan of orbit and skull.
- Neurological investigation.

Systemic Examination

- Complete neurological examination to localize the site of lesion.
- Blood pressure.
- ENT examination.

Investigation

- Blood sugar-fasting and post prandial.
- Thyroid profile.
- CT scan and MRI if indicated.

PARALYTIC SQUINT

Paralytic (incomitant) squint is a condition of dissociation of the ocular movements in which the deviation is irregular and varying in different direction of gaze. It is due to defect in the motor pathway of the binocular reflexes.

A case of a paralytic squint may show the following four characteristic changes:

1. An overaction of the ipsilateral antagonist which later on may result in permanent contracture of the muscle.
2. An overaction of the contralateral synergist muscle.
3. An under action of the antagonist muscle of the contralateral synergist muscle.
4. An over action of the ipsilateral synergist muscle.

Etiology

Any lesion of one or more cranial nerves: third, fourth, and sixth nerves can cause a paralytic squint. The following factors may be responsible for this.

- Injury
- Inflammation like syphilis, encephalitis, meningitis or viral.
- Vascular lesions like hemorrhage, arteriosclerosis aneurysm.
- Neoplasm of brain.

- Degenerative conditions.
- Multiple sclerosis.
- Metabolic factors—diabetes or anemia.
- Myogenic lesions as myasthenia and thyroid ophthalmopathy.
- Orbital apex syndrome.
- Sphenoidal fissure syndrome.

Symptoms

Diplopia

It is the diplopia which makes the patient aware of the disease. Most patients succeed in adopting a posture to neutralize the effect of diplopia.

False Orientation

There is a false orientation when the patient is trying to fix with the paretic eye. The patient tends to past-points towards the field of action of the Paralysed muscle. There is no past-pointing when fixing with the normal eye. It gives difficulty in locating objects or performing routine work which require visual coordination.

Vertigo

Due to diplopia and false orientation the patient may feel a peculiar sensation which manifests in the form of ocular vertigo.

Signs

Abnormal Deviation of Eyes

There is an abnormal deviation of the eyes in the primary position in most cases. Some cases may compensate by the exercise of fusional reflexes. A dissociation of the eyes will manifest the deviation.

Limitation of the Movement of the Eye

There is a limitation of the movements of the eye in the direction of the action of the Paralysed muscle.

Postural Change

The patient adopts a posture which will help him to overcome the distressing symptom of diplopia, false orientation and vertigo. The postural change has two components.

Face Rotation

It is adopted to neutralize the diplopia. To avoid diplopia the face is turned in the direction of field of action of the Paralysed muscle.

Head Tilting

It is adopted to neutralize vertical and torsional displacement of the image. The head tilts towards the shoulder of the side of the higher image.

Clinical Features and Management

1. Paralysed right lateral rectus muscle.
2. Paralysed right medial rectus muscle.
3. Paralysed right superior rectus muscle.
4. Paralysed right inferior rectus muscle.
5. Paralysed right superior oblique muscle.
6. Paralysed right inferior oblique muscle.

Paralysed Right Lateral Rectus Muscle

In Primary Position

In primary position, there is a convergence of the right eye due to over action of the right medial rectus which is the ipsilateral antagonist of lateral rectus.

Ocular Movements

Ocular movements show limitation of the outward movement of the eye. This limitation persists on upward and downward movement of the eye from the primary position and also from the position of right lateral gaze.

Diplopia Charting

- Uncrossed diplopia.
- Maximum separation of images towards the action of Paralysed muscle, i.e. right side.
- Occasionally some vertical displacement may be present.

Hess Charting

- Small field of the right lateral rectus muscle.

- Large field of the right medial rectus muscle.

Posture

There is a simple rotation of the face towards the right side that is towards the Paralysed side.

Paralysed Right Medial Rectus Muscle

In Primary Position

In primary position of the eye, there is slight divergence of the right eye due to over action of the right lateral rectus muscle which is ipsilateral antagonist of right medial rectus.

Ocular Movements

There is limitation of the inward movement of the eye. This limitation persists on upward and downward movement of the eye from the primary position and also from the position of gaze towards the left side.

Diplopia Charting

- There is crossed diplopia.
- Maximum separation of images toward the action of Paralysed muscle that is left side.

Hess Screen Charting

- Small field of affected right medial rectus muscle.
- Large field of normal right lateral rectus muscle.

Posture

There is a simple rotation of the face towards the left side that is towards the Paralysed side.

Paralysed Right Superior Rectus Muscle

In Primary Position

In the primary position, the right eye appears slightly downwards due to over action of the right inferior rectus muscle which is ipsilateral antagonist of right superior rectus.

Ocular Movements

- There is limitation of the movement of the

right eye in an upward and outward (up and right) direction of gaze.

- There is marked upward and inward (up and right) movement of the left eye due to an over action of the left inferior oblique which is a contralateral synergist of the right superior rectus.
- There is hypotropia of the right eye on upward movement from the primary position.
- There is extorsion on right gaze due to over action of two (both) inferior oblique muscles.

Diplopia Charting

- Diplopia is vertical.
- Maximum separation of images towards the action of Paralysed muscle that is in the up and right gaze.
- The image of the right eye is tilted towards left due to torsional effect.

Hess Screen Charting

- Small field of the right superior rectus muscle.
- Large field of the normal right inferior rectus muscle (ipsilateral antagonist).

Posture

There is rotation of face towards up and right side. There is tilting of the head towards the right side.

Paralysed Right Inferior Rectus Muscle

In Primary Position

In the primary position, the right appears slightly upwards due to over action of the right superior rectus which is ipsilateral antagonist of right inferior rectus.

Ocular Movements

- There is limitation of the movement of the right eye in an outward and downward (out and down) direction of gaze.
- There is a marked inward and downward (in and down) movement of the left eye due to over action of the left superior

oblique muscle which is a contralateral synergist of right inferior rectus muscle.

- There is hypertropia of the right eye in primary position of gaze.
- There is intorsion on right gaze due to over action of two (both) superior oblique muscles.

Diplopia Charting

- Diplopia is vertical.
- Maximum separation of images towards the action of Paralysed muscle, i.e. right and down gaze.
- The image of the right eye is tilted towards right due to torsional effect.

Hess Charting

- Small field of right inferior rectus.
- Large field of right superior rectus.

Posture

- There is rotation of face towards down and to right side.
- There is tilting of head towards the left side.

Paralysed Right Superior Oblique Muscle

in Primary Position

In primary position, the right eye appear slightly upwards due to over action of the right inferior oblique which is ipsilateral antagonist of right superior oblique.

Ocular Movements

- There is limitation of the movement of the right eye in downward and inward (down and in) direction of gaze.
- There is a marked outward and downward (out and down) movement of the left eye due to over action of the left inferior rectus muscle which is contralateral synergist of right superior oblique muscle.
- There is hypertropia of the right eye in primary position of gaze.
- There is some extorsion on left gaze due to over action of right inferior oblique muscle and right inferior rectus muscle.

Diplopia Charting

- Diplopia is vertical.
- Maximum separation of images towards the action of Paralysed muscle, i.e. downward and inward direction of gaze of right eye.
- Image of the right eye is tilted towards left because of extorsion of the eye.

Hess Charting

- Small field of right superior oblique muscle.
- Large field of right inferior oblique.

Posture

- There is rotation of face towards down and left.
- Tilting of head towards the left side.

Paralysed Right Inferior Oblique Muscle

In Primary Position

In primary position, the right eye appears slightly downwards due to over action of the right superior oblique muscle which is ipsilateral antagonist of right inferior oblique muscle.

Ocular Movements

- There is limitation of the movement of right eye in upward and inward (up and in) direction of gaze.
- There is marked upward and outward (up and out) movement of the left eye due to over action of the left superior rectus which is contralateral synergist of right inferior oblique muscle.
- There is hypotropia of right eye in primary position of gaze.
- There is some intorsion on left gaze due to over action of right superior oblique and right superior rectus muscles.

Diplopia Charting

- Diplopia is vertical.
- Maximum separation of images towards the action of the Paralysed muscle, i.e. upward and inward direction of gaze of right eye.

- Image is tilted to right side because of intorsion.

Hess Charting

- Small field of right inferior oblique.
- Large field of right superior oblique.

Posture: There is rotation of face towards up and left side. There is tilting of head towards the right side.

MANAGEMENT OF PARALYTIC SQUINT

- Treat the cause.
- Provide relief from annoying symptom of diplopia by occluding the affected eye.
- Wait for at least six months to see the progress. If the palsy has become stabilized then surgery can be done.
- Principle of surgery is to strengthening the partially Paralysed muscle by resection and weakening of the overacting muscle by recession.
- Strengthening of the totally Paralysed muscle is ineffective.
- Muscle transpositioning may be considered.
- Adjustable suture surgery may be tried.

RESTRICTIVE SQUINT

- Restrictive (incomitant) squint is characterized by marked limitation of ocular movements with positive Forced duction test.
- Restriction of ocular movements can be due to
- Muscular contracture
- Persistent abnormal position of globe in the orbit
- Post surgical adhesions or scars

Clinical Features and Management

1. Brown syndrome.
2. Duane's syndrome.
3. Congenital fibrosis of extraocular muscles.
4. Dysthyroid ophthalmopathy.
5. Blow-out fracture orbit.
6. Strabismus fixus.

BROWN SYNDROME
(Superior Oblique Sheath Syndrome)

Clinically, the characteristic feature is limitation of elevation in adduction and V pattern. On adduction the affected eye shoots down and patient is unable to elevate the eye in this adducted position. There is a normal elevation in the primary position and abduction but absent in adduction. This is all due to short sheath of the superior oblique tendon. The sheath is loose when the eye is abducted. The sheath is taut when the eye is adducted. Treat by stripping the sheath. Many cases require tenotomy or tenectomy of the affected superior oblique muscle.

DUANE'S SYNDROME
(Stilling Turk Duane Syndrome)

The clinical features include:
- Limitation of abduction giving an impression of paresis of lateral rectus muscle.
- On the attempt to adduction the affected eye retracts showing a narrow palpebral aperture.
- On the attempt to abduction there is widening of palpebral fissure.
- There is some under-action of medial rectus muscle.
- The eye shoots up if the patient looks above the midline in adducted position of the eye simulating over-action of inferior oblique muscle.
- The eye shoots down if the patient looks below the midline in adducted position of the eye simulating the over-action of superior oblique muscle.

It has been thought that this syndrome is due to fibrosis of the lateral rectus muscle. Other view is that it could be due to abnormal innervation of the lateral rectus muscle. It is to be differentiated from congenital lateral rectus muscle palsy. Under-action of the medial and lateral rectus muscle in the same eye without any previous surgery is diagnostic of Duane's syndrome.

CONGENITAL FIBROSIS OF EXTRAOCULAR MUSCLE SYNDROME

It is characterized by the defect in elevation and ptosis. The patient is unable to elevate the eye to midline neither in adducted nor in abducted position of the eyes. It is an autosomal dominant condition characterized by the fibrosis of ocular muscles. Family history is usually present. Treat by recession of inferior rectus and frontalis sling for ptosis.

DYSTHYROID OPHTHALMOPATHY

In this malady, the restrictive ocular movements are due to muscle fibrosis. Inferior and medial rectus muscles are frequently involved.
   Other clinical features include:
- Proptosis
- Chemosis
- Conjunctival congestion
- Vertical squint
- CT scan shows enlarged ocular muscles
- Manage by steroids, immunosuppressive agents.
- Radiotherapy and orbital decompression.

Refer Chapter 3: A Case with Thyroid Orbitopathy

BLOW-OUT FRACTURE OF ORBIT

Refer Chapter 46: A Case with Blow-out Fracture Orbit

STRABISMUS FIXUS

It is a condition of the eyes in which both the eyes are fixed in the convergent position due to fibrous tightening of the medial recti. Maximal recession of recti provides cosmetic relief.

Other conditions resulting in restrictive squint includes cases following trauma, surgery or myositis.

38

A Case with III, IV and VI Nerve Palsy

History

Record the history with reference to the following:
- Any diplopia.
- Any restriction in the movement of the eyes.
- Any difficulty in coming down-stairs.
- Any trauma that may be insignificant for the patient.
- Any change in hearing power.
- Any associated facial paralysis.
- Any systemic disease like diabetes.
- Any change in his posture.

CLINICAL EXAMINATION

Ocular Movements

Test the ocular movements in all the direction of gaze. Note if there is any restriction of movement of the eyeball.

Pupillary Reaction

The pupil is involved in the third nerve lesion. Test for light reflex and near reflex.

Diplopia Test

It helps to assess the progress of a case.

Hess Chart

It helps to assess the progress of a case. A case of paralytic squint in due course of time becomes a concomitant (non-paralytic) type due to contractures and changes in the antagonist, contralateral synergist, antagonist of contralateral synergist muscle of the paralyzed muscle.

Systemic Examination

It is done to exclude any systemic cause for paralysis. Hypertension, arteriosclerosis and diabetes play an important factor to be considered.

Neurological Examination

The patient must be referred to a neurologist to exclude any neurological factor. Multiple sclerosis is a common factor.

Investigation

X-ray

Sinuses and orbit shall be helpful.

CT Scan

CT scan helps to evaluate a case properly in excluding or diagnosing a lesion behind the orbit.

Laboratory Investigations

- Complete blood picture.
- VDRL.
- Blood sugar-fasting and post prandial.
- Urine examination.

Clinical Features and Management

1. Oculomotor nerve palsy
2. Trochlear nerve palsy
3. Abducens nerve palsy

OCULOMOTOR (THIRD) NERVE PALSY

Etiology

- Encephalitis.
- Orbital cellulitis.
- Cavernous sinus thrombophlebitis.
- Diabetes.
- Superior orbital fissure syndrome.
- Thyroid myopathy.
- Vascular lesions.
- Neoplastic lesions in orbit.
- Trauma.

Symptoms

The patient complains of diplopia, drooping of the lid and inability to move the eyes.

Clinical Features

- Ptosis.
- Eyeball in the abducted position.
- Limitation of movement of the eyeball in the adduction, elevation and depression.
- Pupil is dilated and fixed with no reaction to light or near reflex.
- Intorsion of the globe on attempted down-gaze due to action of superior oblique muscle.

Management

- Treat the cause.
- Surgical treatment only when there is no improvement for a period of six months and the process has stabilized.

Surgical Treatment

- A large resection of the medial rectus muscle along with large recession of the lateral rectus muscle in the affected eye. A recession of the lateral rectus in the opposite eye may be needed to achieve the desired cosmetic results.
- Frontalis sling operation for ptosis.

TROCHLEAR (FOURTH) NERVE

Etiology

Congenital

The position of the one eye is higher than the other either in the primary position or in the field of gaze. There is a head tilt.

Secondary to Closed Head Trauma

Any patient complaining of diplopia after a head injury must be suspected for superior oblique muscle palsy. It is usually a bilateral palsy.

Secondary to Vascular Diseases

It is seen in cases of diabetes, hypertension, and arteriosclerosis. A patient without any apparent cause if complains of diplopia must be suspected for the superior oblique muscle palsy. Presence of diplopia with minimal findings helps to clinch the diagnosis.

Clinical Features

Symptoms: There is diplopia particularly in a downward gaze as in coming down stairs. The patient may present with abnormal posture to avoid diplopia with depression of chin, tilting the head and occasionally turning the face to the opposite side.
- Ipsilateral hyperdeviation and excyclo-torsion.
- Limitation of eye movement in the down and in gaze, i.e. limited depression in adduction.
- An abnormal head posture.
- In a case of bilateral palsy.
  Right hyperdeviation in left gaze and left hyperdeviation in the right gaze.
  There is a V-esotropia, i.e. eyes are converged in down gaze but straight in up gaze.

Management

- Trochlear nerve is the longest of all the cranial nerves. It is very slender nerve. It is the only nerve which emerges from the dorsal aspect of the brain. It is the only nerve which crosses to the opposite side. Usually there is spontaneous improvement in the palsy of this nerve.
- Prescribe prism to help correct the diplopia.

Surgical Management

- Recession of the Inferior oblique— the ipsilateral overacting antagonist muscle—the inferior oblique about 10–12 mm and/or recession of the overacting contralateral synergist the inferior rectus muscle.

- If there is still an under correction then tucking of the paretic superior oblique muscle can be done.

ABDUCENS (SIXTH) NERVE PALSY

History

Ask the patient about any history of trauma, diabetes, loss of hearing. Look for any signs of facial nerve palsy.

Etiology

- The most common causes for an isolated paresis of the sixth nerve are Collier's sphenoidal palsy and Superior orbital fissure syndrome
- Involvement of the seventh nerve indicates a nuclear lesion as the sixth nerve nucleus is closely related to the fasciculus of the seventh nerve. *An isolated palsy of sixth nerve is never nuclear in origin.*
- Any rise of intracranial pressure can cause stretching of the sixth nerve over the petrous tip. In such condition the palsy may be bilateral.
- In its long course it may be affected by acoustic neurinomas, nasopharyngeal tumor, fractures, raised intracranial pressure, otitis media, cavernous sinus thrombophlebitis and superior orbital fissure syndrome.

Clinical Features

- Limitation of abduction.
- Esotropia in primary position.
- Uncrossed diplopia.
- There is turning of face towards the affected side to avoid diplopia (Fig. 38.1).

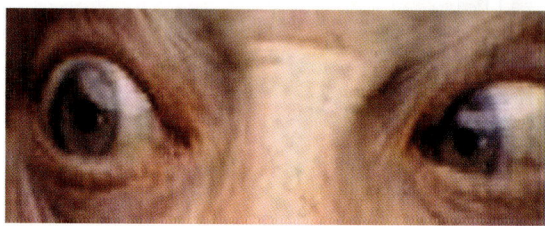

Fig. 38.1: Abducens (VI) nerve palsy

Management

- Treat the cause.
- Surgery after stabilization of the process.

Surgical Management

A recession of medial rectus muscle to 5 mm alone or combined with resection of paretic lateral rectus muscle shall relieve the esotropia. Some case may need recession of the opposite medial rectus muscle also.

39

A Case with Brain Tumor

History

Record the history with reference to the following:
- Headache which is relieved by vomit.
- Headache which increases on coughing and straining.
- Vomit is not accompanied by nausea.
- Any mental symptoms.
- Any history of epilepsy.
- Any history of convulsions.
- Any pain in and around the eye.
- Any change in the level of the eyes.
- Any history of diplopia.
- Any history of hallucination.
- Any loss of vision.
- Any history of missing reading on one side or collusion with people and home furniture without any obvious reason.

CLINICAL EXAMINATION

Inspection

Look for ptosis, ocular movements, nystagmus, squint, conjugate deviation of the eyes, pupillary reaction and proptosis.

Ocular Movements

Test the ocular movements in all the cardinal direction and make a note if there is any involvement of third, fourth, and sixth nerve palsy.

Visual Acuity

Record the visual acuity with and without glasses. Check the refractive error.

Ophthalmoscopy

Ophthalmoscopy may show optic atrophy or papilledema.

Cranial Nerves

Examine all the cranial nerves and note the results.
- Olfactory loss with visual loss is a clue to an olfactory groove meningioma.
- While testing the fifth nerve test all the area covered by the three branches. Test the touch and pin prick sensation separately. Preservation of the touch sensation with loss of pin prick sensation is indicative of an intrinsic brainstem lesion.
- Be careful to differentiate a peripheral and central lesion of seventh nerve. The forehead area has a bilateral innervation.

Neurological Examination

A patient with a suspicion of a brain tumor must be thoroughly checked for any neurological lesion.

CLINICAL INVESTIGATION

Visual Fields

There are several techniques available for charting visual fields. Confrontation method is an easy and quick way of screening. Tangent screen charting for central fields and Lister perimeter or Goldmann perimeter for peripheral fields is advisable.

251

Defect in the visual field is indicative of a supratentorial lesion near chiasma and optic tract.

Photo Stress Test

A patient of brain tumor usually presents with a monocular loss of vision due to affection of optic nerve. In early stage the optic disk appears normal. The photo stress test shows delayed recovery in a case with retinal lesion and normal recovery in a case with optic nerve lesion. Both the eyes should be tested separately for the comparison.

Color Vision Test

A significant defect in color vision is indicative of a diffuse optic nerve lesion due to pressure or demyelination. Normal color vision in a patient with optic nerve disease excludes a pressure lesion of the optic nerve due to tumor.

Opticokinetic Nystagmus

It can be easily tested on a rotating drum with regularly placed alternate dark and white stripes. It helps to diagnose a case of malingering about visual loss. The presence of opticokinetic nystagmus in infants or children who are not able to read or cooperate to read shows that the patient is not blind.

Fluorescein Angiography

Fluorescein angiography in a case of papilledema shows capillary dilation and telangiectatic changes of the disk capillaries. There is leakage of fluorescein from the capillaries over the disk which persists for hours. It is diagnostic of papilledema.

CT Scan

It is the procedure of choice to diagnose intracranial lesion. It is a non invasive procedure and gives quick and reliable results.

Magnetic Resonance Imaging

Magnetic resonance imaging is an imaging technique with the highest sensitivity for characterization of pathology such as tumors, inflammation and infection as well as normal tissue.

Visual Evoked Potential

It helps in diagnosis of optic nerve lesion, localization of lesion in the visual pathway, diagnosis of multiple sclerosis, and monitoring of optic nerve function during intraorbital and intra-cranial surgical procedures.

Cerebral Angiography

It is very helpful in diagnosis of vascular tumors and lesions of brain. It helps to locate even a small vascular lesion when even the computerized tomography scanning may miss the pathology.

GENERAL SYMPTOMS

Headache

Headache is one of the early symptoms. It has no localizing value as its intensity and the site varies. It is due to traction or stretching of structures at the base of the brain like major arteries and veins, the dural sinuses and sensory cranial nerves. A rise in the intracranial pressure or the growth itself can displace the sensitive structure causing headache.

Vomiting

Vomiting is also one of the early symptom caused by the rise in the intracranial pressure or by direct involvement of the brainstem. It has no relation to intake of food and is not accompanied by nausea.

Raised Intracranial Pressure

The rise in the intracranial pressure occurs due to direct effect of the tumor mass, cerebral edema, obstruction to the flow of cerebrospinal fluid, obstruction to venous drainage and interference in the absorption of cerebrospinal fluid. It has no localizing value. There is an early rise of intracranial pressure in the infratentorial tumors.

Mental Symptoms

Patient may show behavior changes, fatigue, irritability, lack of impulse, lethargy, disorientation, depression, euphoria, silly joking and improper judgment.

Epilepsy

Any epileptic attack after the age of 20 must be seen with suspicion. An epileptic attack in the fourth to sixth decade is likely to be due to tumor. Epileptic attacks are more common with supratentorial tumors, tumors which grow slowly and the tumors in the temporal lobe. Tumor is a rare cause of epilepsy in children.

GENERAL OCULAR SIGNS

Ocular Pain

The sensory supply to the eye is by the ophthalmic division of fifth nerve. Any lesion affecting this nerve can give rise to an ocular pain. There is neuralgia and not isolated pain. The following conditions may give rise to neuralgia:

- Superior orbital fissure syndrome
- Cavernous sinus thrombosis
- Neurinoma of trigeminal nerve
- Tumor within gasserian ganglion
- Trigeminal neuralgia
- Tumor in middle fossa
- Tumor in posterior fossa.

Loss of Vision

Loss of vision occurs in the tumors close to optic nerve, chiasma and optic tract. Patient complains of misty vision as if seeing through a veil and continues to deteriorate resulting in complete loss in one eye and affecting the other eye. In early stage the fundus is normal and so can lead to a diagnosis of retrobulbar neuritis. Later the optic disk shows pallor or optic atrophy. A case with raised intracranial pressure may show papilledema.

Optic Hallucination

Formed images of people, animals and objects are seen in a lesion of temporal lobe. Unformed images of light such as flashes, colored spots, circles, flicker lights are seen in the lesion of occipital lobe.

Field Defects

Patient with field defect may experience following:

- Collide to one or both sides with persons or objects without any apparent cause.
- A driver may hit the garrage wall while parking in the garrage or may ride the side path of pedestrians while driving.
- Likely to write beyond the margin of paper.
- Likely to miss words on one or both sides while reading.

All these experiences can be explained by the fact that the hemianopic field defect caused by a tumor is only relative in the sense of so-called Visual inattention. The patient in his daily life is not aware of this but charting will show the field defect.

Visual field defects are caused by supratentorial tumors as these tumors affect the visual pathway.

Papilledema

Papilledema is the passive edema of the optic disk caused by the raised intracranial pressure. The rise in the intraocular pressure occurs early in infratentorial tumors and tumors of third ventricles. As a rule papilledema is bilateral. It may be unilateral in Foster Kennedy syndrome (In a frontal lobe tumor due to compression there may be optic atrophy in one eye and papilledema in other due to raised intracranial pressure) and pre-existing unilateral optic atrophy. Asymmetry of the papilledema does not indicate the side of lesion.

Extrocular Muscle Palsies

The raised intracranial pressure or the tumor mass itself can cause displacement or stretching of the intracranial nerves resulting in the loss of function. Sixth nerve is usually the first nerve to be affected. It has a very long course and thus can be compressed between dura and vessels or at the sharp superior ridge of pterous bone. It has no localizing value. Involvement of other cranial nerves should alert the ophthalmologist and the case must be further investigated.

A palsy of sixth, third, fourth and corneal anesthesia indicates a lesion in the cavernous sinus and orbital fissure.

A sixth nerve palsy with peripheral facial palsy is suggestive of an intra-axial pontine lesion.

A sixth and seventh nerve palsy with ipsilateral unilateral deafness points to a lesion at the cerebellopontine angle.

Proptosis

Proptosis is seen in cases of sphenoid ridge meningioma which extends in the orbit.

Nystagmus

- An isolated nystagmus has no localizing value.
- Seesaw nystagmus with bitemporal field defect indicates a tumor around chiasma.
- Convergence retraction nystagmus is most frequently seen in cases of pinealoma.
- Primary position upbeating nystagmus with increased amplitude on looking upwards suggests a midline cerebellar lesion.
- A lesion in the cerebellum and/or posterior fossa results in horizontal jerk nystagmus.
- Dysfunction of the cerebellum causes ocular flutter and rebound nystagmus.

Clinical Features and Management

1. Frontal lobe tumor
2. Sphenoid ridge meningioma
3. Temporal lobe tumor
4. Parietal lobe tumor
5. Occipital lobe tumor
6. Pituitary adenoma
7. Craniopharyngioma

FRONTAL LOBE TUMOR

The common tumors affecting frontal lobe are glioma, meningioma, ependymomas and vascular tumors.

Mental Symptoms

- Early mental symptoms are silly joking, euphoria, depression, withdrawn behavior, lack of initiative, irritable and apathy.
- Late mental symptoms are memory loss, lack of judgment, disorientation and irrational thinking.

Motor Sign

Forced grasping is diagnostic sign of a frontal lobe tumor. Patient has a violent grasping movement of the hand if an object is placed in hand.

Ocular Signs

- Visual loss in the eye on the affected side. It is due to pressure of the tumor on the optic nerve.
- Papilledema may occur usually on the opposite side if there is a raised intracranial pressure.
- Bitemporal hemianopia if the tumor extends posteriorly and interiorly affecting the chiasma.
- Conjugate horizontal deviation of the eyes with turning of the head away from the side of the tumor.
- Sixth nerve palsy is common due to raised intracranial pressure.

Diagnosis

Frontal lobe tumor grows slowly and symptoms appear late therefore CT scan and MRI is advisable early to detect the tumor.

Treatment

Early surgery to resect the meningioma is rewarding.

SPHENOID RIDGE MENINGIOMA

Sphenoid ridge meningioma affects middle-aged people. It has no localizing signs. Its extension into the orbit through the sphenoidal fissure manifests in form of visual loss, proptosis and varying degree of ophthalmoplegia.

Visual Loss

There is a gradual loss of vision in the eye on the side of tumor. Patient complains of blurring of vision. Fundus examination may show a normal disk leading to a diagnosis of optic neuritis. The patient continues to complain of dim vision. Later the optic disk may show pallor.

Proptosis

Unilateral proptosis occurs due to anterior extension of the tumor in the orbit through the orbital fissure. Obstruction in the venous return causes congestion of the eye and even edema of the optic disk.

Ophthalmoplegia

The sixth nerve is the first nerve to be affected. Later other cranial nerves may be involved including the ophthalmic division of fifth nerve. The clinical picture may simulate an orbital apex syndrome.

Diagnosis

Ocular signs and CT scanning help to locate it early and with accuracy.

Management

Treatment is surgical excision.

TEMPORAL LOBE TUMOR

The common tumors affecting the temporal lobe are glioma, meningioma, metastatic tumors and angioma.

- Symptoms due to raised intracranial pressure appear late.
- Seizures are the most important symptom complex of temporal lobe tumors.
- Olfactory hallucination-feeling of foul or unpleasant odor.
- Gustatory hallucination-feeling of peculiar taste.
- Visual hallucination-as formed images of people, animals, objects, etc. Objects appear smaller or further away.
- Fear and anxiety.
- Aphasia and word deafness.

Ocular Signs

- Homonymous hemianopia which may be complete or incomplete and incongruous. A superior quadrantanopia is also seen.
- Sixth nerve palsy manifests as lateral rectus palsy.

Diagnosis

- Formed visual hallucination.
- Seizure complex.
- CT scanning.

Treatment

It is surgical.

PARIETAL LOBE TUMOR

The common parietal lobe tumors are glioma, meningioma, vascular tumors, ependymomas and metastatic tumors.

Symptoms

- Alexia—inability to read.
- Agraphia—inability to write.
- Acalculia—inability to calculate.

Ocular Signs

- Homonymous hemianopia. The tumor can extend to occipital lobe so one cannot diagnose a parietal lobe tumor only on the basis of field defect.
- Asymmetric opthcokinetic nystagmus.

Diagnosis

- CT scanning.
- Cerebral angiography.

Treatment

Surgical excision and radiotherapy.

OCCIPITAL LOBE TUMOR

Neurologically, the occipital lobe is a silent zone.

The common occipital lobe tumors are glioma, meningioma, metastatic tumors and angioma.

There are no typical neurological features except the visual disturbances which help in the diagnosis.

Ocular Signs and Symptoms

- Complete hemianopia with both splitting and sparing of the macula is the main visual field defect.
- Field defects are congruous.
- Visual hallucination of unformed images such as flashes, flickering lights, colored spots, circles are of diagnostic value.
- Cortical blindness does not occur in the occipital lobe tumors.

- Cortical blindness typically occurs in ischemic lesions of visual cortex.
- There is absence of asymmetric optico-kinetic nystagmus. The presence of opticokinetic nystagmus indicates extension of tumor in the parietal lobe.
- Oculomotor palsies occur due to raised intracranial pressure.
- Papilledema may be seen.
- Patient may complain of periorbital pain.

Diagnosis

CT scanning can locate a mass.

Treatment

Surgical excision and radiotherapy if indicated.

PITUITARY ADENOMA

There are three types of pituitary adenoma:
- Eosinophilic adenoma.
- Basophilic adenoma.
- Chromophobe adenoma.

Eosinophilic Adenoma

There is an increased secretion of growth hormone producing acromegaly in adults and gigantism in young. Patient shows enlarged hands and feet, prominent jaw, thick tongue with amenorrhea in females and impotency in males. No ocular findings.

Basophilic Adenoma

There is an increased secretion of adreno-corticotropin hormone (ACTH) which results in Cushing's syndrome. The clinical features are adiposity, round moon like face, hypertension, hypogonadism and osteoporosis. No ocular findings.

Chromophobe Adenoma

It is one of the most common intracranial tumor. About 50% of cases show endocrine disturbance like delayed growth (pituitary dwarfism), adiposogenital dystrophy, sexual disturbances in form of amenorrhea and impotence, less growth of hairs specially beard, weight gain, dryness and atrophy of skin, hypoglycemia and diabetes insipidus (Fig. 39.1).

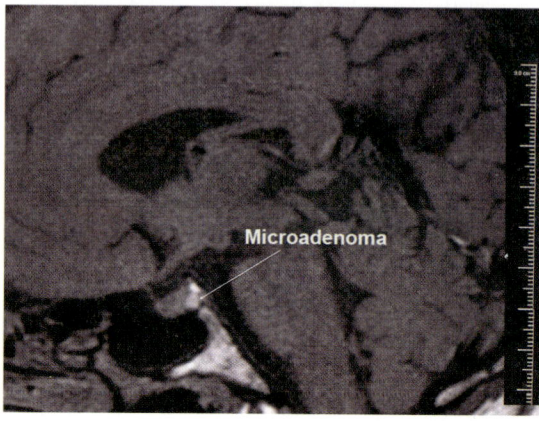

Fig. 39.1: Pituitary adenoma

Headache

The patient may complain of a bursting headache. It is caused by stretching of the major arteries and dura at the base of the brain. The headache may be frontal, bi-temporal or behind the eyeball.

Loss of Vision

The visual loss is gradual affecting one eye first followed by the other. Patient complains of dim and foggy vision as if seeing through a veil. The optic disk is normal so it usually leads to a diagnosis of retrobulbar neuritis.

Field Defect

Bitemporal hemianopia is the pathognomonic visual field defect of chromophobe adenoma. The earliest field defect is the bitemporal superior quadrantanopia followed by lower temporal quadrant then lower nasal quadrant and last to be affected is the upper nasal quadrant. The field defect shows a clockwise rotation in the right eye and counterclockwise rotation in the left eye. The presence of field defect indicates that tumor is of a considerable size.

Optic Atrophy

To begin with there is only pallor of the optic disk. In due course of time one disk may show atrophy while the other only pallor. Presence of optic atrophy indicates poor prognosis.

Ophthalmoplegia

It is rare. It occurs when there is an extrasellar expansion of tumor. The third, fourth and sixth nerve may be involved. Patient complains of diplopia.

Other Findings

Papilledema occurs due to obstruction of third ventricle. Proptosis may occur if there is pressure on the cavernous sinus resulting in stasis of venous return. See-saw nystagmus has been observed in some cases.

Diagnosis

- Plain X-ray skull for pituitary fossa shows ballooning of the sella with enlargement, thinning of the floor of the sella, destruction of the dorsum sella and destruction of the anterior clinoid process.
- Field changes.
- Visual loss with optic atrophy.
- CT scanning.

Treatment

- Surgical excision
- Radiotherapy only or following surgery.
- Medical therapy with bromocriptine.

Bromocriptine causes an increase in the secretion of prolactin-inhibiting factor by the hypothalamus there by blocks the secretion of prolactin by anterior pituitary. It results in shrinkage of prolactin secreting tumor. Many tumors of chromphobe adenoma secrete prolactin and have been referred as Prolactinomas.

CRANIOPHARYNGIOMA

It is a congenital tumor. It originates from the squamous epithelial cell rests which are remnants of Rathke's pouch. It can be primary suprasellar or intrasellar in origin. These are predominantly tumors of childhood. It does occur in the sixth and the seventh decade of life (Fig. 39.2).

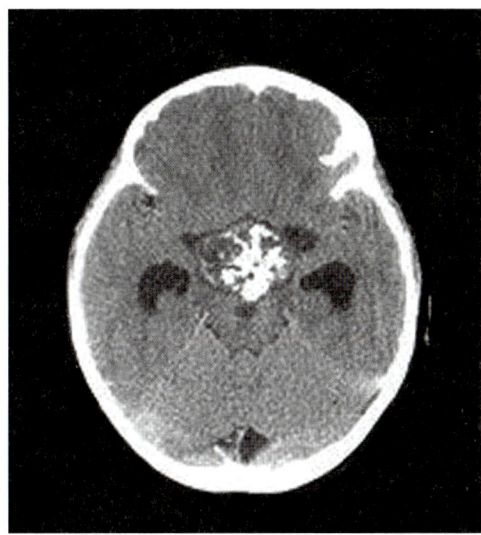

Fig. 39.2: Craniopharyngioma

Symptoms

Symptoms occur early and vary with age. Symptoms are due to endocrine disturbances.

In Children

The common symptoms are adiposogenital dystrophy, obesity, pituitary dwarfism, gonadal atrophy and cachexia.

In Young Adults

Patient presents with infantile body configuration, sparse hairs, amenorrhea, impotence and diabetes insipidus.

In Older

Endocrine disturbances are not conspicuous as in children and young adults.

Ocular Signs

- Headache and vomiting as a manifestation of raised intracranial pressure.
- Loss of vision is due to gradual onset of optic atrophy.

- Bitemporal hemianopia seen in intraseller type of craniopharyngioma.
- Concomitant squint with marked visual loss may be seen in children and may lead to a diagnosis of strabismic amblyopia. Fundus examination shows optic atrophy as the cause of visual loss and thus a need to further investigate the case.

Diagnosis

- A child with endocrine disturbances.
- Headache and vomiting.

- Visual loss and field changes in adults.
- X-ray of skull for pituitary fossa shows suprasellar calcification, a classical finding in craniopharyngioma. In intrasellar type there is ballooning of the fossa.
- Percussion of head in children may result in a resonance of a cracked pot—a sign of suture rupture.
- CT scan helps in early diagnosis.

Treatment

- Excision of tumor and radiotherapy.

40

A Case with Nystagmus

History

Record the history with reference to the following:

In Child

- If the patient is a child, then enquire whether nystagmus was noticed soon after birth or later.
- Any change in his head posture like nodding, torticollis or abnormal head movements.
- Any squint.
- About vision whether normal or reduced.
- Any white reflex from the pupil.
- Any congenital defect in the family members like albinism, Leber's optic atrophy.

In Adult

- Any history of oscillopsia.
- Any history of vertigo.
- Any abnormal feeling.
- Any neurological disease (demyelinating).
- Any vascular accident.
- Usually ophthalmologist is called to examine the case for fundus and then he may notice abnormality in pupil and nystagmus.

CLINICAL EXAMINATION

Inspection

Make the patient sit comfortably and observe the nystagmus and note its rate, amplitude, direction and type of movement.

Ocular Movements

Check the eye movements and simultaneously nystagmus in all the positions of gaze including convergence.

Pupillary Reaction

A normal light reflex in both the eyes helps to exclude sensory lesion to an extent.

Ophthalmoscopy

- Examine the media especially for lens opacities which may be the cause for dim vision and nystagmus in a child.
- Examine fundus for macular and optic nerve lesions in child.
- Examine fundus for any evidence of papilledema.

Radiography

- Radiography of cervical region.
- Laminograms.

CT Scan

CT scan is must in a case who has come to an ophthalmologist first with nystagmus and associated symptoms of oscillopsia and vertigo.

Neurological Examination

It is a must in every case to exclude any demyelinating or other neurological lesions.

Optokinetic Nystagmus Test

It is useful to detect a malingerer.
It is useful to assess vision in small children.

Vestibular Nystagmus Test

It is useful to detect a lesion of vestibule. It is commonly used by ear, nose, and throat surgeon.

NYSTAGMUS

Nystagmus is defined as regular and rhythmic to-and-fro involuntary oscillations of the eyes. It must be differentiated from nystagmoid and myoclonic movements of the eyes.

Nystagmus is characterized by the following:

- Frequency—the oscillations are rapid or slow.
- Amplitude—the oscillations are coarse or fine.
- Direction—the oscillations are horizontal, vertical or rotary.
- Movement—the oscillations are pendular or jerky.
- Pendular nystagmus—the eye movements are of equal velocity in each direction-horizontal, vertical, oblique or rotary.
- Jerk nystagmus—there is a slow movement of the eye in one direction and fast movement of the eye in the other direction. The direction of jerk nystagmus is defined by the direction of the rapid movement.
- Nystagmus may be latent or manifest.

A patient of nystagmus shall show all the above characteristics. The surgeon must make a note of all the characteristics of nystagmus in the case to assess it properly.

Etiology

Nystagmus manifests due to disorder of:
- Sensory visual pathways.
- Vestibular apparatus.
- Semicircular canals.
- Mid-brain and cerebellum.

Clinical Types and Features

1. Physiological nystagmus.
2. Sensory deprivation nystagmus.
3. Motor imbalance nystagmus.
4. Nystagmoid movements.

Physiological Nystagmus

It is of three types: Endpoint, optokinetic and vestibular.

i. *Endpoint mystagmus:* The nystagmus is of jerk type, moderate frequency, fine and horizontal. It is seen when the eyes are in extreme right or left gaze.

ii. *Optokinetic nystagmus:* It is a jerk type of nystagmus. It is induced by moving an object repeatedly across the visual field of the patient. A rotating drum painted with alternate black and white strips is the most common method. It is useful in detecting malingerers and for testing the vision in small children. There is low movement of the eye when it follows the target and fast movement when the eyes move back to refixate the target (Fig. 40.1). Similar phenomenon occurs while looking outside from a moving train.

iii. *Physiological vestibular nystagmus:* It is a jerk type of nystagmus. It is induced by pouring cold or hot water into the ear. It is caused by altered input from the vestibular nuclei to the horizontal gaze centers. If cold water is poured into the right ear the patient will develop a left jerk nystagmus (fast movement towards left side). Now if hot water is poured into the right ear the patient will develop a right jerk nystagmus (fast movement towards the right side). Thus remember as -cold opposite side and warm -same side.

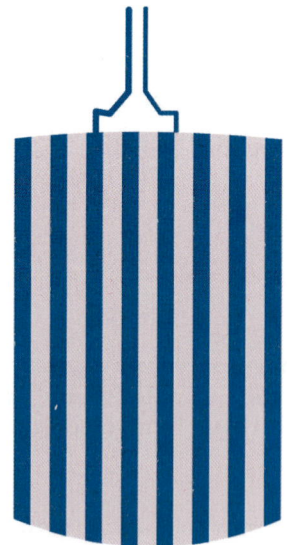

Fig. 40.1: Opticokinetic drum

Sensory Deprivation Nystagmus
(Afferent Defect)

i. *Congenital pendular nystagmus:* Congenital sensory deprivation nystagmus is pendular, slow and horizontal. Patient may develop an abnormal head posture. It occurs due to defect in ocular fixation due to reduced visual acuity. The common causes are congenital cataract, congenital toxoplasmosis, macular hypoplasia, aniridia, albinism, and Leber's congenital optic atrophy. The child develops nystagmus if he loses vision prior to the age of two. The child does not develop nystagmus if he loses the vision after the age of six.

ii. *Miner's rotatory nystagmus:* It is rapid and rotatory type of nystagmus. It is seen most commonly in coal mine workers. It occurs due to fixation problems in dim illumination.

Motor Imbalance Nystagmus
(Efferent Defect)

i. *Congenital nystagmus:* It is apparent at birth or shortly after. It is transmitted as X-linked recessive or autosomal dominant trait. It may be associated with squint or abnormal head movements. It is bilateral, horizontal jerk nystagmus with rapid phase towards lateral side. It is not present during sleep. Vision is variable. The patient does not complain of vertigo, false projection and oscillopsia. He is not aware of it.

ii. *Latent nystagmus:* It is a jerk type of nystagmus, which occurs in the condition of uniocular fixation when one eye is covered. It does not occur when both eyes are open. Nystagmus is seen in both the eyes. It is usually seen in cases of congenital esotropia. The direction of movement is towards the uncovered eye.

iii. *Spasmus nutans:* It is characterized by nystagmus, head nodding and torticollis. The head nodding and nystagmus may be present independently or together. The nystagmus is asymmetrical, pendular, fine and rapid. It is an acquired nystagmus affecting children from the age of four months to one year and resolves within a period of four years. It may be associated with squint. There is no neurological problem associated with it.

iv. *Down beat nystagmus:* It is characterized by the fast phase (movement) of the eye downwards. It is apparent in any position of gaze. Patients with down beat nystagmus may complain of oscillopsia, difficulty in balance and a feeling of being propelled backwards. Down beat nystagmus is associated with a lesion involving the cervicomedullary junction at the foramen magnum.

The common causes are Arnold-Chiari syndrome, platybasia and Klippel-Feil sign. It has been observed with meningiomas at the foramen magnum, and with vascular lesions and demyelinating lesions of the medulla. Clinically a downbeat nystagmus point towards a localized area of pathology. X-ray cervical region including laminagrams are helpful.

v. *Upbeat nystagmus:* It is characterized by fast phase (movement) of the eye upwards. It is associated with lesions at posterior fossa.

vi. *See-saw nystagmus:* It is characterized by a pattern of ocular movements in which one eye moves upwards and intorts while the other eye moves downwards and extorts. An association of bi-temporal hemianopia suggests a lesion of chiasma.

vii. *Periodic alternating nystagmus:* It is characterized by a rhythmic change in the direction and amplitude of jerks of the eyes. A patient who shows a jerk nystagmus to right, on observation shows a decrease in the amplitude and frequency until there is no nystagmus. After a lapse of time the nystagmus begins this time slowly to the left and shows increase in the frequency and amplitude for several minutes and again shows decrease and no nystagmus.

The cycle repeats. This periodic alternating nystagmus may be congenital or acquired. If it is acquired then it may be associated with brainstem lesion which may be vascular or demyelinating. It may be seen following encephalitis and cerebellar degeneration.

viii. *Convergence-retraction nystagmus:* It is characterized by a jerk nystagmus in which the fast phase of the eye movement is inwards. Both the eyes show movement inwards as in convergence movement. This movement of each eye towards each other inwards is associated with retraction of the eyeball in the orbit. This type of nystagmus has been observed in the lesions of pre-tectal area which may be vascular lesions or pinealomas.

ix. *Ataxic nystagmus:* It occurs in the abducting eye in association with internuclear ophthalmoplegia.

x. *Gaze paretic nystagmus:* It is a nystagmus which is the result of the patient's attempt to gaze in the direction affected by neurologic lesion. To begin with there is a gaze palsy. With recovery patient is able to move the eye but is not able to maintain gaze. Gaze paretic nystagmus is a jerk nystagmus which is coarse, of large amplitude and irregular in nature. It is associated with gaze mechanism. It may be seen during recovery from cerebral or pontine lesions which show a horizontal gaze nystagmus. A vertical gaze nystagmus is seen in lesions of pretectal area.

Nystagmoid Movements

There are ocular movements that mimic ocular nystagmus. These are ocular flutter, opsoclonus, superior oblique myokymia and ocular bobbing. These are seen in cases of encephalitis, pontine lesions and dysfunction of brainstem.

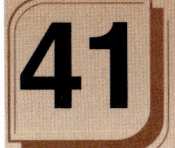

41

A Case with Visual Field Defect

History

Record the history with reference to the following:
- When he noticed first about the defect.
- Any history of collusion with the people on one side.
- Any history of missing lines on one side of paper.
- Any history of riding pedestrians.
- Any associated symptoms like headache, giddiness, vertigo, nausea, vomiting.
- Any change in visual acuity.
- Any change in refraction.
- Any history of seeing a black spot in the field of vision.

CLINICAL EXAMINATION

Visual Acuity

The visual field defect arises due to a lesion of visual pathway. Any lesion of visual pathway is likely to affect the vision. It is essential to record the visual acuity carefully and comparing the vision in two eyes about brightness.

Pupillary Reactions

Elicit the pupillary reactions and make a note about it. Pupillary reaction can give a fair idea about the site of the lesion.

Ocular Movements

Test the ocular movements in all the direction. Any paralysis of a muscle indicates a lesion of the third, fourth and sixth nerve. These can get involved in any intracranial or intraorbit lesion.

Ophthalmoscopy

Direct and indirect ophthalmoscopy is needed to diagnose a lesion of retina and optic nerve which may be responsible for the field defect.

Systemic Examination

The patient with field defect must be thoroughly examined to exclude any systemic lesion especially neurological lesion and to exclude chronic systemic affection especially respiratory and urogenital tract lesions. Dental check up to exclude any septic focus.

Investigations

X-ray skull for any lesion in the pituitary fossa and cranium.
X-ray paranasal sinuses to exclude septic focus.

CT Scan and MRI

If the examination of the patient indicates any intracranial or orbital lesion then it is essential to get CT scan. If there is no positive finding even then it is necessary to get CT scan to exclude any lesion. MRI gives better resolution.

VISUAL FIELD DEFECT

Visual field form an important ophthalmic investigation. If performed carefully it gives a fair indication about the site of the lesion from retina to visual cortex.

Clinical features of visual field defect

1. Methods of visual field charting.
2. Visual pathways.
3. Types of visual field defects.
4. Field defects at various levels of visual pathway and their common causes.
5. Clinical condition and its visual field defect.

Methods of Visual Field Charting

- Confrontation test.
- Perimeter.
- Tangent screen.
- Stereocampimetry.
- Flicker fusion perimetry.
- Multiple pattern test of Harrington and Flocks.
- Ishihara and Amsler charts.

The most commonly used methods for field charting in a clinical practice and hospitals are by the confrontation test, perimeter and Tangent screen.

Confrontation Test for Visual Field Defect

Make the patient sit comfortably in front and at the same level. Explain the patient what you shall be doing and what you expect from him. Ask the patient to cover one eye and fix his gaze at the examiner's opposite eye. Then show fingers to him separately in each of the four quadrants of the field. If the answer is correct then show fingers in two quadrants simultaneously upper and lower. If the response is normal then present the hand simultaneously both upper quadrants, both lower quadrants, upper and lower quadrant on the same side. This last test if normal then one cannot expect a significant field defect on charting with perimeter. This test is simple, quick and can be done even at bed side and effective for screening the cases for the peripheral field defects.

Kinetic Perimetry

In kinetic perimetry a stimulus of known luminance is moved from the periphery towards the center in various isopters. The confrontation test, Lister perimeter, Goldmann perimeter and Tangent screen comes under the kinetic perimetry.

Static Perimetry

In this a stimulus is presented in a predetermined position for a preset duration. Automated perimeters test the visual field by a static method.

Automated Perimetry

In an automated perimeter the computer performs the perimetry and records the results in both the geographical manner and numerical forms.

Tangent Screen Examination

It is done for testing the central visual field defect. It is better to use a 2 meter screen and a white object on a black screen. Patient is asked to sit at 2 meter distance and his one eye is covered. The examiner brings the object from periphery to center in different meridians and make a note of the area of no sensitivity. It is repeated with the other eye.

Lister Perimeter

The most commonly used perimeter is the lister perimeter. After making the patient sit, adjust his chin so that the eye is in level with the fixation point on the perimeter. The other eye is covered. Explain the method and time when he is supposed to notify the target. If in doubt repeat it. Move the arc to a new meridian and move the target and on the sound, click the chart.

Visual Pathways

The visual pathway comprises of retina, optic nerve, optic chiasma, optic tract, lateral geniculate body, optic radiation and occipital cortex.

- The first visual neuron is formed by rods and cones.
- The second visual neuron is formed by the bipolar cells.
- The third visual neuron is formed by the ganglion cells.

The axons from the ganglion cells forms the nerve fiber layer and passes out as optic nerve that crosses at chiasma to emerge as optic tract and ends in the lateral geniculate body.

- The fourth visual neuron emerges from the lateral geniculate body. The axons of fourth visual neuron emerge as optic radiations and ends in the visual cortex in the calcarine area of occipital lobe.

The course of fiber is associated with crossing, shifting, looping and intermingling and final rearrangement in the cortex.

At Retina

The fibers from the nasal part of retina converge on the nasal third of the disk.

The fibers from the temporal retina have an arcuate course due to a horizontal raphe and ends in the upper and lower part of the disk.

The fibers from the macular area form papillomacular bundle and ends in the temporal side of the disk.

In the Optic Nerve

Arrangement of fibers in the optic nerve behind the eyeball is same. After a little distance the Papillomacular bundle occupies the central place.

Chiasma

- The inferior nasal fibers in the optic nerve move anteriorly making a bend and cross to the opposite optic tract to end in the inferior nasal quadrant of the optic tract.
- The superior nasal fibers in optic nerve move posteriorly making a bend and cross to the opposite optic tract to end in the superior nasal quadrant of the optic tract.
- The temporal fibers of the optic nerve pass through the chiasma without crossing in the optic tract of the same side.

Lateral Geniculate Body

The fibers of the optic tract end in the lateral geniculate body. As the nerve fibers travel up towards lateral geniculate body, a nasal rotation takes place so that the horizontal meridian becomes vertical in the geniculate body. Thus the superior fibers are placed medially and the inferior fibers are placed laterally in the geniculate body. The macular fibers are central.

Optic Radiations

The axons of fourth neuron emerge from the lateral geniculate body to form optic radiation. There is a temporal rotation thereby the superior retina fibers occupying the medial position in the lateral geniculate body, now pass in the upper part of the optic radiation and the inferior retinal fibers occupying the lateral position in the lateral geniculate body now pass in the lower part of the optic radiation.

The inferior retinal fibers occupying the lateral position in the geniculate body spread out anteriorly and form a loop known as Meyer's loop around the inferior horn of lateral ventricle towards the pole of temporal lobe before ending in the cortex. Therefore, in a temporal lobe lesion the inferior retinal fibers are involved so the visual defect is in the superior quadrant.

Occipital Cortex

The optic radiations terminate in area 17 of the occipital cortex. The superior retinal fibers occupying the upper part in the optic radiations end in the upper calcarine fissure. The inferior retinal fibers occupying the lower part of the optic radiations end in the lower calcarine fissure. The macular fibers are at the tip of the occipital cortex.

Types of Visual Field Defects
(Figs 41.1 and 41.2)

Central Scotoma

It is a small island of field defect that includes the point of fixation.

Paracentral Scotoma

It is a field defect near the point of fixation but does not include it.

Arcuate Defect

Arcuate-shaped defect is typical of glaucoma.

Cecocentral Scotoma

It is a field defect that includes the point of fixation and the blind spot.

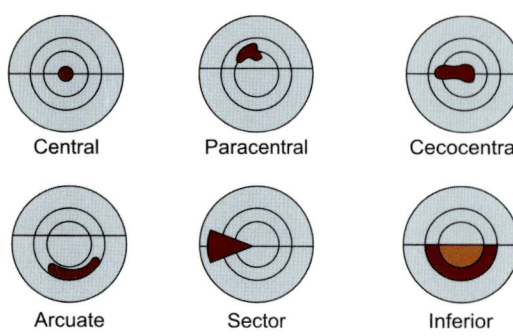

Fig. 41.1: Various types of scotomas

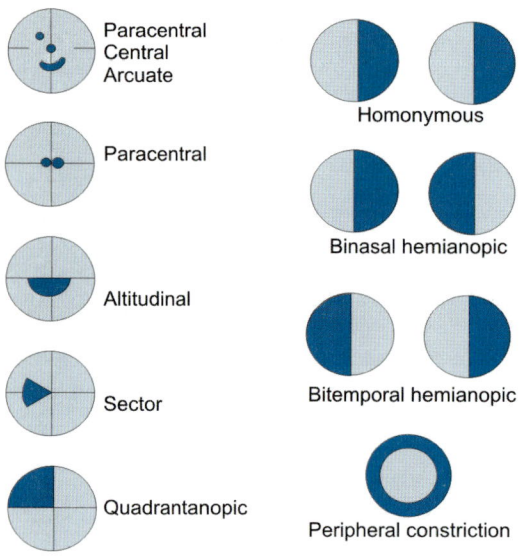

Fig. 41.2: Typical field defects

Altitudinal Defect

It is a field defect that involves either the upper or the lower half of the visual field in one or both the eyes. The line of separation is horizontal meridian.

Hemianopic Defect

The temporal or the nasal half of the field of one or both the eye is involved. It can be either bitemporal or binasal field defect.

Quadrantanopic Defect

It is bounded by a horizontal and a vertical line. A quadrant of the field of one or both the eye may be involved.

Homonymous Defect

In this a corresponding field in each eye is involved. It is a field defect of binocular visual field.

Sector Defect

It is bounded by two radii.

Peripheral Constriction of Field

In this there is peripheral constriction of visual field. It is one of the most common finding of visual field examination. It is seen in wide variety of diseases like optic neuritis, toxic amblyopia, glaucoma, retinitis pigmentosa, bilateral occipital lobe infarction, quinine amblyopia, chronic disk edema, and hysteria or malingering.

Congruous Defect

The field defect is said to be congruous if it is fairly similar in both the eyes.

Incongruous Defect

The field defect is said to be incongruous if there is marked difference in the field defects of both the eyes.

Field Defect with Sparing of Macula

The visual field defect in which the macula is not involved is said to be a defect with sparing of macula. It is typically seen in localized lesions of occipital cortex. This occurs due to a dual blood supply to the cortex and wide representation of macular fibers in the cortex.

Scotoma

A scotoma is an area of decreased visual sensitivity surrounded by an area of normal sensitivity.

Positive Scotoma

When patient can perceive a black spot in his field of vision then this scotoma is said to be positive scotoma. This is a presenting symptom in a case of choroiditis.

Negative Scotoma

In a case of choroiditis in later stages, the affected area which was giving a sensation of a positive scotoma becomes healed with fibrosis and does not give any sensation thus it becomes a negative scotoma. This area of negative scotoma is like blind spot due to optic disk with no sensation.

Relative Scotoma

Some times, a scotoma can be charted by using a small test object. A scotoma which is not charted with a 5 mm object but can be charted with a small object of 1 or 3 mm is said to be a relative scotoma. A scotoma charted with color test object and not with white is also said to be relative scotoma for color, e.g. tobacco amblyopia.

Enlargement of Blind Spot

A blind area in the field of vision due to optic disk is known as Blind spot. Any lesion of retina around the optic disk results in the enlargement of the blind spot. The common cause is papilledema or juxtapapillary choroiditis.

Field Defect with Baring of the Blind Spot

In glaucoma—In some cases the central field defects instead of being concentric around 30 degrees isopter shows a curve inwards to exclude the blind spot. It is not pathognomonic of glaucoma. It can occur due to change in the illumination and the size of the pupil.

Scintillating Scotoma

It is seen in cases of migraine. A positive scotoma appears in the field of vision and covers half of the visual field usually homonymous hemianopia. There is a peculiar shimmering character and patient may see bright spots and rays of various colors. The vision clears in about half an hour followed by severe headache. It is attributed to vasomotor change; vasodilation followed by vasoconstriction in the occipital lobe.

Field Defects at Various Levels of Visual Pathway and their Common Causes

Retina

- A lesion of Rods and Cones results in field defect.
- Field defect due to a lesion of retina takes the shape of the retinal lesion.
- Field defect corresponds to the location of the retinal lesion. A superotemporal retinal lesion shows a defect in the inferonasal quadrant of the chart.
- A lesion around the optic nerve causes an increase in the size of the blind spot like juxtapapillary choroiditis.
- Arcuate scotoma occurs due to affection of arcuate fibers as in glaucoma, temporal arteritis and collagen vascular disease, ischemic optic neuropathy and congenital optic disk and drusen.
- A central scotoma occurs in optic neuritis.
- A cecocentral scotoma occurs in tobacco amblyopia, Leber's optic neuropathy and in inflammatory conditions.
- A sector defect may occur if a segment of fibers passing from the retina into the optic nerve are interrupted.
- A ring scotoma is seen typically in retinitis pigmentosa.

Optic Nerve

- Enlargement of the Blind spot in papilledema.
- Peripheral constriction of field in optic atrophy, post neuritic optic atrophy, post papilledematous optic atrophy.
- Cecocentral scotoma in retrobulbar neuritis and tobacco amblyopia.
- Peripheral constriction of field in quinine amblyopia.
- Field defect is due to a lesion anterior to chiasma. It may be unilateral or bilateral depending on the site of affection of the optic nerve.

Chiasma

- Bitemporal hemianopia is a typical field defect of chiasma. To begin with there is a field defect in temporal superior quadrant, followed by the temporal inferior quadrant, followed by nasal inferior quadrant and last to be affected is the superior nasal quadrant. Thus there is clockwise loss of field in the right eye and anti-clockwise in the left eye. Pituitary adenoma is the common cause.
- Cecocentral or paracentral scotoma develops in a case of chiasmal arachnoiditis or vascular lesions of the chiasma.

Optic Tract

- The typical defect is homonymous hemianopia.
- The defect is incongruous due to crowding of fibers.
- Incongruous field occurs mostly due to lesions in optic tract and lateral geniculate body.

Lateral Geniculate Body

- The typical defect is homonymous hemianopia.
- The field defect is incongruous due to crowding of fibers.
- A geniculate lesion is indicated when the homonymous hemianopia involves the central portion of the field as the geniculate body represents the macula predominantly.

Optic Radiations

- The field defect is fairly congruous.
- Homonymous quadrantanopia is almost pathognomonic of lesions of optic radiations.
- Homonymous superior quadrantanopia is the result of the involvement of the inferior fibers of the optic radiation. The usual cause is a temporal lobe lesion.
- Homonymous inferior quadrantanopia is the result of the involvement of the superior fibers of the optic radiation. The usual cause is parietal lobe lesion.

- A large lesion of either temporal lobe or parietal lobe causes a homonymous hemianopia.
- Enquire about the associated symptoms of the temporal lobe lesion like olfactory and gustatory symptoms and hallucinations.

Occipital Cortex

- The field defect is congruous.
- There is sparing of macula. Macula sparing is due to dual blood supply of the visual cortex by the middle and posterior cerebral arteries and also due to extensive representation of the macular fibers in the cortex occupying half of the total area of the calcarine fissure thus some fibers are always left for the function of the macula.
- Involvement of the macula does not exclude the lesions of the occipital cortex. A macula sparing with good fixation is indicative of occipital lobe lesion. Most occipital lesions are vascular.
- A field defect due to occipital lobe lesion is usually associated with normal opticokinetic nystagmus response while parietal lobe lesions are associated with abnormal opticokinetic response.

Clinical Condition and Field Defects

Glaucoma

Scotoma with baring of blind spot.

Seidel's sign—there is a sickle-shaped extension of the blind spot above or below or both with concavity towards the fixation point.

Bjerrum's scotoma—the scotoma is in direct continuity with blind spot and may extend above or below the fixation point or may form a complete ring.

Roenne's step—there is upper or lower sectorial defect with a horizontal edge.

Peripheral constriction of visual field leaving only a small patch of paracentral visual field in the temporal area.

Retinitis Pigmentosa

A ring scotoma at the equatorial region with a tendency to spread towards the periphery and centre leaving small tubular visual field.

Papilledema

There is enlargement of the blind spot in early stage of papilledema. Peripheral constriction in later stage as the optic atrophy sets in.

Retrobulbar Neuritis

Central or paracentral scotoma in early stage.

Leber's Optic Neuropathy

Central or cecocentral scotoma.

Tobacco Amblyopia

Central scotoma involving fixation area causing loss of central vision. The peripheral field remains unaffected. It is due to degeneration of ganglion cells of retina involving papillomacular bundle.

Methyl Alcohol Amblyopia

Absolute central scotoma and later peripheral constriction resulting in complete loss of vision. It is due to degeneration of ganglion cells of retina, later optic atrophy sets in.

Quinine Amblyopia

Peripheral constriction of field almost to blindness.

In some cases central vision may be there giving the patient a tubular vision.

Ethambutol Amblyopia

Central scotoma which is reversible if drug is disontinued. It is due to optic neuritis.

Thiamine Deficiency

Central sctoma. It is due to optic neuritis.

Optic Atrophy

Peripheral constriction of the field to cause complete blindness.

Medullated Nerve Fibers

Enlargement of the blind spot.

Central Retinal Artery Occlusion

A small cuff of field remains around the blind spot.

Central Retinal Vein Occlusion

Central scotoma.

Superior Temporal Vein Occlusion

Sector defect.

Detachment of Retina

Field is lost opposite to the retina detached.

Coloboma-retina and Choroid

Sector defect in correspondence with retinal area involved.

Ischemic Optic Neuropathy

Altitudinal field defects, arcuate defects, and central scotoma.

Juxtapapillary Choroiditis

Enlargement of the blind spot.

Pituitary Adenoma

Bitemporal hemianopia.

Chiasmal Archnoiditis

Cecocentral or paracentral scotoma.

42

A Case with Sudden Loss of Vision

History

Record the history with reference to the following:
- Loss of vision was gradual or sudden.
- Any pain associated with loss of vision.
- Any associated signs and symptoms such as seeing flash of light, floaters and loss of visual field.
- Any history of seeing a shadow or a curtain like thing which obscures peripheral visual field.
- Any feeling of observing a change in the size and shape of the objects.
- Any feeling of a positive scotoma.
- Any pain on the movement of the eyeball
- Any history of systemic diseases like diabetes and hypertension.
- Any family history of retinal detachment
- Any addiction to tobacco and alcohol.
- Any history of intake of oral drugs such as chloramphenicol, quinine, ergot, salicylates, aspirin and oral contraceptives.
- Any septic focus in the system especially throat, teeth and genitourinary tract.
- Any history of trauma even insignificant.

CLINICAL EXAMINATION

Record Visual Acuity

Record the visual acuity.

Ocular Movements

Test the ocular movements in all the cardinal direction. Note if there is any pain on the movement of the eyeball especially movement in the upward gaze. In optic neuritis patient may complain of pain on the movement of the eyeball in upward direction.

Pupillary Reaction

A careful test for pupillary reaction direct and consensual light reflex shall give important information. An afferent pupillary defect indicates a lesion of optic nerve and macula. The pupil reacts normally in a case of vitreous hemorrhage, retinal detachment, central retinal vein occlusion and hysteria.

Refraction

Examination by plane mirror gives information about the refractive state of the eye. In a case of high myopia there is sudden loss of vision due to macular hemorrhage-'Fuch's spot'. There is no red reflex in a case with vitreous hemorrhage. There is a grey white reflex in a case with retinal detachment.

Ophthalmoscopy

Perform direct and indirect ophthalmoscopy to assess lesion in the retina and optic nerve.

Slit Lamp Biomicroscopy

It helps to detect early macular pathology which may be responsible for loss of vision.

Causes of sudden loss of vision
1. Central retinal artery occlusion.
2. Optic neuritis.
3. Arteric anterior ischemic optic neuropathy.
4. Toxic optic neuropathy.
5. Central retinal vein occlusion.
6. Central serous chorioretinopathy.
7. Retinal detachment.
8. Inflammatory maculopathies.
9. Macular hemorrhage.
10. Vitreous hemorrhage.
11. Berlin's edema (commotio retinae).
12. Sun-eclipse maculopathy.

CENTRAL RETINAL ARTERY OCCLUSION

Central retinal artery occlusion results in irreversible loss of vision. Its frequency is 1 in 10000 out-patients cases. It is a branch of ophthalmic artery and supplies the inner retina. Its sudden occlusion results in edema of inner layers of retina. The edema gives an opaque or yellow-white appearance of the retina. The fovea appears red as the retina is thin allowing visualization of normal retinal pigment epithelium and choroid in presence of surrounding white or opaque retina. This typical appearance has been labeled as "Cherry red spot" at macula.

Etiology

- High blood pressure.
- Cardiac valvular disease.
- Emboliform heart is the most common cause.
- Giant cell arteritis.
- Atherosclerosis.
- Oral contraceptives.

Embolization

This is the most common cause of retinal artery occlusion. As the ophthalmic artery is the first branch of the internal carotid artery therefore the emboliform the heart and/or the carotid arteries has a direct and easy entry in the ophthalmic artery.
- *Vegetation emboli:* It is common in patients with subacute bacterial endocarditis.
- *Thrombus emboli:* It is common in cases with myocardial infarction.

- *Calcific emboli:* It arises from calcified aortic valves and from atheromatous plaques in the ascending aorta and carotid arteries.
- *Cholesterol emboli (Hollenhorst plaques):* It occurs due to necrosis of an atheromatous plaque with discharge of its contents into the circulation.
- *Fibrinoplatelet emboli:* It occurs due to loss of continuity of the endothelial cells lining an atheromatous plaque. Platelets become adherent to it and form a fibrinoplatelet plug. This fibrinoplatelet plug is discharged in the circulation causing occlusion.

Vessel Obliteration

It occurs due to arteritis. Disorders causing arteritis are giant cell arteritis, systemic lupus erythematosus, polyarteritis nodosa, dermatomyositis and scleroderma.

Increased Intraocular Pressure

An increased intraocular pressure can cause obstruction to flow of retinal circulation.

Clinical Features

- There is marked loss of vision. The vision may be reduced to even perception of light only.
- There is an ill-sustained pupillary reaction to direct light reflex.
- Fundus examination shows marked narrowing of the retinal arterioles with irregular caliber, sludging and segmentation of the blood column in both the arterioles and venules and "Cherry-red spot" at macula. The foveal reflex appears as a red spot in the surrounding white retina at the posterior pole. This appearance is known as "cherry-red spot".
- Some cases later develop rubeosis iridis followed by neovascular glaucoma.

Investigations

- Complete blood picture, ESR.
- Blood sugar fasting and post-prandial.
- Lipid, thyroid and renal profile.
- Fluorescein angiography.

- Electroretinogram.
- Echocardiography.
- Carotid imaging.
- MRI.

Management

- Urgent and energetic treatment to dislodge the emboli or thrombus by manual massage of the globe and by lowering the intraocular pressure with fast I.V mannitol followed by oral acetazolmide and topical beta blockers.
- Vasodilators and inhalation of a mixture of 5% carbon dioxide and 95% oxygen may help by relieving the factor of angiospasm.
- Anticoagulants may be helpful in some cases.
- Steroids are indicated in cases of giant cell arteritis.
- Subject patient to a thorough cardio-vascular check up.
- Laser photocoagulation to prevent neo-vascularization.

Prognosis

- Most of the patients end with severe loss of vision.
- About 10% patients retain good central vision due to presence of a cilioretinal artery.
- Retinal embolus is associated with high mortality—about 56% over 9 years.

INFLAMMATORY MACULOPATHY

Most of the inflammatory maculopathies are associated with inflammation of choroid. Inflammation involves both the tissues to form a chorioretinitis. The most common source for inflammation is endogenous. The most frequent causes are choroiditis (granulomatous and non-granulomatous), septic emboli, toxoplasmosis and viral infections.

MACULAR HEMORRHAGE

Macular hemorrhage shall cause sudden loss of vision. It can occur in the follwing conditions

- High myopia.

- Trauma.
- Chorioretinitis.
- In degenerative maculopathies.
- Retinal vein branch occlusion.
- Systemic diseases like leukemia, anemia, diabetes, and hypertension.

VITREOUS HEMORRHAGE

Etiological Factors

- Proliferative retinopathies occurring in:
  - Diabetes.
  - Sickle cell anemia.
  - Retinal vein occlusion.
  - Eales' disease.
- Retinal tear:
  - Posterior vitreous detachment with traction on retinal vessel.
  - Trauma.
- Blood dyscrasia:
  - Leukemia.
  - Purpura.
- Dysproteinemia.

Hemorrhage in Healthy Vitreous

The blood clots early in a healthy vitreous. The blood clots along the vitreous fibers and so shows finger like projection into the vitreous from the site of bleeding. A massive hemorrhage into the vitreous has a tendency to diffuse anteriorly and centrally thereby obscuring the view of fundus and causes marked loss of vision. A slit lamp bio-microscopy shows hemorrhagic debris in the anterior vitreous and on the posterior lens capsule. The blood remains stationary in a formed vitreous and moves slightly on the movement of the eyeball. It takes a long time to resolve thereby the visual loss is for a long period. Later there appear yellowish fluffy opacities in the vitreous.

Hemorrhage in the Liquified Vitreous

Blood in the lacuna of vitreous appears similar to preretinal hemorrhage. The blood remains unclotted and shifts with gravity. It has a tendency to resolve early in comparison to the blood in a healthy vitreous.

BERLIN'S EDEMA (COMMOTIO RETINAE)

The common cause is a blow on the eyeball. Any contusion injury can cause Berlin's edema. It is a contrecoup type of lesion as the blow on the eyeball causes edema of the retina at the posterior pole. There is a marked loss of vision. On ophthalmoscopy there is a cherry-red spot at the macula. An injury causes edema of the retina at the posterior pole thereby the retina appears as milky-white. In this area the foveal reflex shows up as red spot known as "cherry red spot". If edema is more and treatment is delayed then the organic changes at the macula occurs in the form of pigment deposits, macular cyst and macular hole.

SUN-ECLIPSE MACULOPATHY

Looking at the sun-eclipse without protective goggle results in sun-eclipse maculopathy. Patient complains of loss of vision, after image, positive scotoma and metamorphopsia. On ophthalmoscopy there is edema at the macula. Later there may be degenerative changes at the macula in form of pigment deposits, cystic degeneration and formation of macular hole.

It can be prevented by use of protective goggle.

OTHER DISORDERS

- Optic Neuritis *refer Chapter 33.*
- Arteric anterior Ischemic Optic Neuropathy *refer Chapter 33.*
- Toxic Optic Neuropathy *refer Chapter 33.*
- Central Retinal Vein Occlusion *refer Chapter 31.*
- Central Serous Chorioretinopathy *refer Chapter 28.*
- Retinal Detachment *refer Chapter 27.*

43

A Case with Low Vision

History

Record the history with reference to the following:
- Low vision is acquired or congenital.
- Any disease known to have caused the low vision.
- Any diagnosis made by ophthalmologist.
- Visual requirement for daily routine work.
- Can see better in what kind of illumination, dim, normal or bright.
- Any educational qualification.
- His past vocation.
- His present aspiration.
- In a child enquire about his relations with other children.
- Is he attending a regular school or not.
- Assess his reaction to his handicap and readiness to use low vision aids.
- Assess general health and enquire about it.
- Is his vision is stationary or falling gradually over a period.
- His hobbies if any.
- Economic status and family life.

CLINICAL EXAMINATION

Clinical examination in a patient of low vision needs great flexibility in the approach, in conducting various tests to assess his vision and help him with low vision aids.

Visual Acuity

Determine carefully, the visual acuity for distance and near with and without currently worn glasses.

Refraction

Try to assess correct visual acuity rating after retinoscopy and subjective testing.

Slit Lamp Biomicroscopy

It shall provide information about the pathology in the anterior segment of the eyeball as well in the posterior segment.

Ophthalmoscopy

Examine the patient with direct and indirect ophthalmoscope to assess the pathology in the fundus.

Fundus Contact Lens

It shall help to examine the angle of the anterior chamber and fundus under high magnification especially macula and peripheral fundus.

Ophthalmometry

It shall help in all the cases where retinoscopy may be difficult, because of small pupil, opacities in media and irregular corneal surface. Ophthalmometry shall provide information about presence of keratoconus or irregular corneal surface. It also helps to prescribe any cylinder including its power and axis. It also helps to determine the need to prescribe contact lens.

Visual Field

It is essential to assess the central and peripheral visual field. It shall help us to establish the type of low vision aid needed by the patient.

Tonometry

Record the intraocular pressure in all the cases. It helps to assess the prognosis of the pathology by which the patient is suffering from.

Clinical Conditions with Low Vision

- Macular degeneration.
- Diabetic retinopathy.
- Albinism.
- High myopia.
- Nystagmus.
- Coloboma.
- Optic atrophy.
- Macular holes.
- Achromatopsia.

Spectacle Types of Low Vision Aids

- Contact lenses.
- Hand held and stand mounted magnifying devices.
- High plus reading additions.
- Microscopic lenses.
- Telescopic lenses.
- Projection devices.
- Night telescope for night blind patients.
- Color gain lens for color blind patients.
- Iridium lens for aniridia.

Non-spectacle Types of Low Vision Aids

- Large print and typewriters.
- Talking books.
- Line guides.
- Reading stands as per requirement of patients.
- Special arrangement for illumination needed by the patient.

Contact Lenses

It is useful in cases of keratoconus, irregular corneal surface, irregular astigmatism, aphakia, high myopia and high astigmatism. The use of the pinhole in contact lens provides another use of contact lens in low vision aids. Such contact lenses are known as "controlled-pupil corneal contact lens". Such lenses have

been beneficial in cases of low vision due dilated pupil, distorted pupil, corneal scar, corneal opacity, coloboma of iris, aniridia, and opacities in media.

Hand and Stand Magnifiers

Hand held magnifier lens are available in almost all the size and power. The patient can vary the distance between eye and lens depending upon reading distance and magnification required by the individual. It does give problem in maintaining constant focus. Stand magnifiers having a fixed object-to-lens distance are used with the eye close to lens. It provides a large field and little aberration. Stand magnifiers which can be focused with variable object-to-lens distance allows variation in magnification.

Indication

- Visual field less than ten degrees.
- In cases of hand and head tremor as associated with parkinsonism, multiple sclerosis and cerebral palsy.
- In cases where spectacle cannot be used.

Pin-hole Spectacles

Pinhole spectacles are useful in cases with opacities of ocular media and corneal irregularity. Pinhole improves vision provided the macular function is normal. The reading slit or typoscope is a further improvement in which one or more lines of reading material is visible at a time. It is useful in cases with early cataract who finds problem in reading.

High-plus Reading Lenses

These lenses have an advantage over other low vision aids as these provide a large field of view and greater depth of focus. Patient feels comfortable with these lenses. These can be made either in a single vision or in a bifocal form.

Telescopic Lenses

The simple telescopic lens consists of two lenses: a minus ocular and a plus objective mounted coaxially and separated by a distance equal to the sum of their focal lengths. There is no focus therefore the entire unit of telescopic lenses is termed as "afocal". The system is afocal for distance objects. It needs reading addition for viewing near objects.

- Spectacle mounted distance vision telescope.
- Spectacle mounted near vision telescope.
- Spectacle mounted telescope for enhancement of visual field.

Microscopic Lenses

These lenses are of short focal length so used for viewing near objects. These can be designed as a single vision, double or in triplet.

Projection Devices

An enlarged image of the object is formed on the screen therefore adaptation by the patient is easy. Closed-circuit television (CCTV) magnification system shall provide more relief to low vision patients. Its other advantages are good range of magnification, better contrast, less aberration, less distortion, and almost normal reading distance.

Illumination

Illumination plays an important role in providing good visual acuity. Advise the patient to use the light with proper angle and intensity to give him the best vision possible.

Individual and Social Acceptance

It is very essential that the low vision patients are accepted by the individual, the family and the society as any normal person. This will help him to get rehabilitated early and accept the low vision aids with confidence. The patient needs regular counseling.

44

A Case with Contusion/Concussion Injury

History

Record the history with reference to the following:
- **Closed-globe injury**
- **Contusion injury** is caused by direct hit of the globe by a large blunt trauma.
- **Concussion injury**

Assess the type of closed-globe injury sustained whether it is contusion or concussion injury.

Closed-globe injury denotes wherein the eyeball—the cornea and sclera does not show full thickness wound. But there is an intraocular damage due to direct-contusion or indirect concussion trauma.

Contusion injury is caused by direct hit of the globe by a large blunt trauma.

Concussion injury occurs due to indirect hit of the globe either by tissue conduction or by air conduction of the compression wave.

- Duration of the injury.
- Any first aid treatment received. A proper first aid attention can prevent complication and therefore help to save the vision.
- Any previous history of an eye disease.
- Any systemic disease like diabetes.
- Any history of allergy to any drug.
- Any previous record of visual acuity so that the loss of vision can be assessed properly.
- Any specific visual disturbance or symptoms like diplopia, flashes of light, positive scotoma, floaters, red vision, half vision, etc.
- Any associated pain in the eye when resting or on movement of the eyeball.
- Any hemorrhage or discharge from the eye or nose.
- Any previous injury to the eyeball prior to this present injury.

CLINICAL EXAMINATION

Visual Acuity

Record the visual acuity in each eye with and without glasses carefully. A proper assessment of the visual acuity is important for the diagnosis, management and medico-legal aspect of a case.

Ocular Movement

Test the ocular movements in all the cardinal direction. Make a note if there is any restriction of movement in any direction. If a patient complains of diplopia then conduct a diplopia test and also perform a hess screen test.

Lid Movement

Test the movement of the lids by asking the patient to open and close the eye repeatedly. Look for any erythema, ecchymosis and edema. Palpate the lids for subcutaneous emphysema. Evert the lid to look for any foreign body or mild laceration.

Orbital Margin

Palpate the orbital margin for any localized tenderness and defect in the orbital margin. Palpate for subcutaneous emphysema.

Eyeball

- Look for any exophthalmos or enophthalmos. If any doubt then perform the exophthalmometry by Hertel's exophthalmometer.
- Examine the conjunctiva and sclera for any laceration, chemosis and sub-conjunctival hemorrhage.
- Examine the cornea for any abrasion or even tear. Use fluorescein strip to stain the cornea to detect minute abrasions likely to be missed.
- Examine the anterior chamber, iris, pupil and lens for any abnormality.

Slit Lamp Biomicroscopy and three Mirror Contact Lens

Examination with slit lamp shall help to look for rupture in Descemet's membrane, keratic precipitates, tear in lens capsule and any changes in the posterior lens capsule.

Examine the angle of the anterior chamber especially for any recession of the angle.

Examine the macula and the peripheral fundus for any lesion.

Refraction

A good red reflex is a healthy sign. A change in the reflex indicates a lesion which may be involving the lens, vitreous or retina. Assess the refractive state of the eye.

Ophthalmoscopy

Examine the fundus thoroughly with direct and indirect ophthalmoscopy under full mydriasis to exclude any lesion in the posterior segment of the eyeball such as hemorrhage, tear, retinal detachment, macular pathology, and changes in the vitreous.

Tonometry

Measure the intraocular pressure in every case. A normal pressure is a good omen. A low pressure indicates damage to the ciliary body or rupture of globe which warrants further careful examination. It is advisable to keep watch on the intraocular pressure for at least six months after the injury.

Field of Vision

With good vision testing the visual field with confrontation test may be sufficient. It is essential to record the visual fields in a case having associated neurological disorder.

INVESTIGATIONS

X-ray Orbit

It is always advisable to exclude any fracture of the orbital margin.

CT Scan

It provides excellent delineation of the soft tissue injury. With this one can study the whole eyeball and orbit.

Magnetic Resonance Imaging

It is a very sensitive test for detecting difference between the normal and abnormal tissue.

Ultrasonography

B-scan is a complimentry to CT scan. It is useful in cases where there is a concern about the dislocation or subluxation of lens, vitreous hemorrhage and retinal detachment.

CLOSED AND OPEN-GLOBE INJURY

The strong bony orbital margin prevents many injuries of the eyeball. The lids and the eyelashes are very sensitive and the lids get closed quickly through the reflex stimuli. The Bell's phenomenon, i.e. the upward rotation of the eyeball is an additional protective reflex action which further helps to protect the globe from injuries.

Closed-globe injury denotes that the eyeball does not have a full thickness wound of cornea or sclera but there is an intraocular damage. It includes contusion and lamellar laceration.

Open-globe injury denotes full thickness wound of the sclera or cornea or both. It includes rupture and laceration of the eye wall.

It can be caused by contusion-concussion injury.

Contusion and concussion injury can result in either a closed-globe injury or an open-globe injury, depending on the impact. And many associated factors.

CONTUSION INJURY

A contusion injury of the eyeball occurs due to direct hit of the eyeball by any kind of large blunt object. The most common case belongs to the injury by a stone thrown by someone or a direct hit by a fist in a quarrel between people. The other common way of injury is striking against a blunt object unknowingly in dark area, e.g. against a pile of burning wood, a leg of wooden bed or the handle of the door.

CONCUSSION INJURY

A concussion injury is an injury which is not due to a direct hit of the eyeball. A concussion injury results due to creation of *compression wave force* transmitted through tissue conduction or by air conduction.

Tissue Conduction Concussion Injury

The concussion injury due to tissue conduction occurs due to a force striking the head, orbit, orbital margin or any structure close to the orbit. The waves created by the striking force are conducted to the eyeball through the tissue namely the bone and the orbital fat.

Air Conduction Concussion Injury

The concussion injury due to air conduction occurs due to explosions far away from the eyeball.

Compression wave force strikes the cornea and the force is transmitted to the ocular tissues giving rise to many kinds of injuries to the eyeball.

Mechanism of Concussion Injuries

The precise mechanism is not yet completely clear and understood.

- The effect of an impinging force usually acting in the anterior-posterior direction thereby forcibly expanding the globe around the equator has been attributed to produce the damage to the eyeball.
- The impact of the compression wave of pressure passing through the fluid contents of the eye which results in cornea being pushed in, the aqueous forced backwards pushing the iris and lens and vitreous against the posterior pole of the eyeball has been attributed for the damage caused. This type of injury comes under the *"contrecoup"* injuries to the eyeball. Thus a line of force traversing the eye causes damage to all interfaces. The extent of the damage depends upon the force created by the injury.

The injuries caused are due to three factors:

- The immediate damage to the tissue cells causing disruption of their physiological activity.
- The remote effects of the vascular reaction.
- The mechanical tearing and laceration of the intraocular tissues.

The injuries tends to be diffuse, multiple and variable in their effect. The damage to the eye shortly after the injury may appear to be almost negligible. The damage caused may be a small hemorrhage or complete rupture and disorganization of the globe. The damage caused may be to the anterior segment of the eyeball or the posterior segment of the eyeball or to both the segments. Considering the variability of the damage and its late manifestation, a careful follow up is very essential in a case especially with negligible signs and symptoms. Always give a guarded prognosis and follow-up the case for at least six weeks before declaring him normal with no damage.

LESIONS OF CONTUSION OR CONCUSSION INJURY

Lids

- Ecchymosis.
- Traumatic ptosis.

Conjunctiva

- Conjunctival ecchymosis.

Cornea

- Blood staining of the cornea.

Pupil

- Traumatic miosis and spasm of accommodation.
- Traumatic iridoplegia and cycloplegia.

Anterior Chamber

- Traumatic hyphema.
- Recession of angle of the anterior chamber.

Lens

- Concussion cataract.
- Subluxation and dislocation of lens.

Vitreous

- Liquefaction of vitreous.
- Vitreous hemorrhage.
- Herniation of the vitreous into the anteror chamber.

Retina-optic Nerve

- Traumatic retinal tear.
- Traumatic retinal detachment.
- Concussion changes at the macula.
- Choroidal hemorrhage and detachment.
- Optic atrophy.

Refractive Error

- Traumatic myopia.
- Traumatic hypermetropia.

Tension

- Changes in the ocular tension.

Globe

- Rupture of the globe.

Clinical Features and Management

1. Ecchymosis lid.
2. Traumatic ptosis.
3. Conjunctival ecchymosis.
4. Blood staining of the cornea.
5. Traumatic miosis and spasm of accommodation.
6. Traumatic iridoplegia and cycloplegia.
7. Traumatic hyphema.
8. Recession of the angle of the anterior chamber.
9. Concussion cataract.
10. Subluxation and dislocation of lens.
11. Liquefaction of vitreous (Syneresis).
12. Herniation of vitreous in anterior chamber.
13. Traumatic retinal tear.
14. Traumatic retinal detachment.
15. Concussion changes at macula.
16. Choroidal hemorrhage and detachment
17. Traumatic myopia.
18. Traumatic hypermetropia.
19. Changes in ocular tension.
20. Rupture of globe.

Ecchymosis Lid

Echymosis of lids is very common in concussion injury. The blood tends to diffuse through loose connective tissue of the lids. It is checked from further spread to cheek, upper lip and forehead by the firm adhesion of the fascia at the eyebrows and at the naso-jugal and malar folds. The lids appear swollen and the eye is closed. The upper lid may overhang the lower lid. The blood from one upper lid crosses over to the lid of the opposite side across the nasal bridge thereby there appears an ecchymosis of the other un-injured eyelid. There is no continuity of the ecchymosis of one eye to the other eye. This is due to the fact that the skin over the nasal bridge is thick so the blood underneath is not visible and the skin over the nasal bridge appears normal. The patient is alarmed of this phenomeon seeing the black circle in the opposite un-injured eye. Explain to the patient that this is normal and natural process to diffuse the blood early.

An ecchymosis of the lids is mostly accompanied by the ecchymosis of the conjunctiva. Even a minor insignificant trauma to the eye can cause a sub-conjunctival hemorrhage. Seeing a red patch in the eye the patient seeks an opinion of an eye surgeon. Assure him that it shall take about 1–3 weeks to get absorbed and it shall cause no harm to his vision.

Traumatic Ptosis

It is common with injury to the orbital margin. It occurs due to damage to the levator tendon or to the palpebral branch of the oculomotor nerve. On recovery some cases may show a phenomenon of a paradoxical elevation of the upper lid (Marcus Gunn phenomenon). Injury to the orbital margin is likely to develop periostitis at the site of the injury. If not treated early and carefully it may be followed by caries and necrosis probably due to activation of tuberculous or syphilitic periostitis in susceptible persons usually younger in age.

Conjunctival Ecchymosis

Conjunctival ecchymosis is common and vary in degree from a minute petechial to extensive spread in the exposed part of the bulbar conjunctiva (Fig. 44.1).

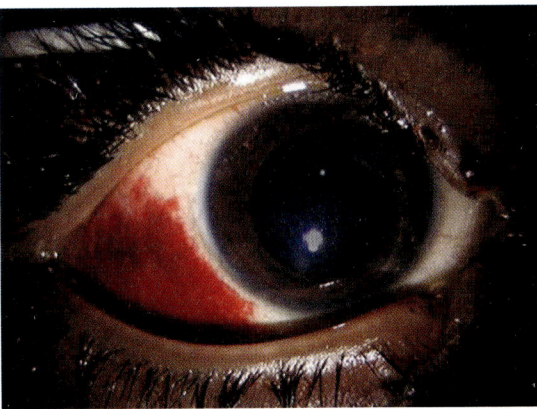

Fig. 44.1: Conjunctival ecchymosis

Causes

- Local trauma to the conjunctiva by foreign body, hand, postoperative.
- Injury to orbital structures.
- In fracture of roof of orbit—the blood tracks along the levator muscle to upper fornix and lids.
- In fracture of floor of orbit—the blood tracks along in lower fornix and lids.
- In fracture of apex of orbit—the blood tracks along the lateral rectus muscle.
- In fracture of orbital plate of sphenoid— the blood tracks along the temporal aspect of the globe.

- In fracture of base of skull—the blood tracks along the floor of orbit then fornix and then to conjunctiva.
- Usually it takes 12–24 hours for the blood to reach the subconjunctival tissue.
- Petechial hemorrhage in pneumococcal conjunctivitis.
- Sudden severe venous congestion of head as in whooping cough, vomiting, blowing the trumpet, fits, strangulation, violent compression of thorax in stampede or accidents.
- Systemic vascular disease like arteriosclerosis, hypertension, nephritis and diabetes. A patient with a small tiny hemorrhage should be subjected to a meticulous check up of cardiovascular system.
- Blood dyscrasias such as purpura, thrombocytopenia, leukemia.

Investigation

Angiography, platelet count, complete blood picture, complete systemic check up specially CV system.

Treatment

Assurance, cold packs, vitamin C and evacuate blood if large.

Blood Staining of the Cornea

The blood staining of the cornea is due to absorption of the disintegrated produce of the erythrocytes which have broken down in the anterior chamber in a case of total hyphema associated with raised intraocular pressure. Most likely the blood products enter the cornea through the damaged endothelium. The most common cause for the blood staining of the cornea is the contusion injury to the eyeball.

Clinically

- There is a wide spread staining of the corneal stroma involving entire cornea leaving a clear ring round the periphery.
- The cornea appears red rusty brown which later changes to greenish yellow or grey.

- It can be prevented by an early treatment of total hyphema by evacuation of blood from the chamber and early control of raised inraocular pressure.
- A blood stained eye is usually lost and eventually needs an excision if associated with pain.

Traumatic Miosis and Spasm of Accommodation

The traumatic miosis is the immediate reaction to the trauma of the eyeball. There is a marked constriction of the pupil but transient. It is usually associated with the spasm of the accommodation. It is relieved by the instillation of the atropine eyedrop topically.

Traumatic Iridoplegia and Cycloplegia

A traumatic dilation of the pupil is common sequelae of the concussion injury to the globe. It is usually associated with the paralysis of the accommodation. The pupil is usually moderately dilated and quite often eccentric with abolished or diminished reaction to the light both the direct and consensual and accommodation. The pupil may dilate slowly with atropine. It may show slight constriction with instillation of topical eserine. Other miotics have no effect on it. There is an associated paralysis of accommodation. It causes discomfort on reading and sometimes pain and early fatigue. Treat by prescribing full correction for the distance and near.

Traumatic Hyphema

An occurrence of hyphema following trauma to the eyeball is of common occurrence especially in childern even with mild concussion. The hyphema may be just a small sediment of 1–2 mm in height or may completely fill the anterior chamber causing loss of visual acuity to just perception of light (Fig. 44.2). The hyphema usually absorbs rapidly in 1–7 days. A severe injury with hyphema may result in complications like secondary glaucoma and blood staining of the cornea. Keep a watch on the intraocular pressure. Evacuate the hyphema early if there are no signs of absorption.

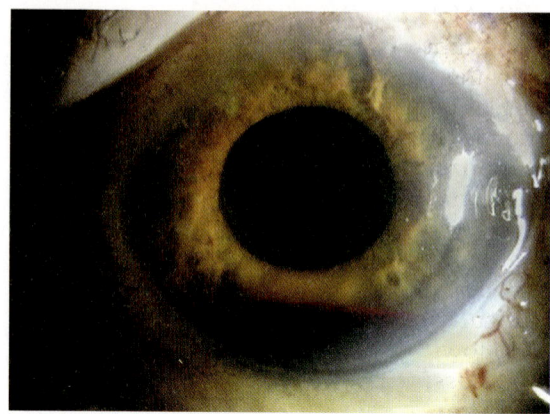

Fig. 44.2: Hyphema

Recession of the Angle of the Anterior Chamber

The lesion of the recession of the angle of the anterior chamber is produced by a concussion force which tears into the face of the ciliary body thereby causing separation of the circular and radial fibers from the longitudinal muscles.

The longitudinal fibers remain intact attached to the scleral spur. The separated circular and radial fibers along with the root of the iris tend to retract posteriorly therefore the anterior chamber gives an appearance of abnormal depth. On gonioscopy the recess of the chamber appears well behind the scleral spur. This recession of the angle causes the interference with the function of the outflow of aqueous. It is essential to examine every case with trauma and/or hyphema with gonioscopy so as to diagnose the recession of the angle of anterior chamber early. Keep watch on the intraocular pressure and treat like a case of simple chronic glaucoma if there is a rise of intraocular pressure.

Concussion Cataract

The concussion cataract occurs due to the concussion effects on the cells of lens and tear of the lens capsule. Thus the concussion cataract can be divided into two categories.

    i. Associated with a tear in the lens capsule.

ii. Not associated with any tear in the lens capsule.

In the first category—the opacification of the lens occurs due to free entry of the aqueous into the lens and in the second type-the opacification of the lens occurs due to derangement of the normal semipermeability of the lens capsule. Clinically the two types of opacification is almost similar. The opacification may be diffuse or may remain segmental. The lenticular opacities due to concussion can be as follows:

- *Vossius's ring opacity:* In this condition, there is a formation of a ring corresponding to the pupillary aperture. The ring is about 1 mm in breadth and is comprised of reddish-brown granules of pigment deposited flatly on the anterior lens capsule. There is a single layer of pigment granules. The Vossius's ring is due to an imprint of the pupillary border of the iris upon the capsule due to concussion injury. The imprint occurs at the time of the injury and is due to the iris being suddenly forced against the lens and the pigment gets adhere to the surface of the lens capsule.
- *Localised opacities due to subcapsular changes:* These opacities may be discrete, punctate, scattered, zonular or rosette shaped. It may assume any form. It may remain localised for a long time and may precipitate the development of pre-senile or senile changes.
- *Diffuse lens opacities are common*

Treatment

- Conservative treatment is best if the eye is quite and there is minimal loss of vision.
- Treat the complications if any or treat to prevent the occurrence of complications.
- Correct refractive error.
- Surgical removal of lens.

Subluxation and Dislocation of Lens

Subluxation

The subluxation of the lens occurs following damage to the zonular attachment. The lens may remain in its place retained by its attachment to the vitreous. The lens is tremulous and usually sinks downwards a little due to gravity. The refraction tends to be myopic with astigmatism. There is loss of accommodation. The vitreous may herniate in the anterior chamber through the pupil. With more subluxation the equatorial edge of the lens may appear as a cresent in the pupillary area with phakic and aphakic part. There is iridodonesis and the anterior chamber is of unequal depth in its circumference. In some cases there may be an axial subluxation with the equator of the lens presenting in the anterior chamber through the pupil.

Dislocation

In complete traumatic dislocation, the lens may be dislocated into the anterior chamber, the vitreous, the inter retinal space, the subscleral region and outside the eye on rupture of the globe to rest under the subconjunctival space or subtenon's space or thrown out and away.

Complications

The following complications are usually seen.
- Traumatic opacities of lens.
- Uveitis usually phaco-anaphylactic type.
- Secondary glaucoma.
- Retinal detachment.

Liquefaction of Vitreous (Syneresis)

The liquefaction of the vitreous is common sequelae of a concussion injury. It can be seen by slit lamp biomicroscopy. The beam of the slit lamp as it traverses the vitreous shows a plasmoid diffusion rich in protein in the vitreous. There is disruption of the frame work and liquefaction of the vitreous. There are colorless cells, erythrocytes and granules of the pigment visible in the vitreous. It needs no treatment as such but careful and regular follow up for any further complications which may arise.

Vitreous Hemorrhage

The commonest cause of the vitreous hemorrhage is a tearing of the retina with or without a retinal detachment. Even a minor contusion is enough to produce a tear in a retina associated with degenerative changes especially in high myopic. With an extensive hemorrhage in the vitreous there is no red reflex. If the hemorrhage is localized then one can see by the slit lamp the disruption of vitreous gel. The hemorrhage may absorb completely. It may get organized in bands. It can also cause hemosiderosis and hemolytic glaucoma. Treat by conservative methods until one can visualize the fundus and thereafter treat accordingly.

Herniation of Vitreous in Anterior Chamber

The herniation of the vitreous into the anterior chamber is always a post-traumatic or a post-operative condition. It occurs after the injury to zonules and with luxation or subluxation of the lens. The herniation may be relatively solid forming a bead which shows movement with the movement of the globe. There is always a dispersion of pigment granules in this herniated vitreous. If the herniated vitreous is fluid then it may fill the anterior chamber. This can lead to secondary glaucoma.

Traumatic Retinal Tear

An occurrence of a retinal tear after a concussion even of a very mild nature is not uncommon. The patients having myopia with degenerative changes are more prone to it the trauma acting as a precipitating factor. The retinal tear is usually near the periphery and of horseshoe shape. The mechanism is the sudden thrust and recoil of the vitreous to which the retina is firmly adherent. An examination of the fundus by a binocular indirect ophthalmoscope shall help to locate the tear and immediate treatment shall prevent the occurrence of impeding retinal detachment.

Traumatic Retinal Detachment

It is important to remember the fact that a traumatic retinal detachment in a healthy eye is a rare phenomenon. From the pathological point of view the traumatic retinal detachment can occur in the following conditions:

- The detachment occurs in a case with a collapse of globe following rupture due to contusion.
- The detachment occurs following choroidal hemorrhage or exudation due to contusion.
- Detachment occurs following a tear in the retina due to trauma.
- A detachment occurs secondarily to contraction of organized bands in the vitreous.
- A detachment occurs in a case with senile or post-inflammatory degeneration or myopic degeneration, the trauma playing a precipitating etiological factor.

Keeping the above facts in mind it is important to examine the retina by a binocular indirect ophthalmoscopy soon one can visualize the fundus so that if there are degenerative changes in the retina or a hole or tear is detected then one can start treatment early to prevent subsequent detachment.

Concussion Changes at Macula

Concussion can cause the following changes at the macula
- Macular edema.
- Macular cyst and hole.
- Traumatic macular atrophy.
- Commotio retinae.

Macular Edema

The occurrence of the macular edema is the most common lesion following a concussion of the eyeball. Many factors are responsible for this:

- The posterior pole is in the line of indirect contrecoup for the force impinging on the eyeball.
- Any injury on the face excites throughout the soft tissue the waves of pressure which enter the orbit through the pterygo-maxillary fissure and strikes at the vulnerable posterior part of the globe.
- The anatomical factors: rich choroidal capillary bed at the macula, the thick fiber layer of Henle can absorb more fluid and the avascularity does not allow early resolution of fluid.

On ophthalmoscopy, the macular edema is characterized by dullness at the macula and a halo-reflex or radial striae. In severe degree of macular edema the fovea stands out as a cherry-red spot surrounded by an area of milky white retina.

Macular Cyst and Hole

The macular edema results in formation of macular cyst which later on rupture to form hole. On ophthalmoscopy, the picture is characteristic. It appears as a dark red spot at the fovea as if it has been punched out. At the bottom of this dark red spot one can see finely granular surface of the choroid and a parallax can be elicited between the floor of the dark red spot and the surrounding retina. A clinical differentiation between a cyst and a hole can be best assessed by slit lamp biomicroscopy using a three mirror contact lens in which the optical section of the area gives the clear picture. The optical line of the surface of the retina is seen to be continuous over a cyst, while it is interrupted in a case of a hole.

Traumatic Macular Atrophy

The macular atrophy follows edema at the macula usually the Berlin's edema due to concussion injury. In course of time the edema disappears, the fovea appears more red with dull reflex. Later there occurs a pigmentary stippling along with fine hemorrhages. Some cases may show white patches with proliferation of pigment.

Commotio Retinae (Berlin's edema, concussion edema of retina)

A commotio retinae is a condition of edema of the retina due to simple concussion, the changes are reversible and transient, though frequently it may involve permanent visual loss to a marked degree. Ophthalmoscopically the fovea stands out as a red spot against the background of milky white appearance of surrounding retina due to edema. The clinical picture resembles the appearance seen after occlusion of the central retinal artery. The picture varies considerably depending on the force impinging the posterior pole and

therefore the eventual outcome which may be a normal fundus with normal vision or reduced vision with changes at the macula in the form of macular cyst, macular hole or macular degeneration.

Choroidal Hemorrhage and Detachment

A hemorrhage in the choroid is a frequent occurrence following a concussion injury. The hemorrhage may be small and intrachoroidal, may appear under retina, may be between the choroid and the sclera, and if the retina is torn then the blood may escape in the vitreous. A localized choroidal hemorrhage appears as a round dark blotch with blurred margins crossed over by the retinal vessels on ophthalmoscopy. The blood tends to absorb leaving a patch of atrophy and pigmentation. A collection of blood between the choroid and sclera results in the detachment of the choroid. A detachment of the choroid may follow a tear of the posterior ciliary artery.

Traumatic Myopia

A concussion to the globe can cause a change in the refractive error the commonest being the myopia. There is an increase of myopia from one to six diopter but usually this change is reversed back to normal within a week to four weeks. The ciliary spasm is the main factor responsible for this change in refraction to myopia. The ciliary spasm is due to irritation of the muscle fibers or the third nerve. The ciliary spasm is associated with miosis. The ciliary spasm is associated with a change in myopia from one to four diopters. There is loss of accommodative amplitude. In most cases the ciliary spasm is temporary and also disappears under the effect of topical atropine instillation.

The other factor for myopic change is damage to the suspensory ligaments of the lens and anterior dislocation of the lens. Damage to suspensory ligaments of the lens results in permanent change in the refraction to myopia as it involves an increase of lenticular curvature. The change may amount to about five to six diopters. An anterior dislocation of the lens shall produce higher degree of myopic change. Treat by correcting the refractive error.

Traumatic Hypermetropia

The traumatic hypermetropia is associated with paralysis of the accommodation which may be either temporary or permanent. This is due to an injury to the ciliary nerves or ciliary muscle itself. The posterior dislocation of the lens also gives rise to hypermetropic change in refraction. Treat by prescribing glasses for near work.

Changes in Ocular Tension

Some cases may develop an alarming rise in the ocular pressure due to damage to structures of the angle of the anterior chamber along with other lesions of concussion. Other cases may show a permanent hypotony which may ultimately lead to an atrophic bulbi. As there is a change in the ocular pressure it is advisable to record the intraocular pressure in all the cases of injury, however, mild it may look and follow it up for at least three months. Treat the case as per its requirement.

Rupture of Globe

Direct Rupture of Globe

The rupture of the sclera occurs due to a gross injury usually due to a large and blunt object being driven into the orbit between the globe and the orbital walls. The common cause is an injury by cow horn and stick. A diseased eye like having staphyloma, buphthalmos or absolute glaucoma shall give way easily with less severe trauma.

Indirect Rupture of Globe

The site of an indirect rupture of the sclera is almost constant. The rupture occurs concentric with the limbus about 2 to 4 mm behind the corneo-sclera junction, situated above the horizontal meridian in the upper and inner quadrant of the globe (**Contrecoup effect**) in vast number of cases. Usually it extends to about 10 to 14 mm in length.

Common Clinical Features and Management

- Orbital hemorrhage and proptosis.
- Lids are swollen and bruised.
- Ecchymosis and subconjuctival hemorrhage.
- Tear in the conjunctiva.
- Tear in the sclera with gapping edges with uveal tissue bulging.
- Subconjunctival dislocation of the lens.
- With a large tear in the sclera the lens and vitreous may be extruded.
- Anterior chamber is full with blood.

Prognosis is poor. A severely damaged globe should be enucleated. A moderately damaged globe should be repaired and treated energetically to save the eye by use of antibiotics, steroids and all the supportive treatment needed.

Usually it ends in phthisis bulbi or atrophic bulbi.

45

A Case with Retained Intraocular Foreign Body

History

Record the history with reference to the following:
- The time of injury.
- How the patient got injured whether accidental or during occupation.
- Nature of foreign body magnetic or non magnetic, glass, wood, plastic, concrete, thorn, branch of a thorny bush, pencil, pen, knife, etc.
- Any history of previous eye disease.
- Vision prior to injury if there is any record.
- Treated by any ophthalmologist.

OPEN-GLOBE PENETRATING INJURY WITH RETAINED INTRAOCULAR FOREIGN BODY

Inspection

Open-globe injury denotes wherein full thickness wound of the eyeball—the cornea or sclera or both are involved

It includes
- **Rupture of the eyeball** refers to wound that is caused by impact of trauma. It occurs due to raised intraocular pressure with inside-out mechanism that is **contrecoup** effect.
- **Laceration of the eyeball** refers to full thickness wound that occurs at the site of impact by outside-in mechanism that is by sharp object.

It includes:
i. *Penetrating injury:* It refers to a single laceration of the eyeball by sharp object.
ii. *Perforating injury:* It refers to two full thickness laceration: one entry and one exit wound of the eyeball by the same object of trauma.
iii. *Intraocular retained foreign body:* It refers to penetrating injury associated with retained intraocular foreign body.

CLINICAL EXAMINATION

Visual Acuity

Record the vision carefully. Make a note about the perception and projection of light if vision is markedly reduced.

Torch and Loupe

Examine the eye with a torch and loupe. Quite often one can localise a foreign body on cornea easily due to the reflex from the foreign body.

Eversion and Double Eversion of Upper Lid

Examination of upper lid is very important in a routine search for small foreign bodies. A double-eversion of lid may be rewarding in some cases. It should be a routine in all cases of injury.

Slit Lamp Biomicroscopy with Gonioscopy

Examine the bulbar conjunctiva and fornices for any foreign body or mark of entry. Examine the anterior segment of the eye. Direct focal illumination is useful in examination of cornea, iris and lens. A retro-illumination can show a red fundus reflex through the iris hole created by entry of foreign body. Look for bedewing of cornea, epithelial edema, endothelium of cornea, any changes in the iris and any tract visible in cornea, lens and vitreous. Gonioscopy helps to examine the angle of anterior chamber.

Ophthalmoscopy

A foreign body in the vitreous and retina can be easily visualized by ophthalmoscopy provided the media is clear. The media may be clear in early hours after injury so examine the case immediately for ophthalmoscopy. Indirect ophthalmoscopy is useful in locating the exact position and nature of foreign body and assessing any lesion of posterior segment of the eye such as trauma to disk, macula and retina, track in the vitreous, hemorrhage and detachment.

X-ray Orbit

X-ray orbit-antero-posterior and lateral views are helpful in localization of intraocular or intraorbital foreign bodies.

CT Scan

A computerized tomography scanning with axial and coronal cuts is the best method for intraocular foreign body localization.

Ultrasonography

Ultrasonography may demonstrate a foreign body even though the X-ray is normal. It reveals the exact length of the eyeball thus helps in exact localization by the sweet localization technique. It helps to detect presence of retinal detachment, vitreous hemorrhage, bands and membranes and the magnet-induced movability of a foreign body. Both A-scan and B-scan ultrasonography should be performed to arrive at proper diagnosis. It shall benefit to use both the radiographic and ultrasonography technique to locate the foreign body.

Therefore, it is mandatory to examine every case with care and precision.

RETAINED INTRAOCULAR FOREIGN BODY

Types of Intraocular Foreign Body

Usually it is iron, steel, brass, copper, bronze, zinc, lead and aluminium or any combination of these. It can be piece of stone, glass, coal, concrete, and fiber glass, plastic and wood. It can be anything.

The most common is iron particle with use of hammer and chisel, or grinder. The size of the foreign body varies. A large particle may completely disorganize the eye. A small particle penetrates the globe and may lie in the lens or vitreous.

There may be multiple foreign bodies in the eye when it is due to a blast injury.

Modes of Damage

Mechanical Effect

A flying particle may have sufficient velocity to traverse the anterior chamber, lens and vitreous to reach the retina. It may cause double perforation and lie in the orbit. It may get embedded in retina. It may remain lodged in the vitreous. It may enter lens and remain there. The mechanical effect shall vary depending on the size, velocity and the site of entry. An inert particle may remain without much effect.

Intraocular Infection

An infected particle may induce suppuration. Intraocular suppuration usually results in endophthalmitis or even panophthalmitis.

Uveitis

Most cases do develop uveitis which leads to atrophic bulbi.

Intraocular Hemorrhage

A hemorrhage in the vitreous induces fibrosis and later retinal detachment.

Specific Effects of Foreign Body Retained in the Eye

The reaction of the eye varies with the composition of the foreign particle. An inert and aseptic foreign body may not cause any reaction except mechanical effect.

- Non-organized substances usually do not cause any reaction except mechanical effect coupled with exudation and fibrosis which isolates the foreign particle by encapsulation.

- Non-organized substances which interacts with the tissue and cause a non-specific damage.
- Organized material tends to set up a proliferative response.

Clinical Features and Management

1. Siderosis bulbi.
2. Chalcosis.
3. Intraorbital foreign body.

SIDEROSIS BULBI

Siderosis bulbi refers to degenerative changes induced by an iron foreign body. It occurs due to retained iron foreign body in the eye even from a very small particle. In direct siderosis the iron is deposited in the nearby structures. In the indirect siderosis most of the ocular tissue is involved.

Pathogenesis

The spread of the metal is due to electrolytic dissociation by the constant current of rest present in the eye. The ions disseminate throughout the eye in a postero-anterior direction. The ions combine with intracellular proteins and induce degenerative process especially in the epithelial structures of the eye. In the cell, the ions combine with protein to form an insoluble protein salt. It interrupts the cellular activity thus causes the death of cells rather than affecting the metabolic activity.

Symptoms

- Dim vision due to changes in the cornea, lens and retina.
- Concentric contraction of visual fields.
- Night blindness is a prominent feature.
- Complete blindness gradually occurs.

Signs

Slit lamp biomicroscopy and ophthalmoscopy
- Cornea shows a rusty stain in the beam of slit lamp. The coloration is deeper in the periphery and lighter in center. Interstitial keratitis and vascularization of cornea has also been noticed.
- The iris also takes a rusty color from brown to yellow, green, red or reddish brown. It shows a good contrast with the opposite iris. Synechia has been observed indicating occurrence of silent inflammatory reaction.
- The pupil is dilated with no reaction to light probably due to atrophy of muscle fibers of pupil, the sphincter and dilator.
- In the lens there are innumerable minute brown dots in the sub-capsular region. Gradually the whole lens appears yellow tinted. Examine the lens after dilation of pupil to appreciate the changes better. It becomes opaque.
- The vitreous shows brown spots all over and degenerates.
- In the retina there is a pigmentary degeneration in the periphery. The macula may show changes with fine pigmentation, loss of foveal reflex and change in the color of paramacular region.
- The optic disk may show a rusty color.
- Later, there is retinal detachment.
- There is a secondary glaucoma, which does not respond to medical or surgical therapy.
- The electroretinogram is of negative plus type which becomes negative minus type and ultimately no response.

Treatment

An early removal of foreign body is the only treatment to prevent occurrence of siderosis. The end result is atrophic bulbi.

CHALCOSIS

Chalcosis occurs with a retained foreign particle in the form of an alloy containing little pure copper. There is a slow diffusion of copper. The metal deposition occurs in the limiting membranes of the eye. A reaction to pure copper is very severe and suppurative type. The clinical picture is classical.

Pathogenesis

There is electrolytic dissociation of the copper ions from the alloy and these ions are deposited under the membranous structures of the eye. The copper ions do not combine with the proteins of the cells and thus do not induce degenerative changes.

Clinical Manifestations

Slit lamp biomicroscopy and ophthalmoscopy shows

Kayser-Fleischer Ring

There is a golden brown ring in the periphery of cornea located mainly in the Descemet's membrane.

Sunflower Cataract

It is brilliant golden green in color and arranged like petals of sunflower under the posterior capsule of the lens.
- Zonular fibers are also affected by deposits of copper.
- Many particles may be seen in the aqueous humor.
- The iris shows a greenish color.
- Vitreous may show deposits in its framework.

Metallic sheen in Retina

There are refractile deposits on the retina covering macula and vessels also.

Differential Diagnosis
- Hepatolenticular degeneration.
- Copper poisoning.

Treatment

The only treatment is to remove the intraocular foreign body to prevent the occurrence of chalcosis.

OTHER COMPLICATIONS OF FOREIGN BODY

Intraocular Hemorrhage

The hemorrhage may be little or massive. A massive hemorrhage leads to proliferative retinopathy eventually to detachment and atrophic bulbi.

Endophthalmitis

The infection may be introduced with the foreign particle. Once the endophthalmitis develops it is difficult to cure. An early vitrectomy is advisable to save the eye and some vision. Antibiotic by all the routes is helpful.

Sympathetic Ophthalmitis

It is more common if the foreign body is lodged in the ciliary body or has damaged it extensively. If there is a chance for a useful vision then treat the case with all the aseptic precautions, repair with removal of foreign body along with topical and systemic antibiotics and steroids.

Treatment
- The bst treatment is removal of a foreign body from the eye.
- Anterior segment foreign bodies can be removed easily either through the wound of entry or by limbal incision.
- Magnetic foreign bodies can be manipulated and removed through the scleral incision from the posterior segment.
- Non-magnetic foreign bodies can be removed from the posterior segment through pars plana route using vitrectomy.
- For an intralenticular foreign body perform a cataract extraction.

INTRAORBITAL FOREIGN BODY

Specific effect of a foreign body in the orbit is much less harmful than in the eye. The main effect is mechanical trauma. Most metals, like iron, steel, aluminium, are inert and cause no effect, and lie quietly. A copper foreign body has a tendency to excite a suppurative inflammation. Other foreign body such as glass and stone are also inert. Organic foreign body causes a granulomatous reaction.

Complications

Emphysema

Emphysema results due to fracture of orbital wall, thereby opening the aircells. It is an immediate complication following trauma.

There is marked swelling of the lids. It can be diagnosed easily, by mild pressure on the swollen lids. The air in the lids give feeling of being displaced. Large emphysema may be treated by an incision and release of air.

Hemorrhage

A tear of a large vein may cause proptosis and ecchymosis. A pressure bandage is enough to stop further bleeding. The hemorrhage shall absorb in 3–4 weeks.

Infection

Though the foreign body in the orbit remains inert yet if it is infected then it shall cause infection resulting in cellulitis. A retained piece of wood is most likely, to set up cellulitis. Treat by antiobiotics and removal of foreign body at the earliest.

Other

Proliferating mass of granulation tissue around the foreign body. Infraorbital neuralgia, due to injury to infraorbital branch the maxillary nerve.

- Sinusitis due to involvement of a sinus in injury.
- Traumatic cyst
- Fibrous bands.

Management

- It is advisable to leave the foreign body in place if there is no definite indication for its removal. As its removal may cause further trauma to important structures in the orbit.
- It is advisable to remove a foreign body of wood or of any organic matter.
- Suitable antibiotic cover for infected foreign body.
- A lateral orbitotomy may be needed for a foreign body at the apex of orbit.

A Case with
Blow-out Fracture Orbit

History

- Any history of a blunt trauma to the orbit. Ask details about blunt trauma.
- Any diplopia.
- Any change in the position of the eyeball.
- Patient complains that his eyeball has shrunk in the orbit after injury.
- Patient complains that there is a relative change in the position of the two eyes after injury.

CLINICAL EXAMINATION

External Examination

The affected eye and the opposite eye should be thoroughly examined. The external examination will show varying degree of edema, hemorrhage, ecchymosis and proptosis. The real picture manifests after subsidence of edema and hemorrhage. In a case with mild edema there may be noticeable enophthalmos and inferior displacement of the globe, "globe-ptosis". The movements of the eyeball may be restricted with complain of diplopia.

Palpation of the Orbital Rim

The orbital rim should be palpated to detect any deformity, discontinuity and tenderness.

Sensation of Skin around the Inferior Orbital Margin

There may be anesthesia in the area supplied by the infraorbital nerve if the fracture has involved the infraorbital canal.

Exophthalmometry

It will show the degree of enophthalmos.

Assess the Globe-ptosis

It can be assessed by placing a scale across the medial canthi. The edge of the scale will show the degree of inferior displacement of the affected eye in comparison to the normal eye.

Motility of the Eyeball

Assess the motility of the eyeball in all the cardinal position of gaze and note if there is any restriction. Repeat the test every 3rd day for at least two weeks.

Diplopia Field Charting

It is an easy, precise and graphic method of following gaze limitation. Make the patient seated at a Goldmann perimeter with both eyes open. The perimeter is centered on the bridge of the nose. Move a large test object outward from the fixation point in eight meridians. Ask the patient to respond when he notices diplopia. By this an island of single vision is outlined surrounded by a field of diplopia. The diplopia field should be charted out every seventh day. Any enlargement of the island of single vision is a clear sign of improvement.

Forced Duction Test

The forced duction test should be performed when there is restriction of motility of the eyeball under topical anesthesia. The forced duction test is helpful when the test is either positive or negative.

CT Scan

CT scan in both axial and coronal plane helps to determine the location of fractures and soft tissue deficit.

CLINICAL FEATURES AND MANAGEMENT

Etiology

A blow-out fracture occurs following an injury to the orbit by a blunt object that is bigger in size than the diameter of the orbital margin. An injury by a smaller object shall produce a severe contusion or concussion causing even rupture of the globe. The most common mode is a blow from a fist, a tennis ball or rounded blunt object.

Pathogenesis

There are two ways in which a blow-out fracture of the orbit can occur.

Hydraulic Theory

Smith and Began in their "Hydraulic theory" postulated that when a blunt object strikes the orbit, the eyeball along with its soft tissues are pushed posteriorly thereby suddenly increasing the intraorbital pressure. This increased intraorbital pressure is relieved by fracture of the posterior orbital floor. The posterior orbital floor is very thin (0.5 to 1.0 mm), has a slight convexity and is inclined superiorly and is further weakened by infra-orbital groove and canal. All these factors contribute to its fracture.

Buckling Force

A blow to the inferior orbital margin produces a "Buckling force" on the floor of the orbit. The force is transmitted directly to the thin orbital floor buckling it and fracturing it downwards into the maxillary antrum.

CLINICAL FEATURES

Proptosis

Immediately after the injury, there may be proptosis due to marked orbital hemorrhage and edema. The real picture manifests after the subsidence of edema and absorption of hemorrhage.

Enophthalmos

There is enophthalmos due to fracture of the floor of the orbit and damage to supporting ligaments of the globe. The herniation of the soft tissues of the orbit in the maxillary sinus further contributes to an appearance of eno-phthalmos. If the enophthalmos is marked then there is a noticeable superior sulcus deformity.

Globe-ptosis

The eyeball may be displaced inferiorly in a large fracture of the floor of the orbit. The ptosis of the globe can be assessed by placing a scale across the medial canthi and compare the position of the two eyes. The lateral canthus of the affected eye is displaced inferiorly even with slight degree of globe-ptosis in orbital floor fracture. The inferior displacement of the lateral canthus is a classical sign in a zygomatic fracture due to separation of fronto-zygomatic suture. The inferior displacement of the lateral canthus is due to a pull by the check ligaments of the lateral rectus muscle and Lockwood's ligament of the eyeball. The displacement of the lateral canthus is comparable to the globe-ptosis. In a large fracture of the orbital floor there is also a displacement of the medial canthus.

Diplopia

Diplopia is the most common symptom present in all the cases. Any patient who complains of diplopia in any field two weeks after injury must be explored for orbital floor fracture. Diplopia occurs due to the following causes
- Incarceration of the inferior rectus and inferior oblique muscle in the fracture site.
- Orbital hemorrhage and edema of the orbit may produce diplopia by taugh-tening the fibrous septa which connects the inferior rectus and inferior oblique muscles to the periostium.
- Incarceration of the orbital fat in the fracture site.

- Direct injury to the extraocular muscles
- Trauma to the motor nerves—third, fourth and sixth nerve.
- Decompensation of phoria due to patching of the affected eye may disrupt the binocular vision resulting in diplopia.

MANAGEMENT

Indications for Repair

The indications for repair of blow-out fracture depend on the degree of enophthalmos, globe-ptosis and diplopia.

- An enophthalmos of 3 mm or more is an indication for repair as it becomes cosmetically embarrassing more so if associated with a globe-ptosis.
- A large defect in the orbital floor is an indication for repair.
  A fracture involving more than half of the orbital floor is considered as a large defect. A large defect results in a large inferior displacement of the globe along with marked enophthalmos.
- A troublesome diplopia with positive forced duction test is an indication for repair. Watch the case for any improvement in the motility and decrease in diplopia. If there is an improvement then wait until the case gets stabilized.
- Every individual case must be assessed depending on his vocation and signs of improvement.

Surgical Management

A transconjunctival approach is easy and provides excellent visualization of the operation field and leaves no scar on the skin.

COMPLICATIONS

Persistent Diplopia

The diplopia persist either due to entrapped tissue by the implant or fibrosis of the extra-ocular muscles.

Loss of Vision

There may be complete loss of vision due to injury to the optic nerve or compression of the optic nerve by an implant. The surgery should be taken only after subsidence of edema and absorption of hemorrhage. If the visual loss has followed the surgery then it is advisable to remove the implant to relieve the compression of the optic nerve. Give steroids.

Extrusion of Implant

The implant is thrown out if it is of large size or becomes infected.

Chronic Maxillary Sinusitis

There may be a chronic infection of the maxillary sinus. Treat it with appropriate drugs.

A Case with Sympathetic Ophthalmitis

History

- Duration of injury.
- Vision in the injured eye.
- Any blurring of vision.
- Any pain or tenderness in the eye.
- Any history of intraocular operation.
- Any investigations or treatment.

CLINICAL EXAMINATION

Visual Acuity

The vision varies with severity of the onset. Record the vision carefully with and without glasses. Assess the refractive error.

Slit Lamp Biomicroscopy

Examine the anterior segment and also posterior segment by gonio lens and make a note.

Ophthalmoscopy

Fundus examination is a must to diagnose lesions in retina, optic nerve and vitreous.

Fundus Fluorescein Angiography

In acute phase-fundus fluorescein angiography shows points of hyper fluorescence followed by leakage and even pooling.

Optical Coherence Tomography (OCT)

It is very useful to assess the condition of macula especially serous macular detachment.

Ultrasonography

It may show thickening of choroidal layer.

CLINICAL FEATURES AND MANAGEMENT

Sympathetic ophthalmitis is a bilateral granulomatous panuveitis which occurs after a penetrating ocular injury involving incarceration of the uveal tissue. Sympathetic ophthalmitis has been also reported after cataract and glaucoma surgery, proton beam irradiation, Nd:YAG cyclophotocoagulation and cyclocryotherapy.

The eye which suffered trauma is known as the *inciting eye* and the fellow sound eye which develops inflammation is known as *sympathizing eye*.

Incidence

The onset has been reported after nine days of injury and may be delayed for months and years. The enucleation of the injured eye after 14 days even if the fellow eye is not inflamed is not absolutely protective. Incidence has tremendously decreased due to microsurgical technique and steroids.

Etiology

Though it is considered to be an autoimmune disease, the actual antigen inciting bilateral pan uveitis has been poorly identified. Retinal antigens S-protein and Inter photoreceptor binding have been implicated as antigens.

Pathogenesis

Dalen-Fuch nodules: The nodular aggregation formed by proliferation of pigment epithelium of iris, ciliary body and choroid are characteristic. The entire uveal tract is invaded by the nodular aggregation of lymphocytes, plasma cells, epitheloid cells and giant cells.

CLINICAL FEATURES AND MANAGEMENT

Inciting Injured Eye

The inciting injured eye shows mild plastic iridocyclitis with ciliary congestion, lacrimation, tenderness and keratic precipitates.

Sympathizing Sound Eye

It manifests as an acute pan uveitis and also as neuroretinitis.

In prodromal stage the patient complains of photophobia and difficulty in reading or any near work due to weakness of accommodation and mild tenderness on movement of the eyes. Slit lamp bio-microscopy shows mild circumciliary congestion, aqueous flare, cells and keratic precipitates, fine vitreous haze and optic neuritis or neuroretinitis.

The ophthalmologist must clinch the diagnosis with prodromal symptoms of photophobia, problems with near vision and mild tenderness and presence of aqueous flare with one or two keratic precipitates. Treatment at this stage shall cure the patient in no time.

In a day or two the patient develops characteristic acute pan uveitis in both the eyes.

Anterior segment shows circumcorneal congestion, large granulomatous kp's, aqueous flare and cells, muddy iris, sluggish pupil, and posterior synechia.

Fundus examinations shows vitreous haze, hyperemic and blurred optic nerve head, localized yellow lesions (Dalen-Fuch nodules) at deep level.

Management

Manage with topical instillation of antibiotic, steroid and cycloplegic eye drops. Add systemic steroids in high doses (1–2 mg/kg body weight) daily in divided dose and taper gradually to a maintenance dose of 10 mg daily for long time.

In an acute phase: manage with topical instillation of antibiotic, steroid and cycloplegic eye drops and intravenous steroids-Methyl prednisolone or Dexamethasone for 3–5 days followed by 100 mg of prednisolone daily in divided doses for few days. Taper the steroids gradually depending on the response. Keep the patient on maintenance dose of 10–20 mg daily for few months.

In steroid resistance cases and cases showing severe side effects to steroids; manage with immunosuppressive therapy.

A Case with Migrainous Headache

History

Record the history with reference to the following but carefully avoiding the leading questions:

- Location of headache—frontal, temporal, occipital, vortex or generalized.
- It is unilateral, bilateral, half headache or the area of headache is shifting with each attack.
- It is dull ache, throbbing, piercing, bursting, boring or any specific description given by the patient.
- It is worse in morning or evening or gradually increases with the day, i.e. starts with mild headache which increases with the day as the sun rises and settles down with sunset.
- Any association with typical visual symptoms like rainbow color halos, scintillating scotoma, blurring of vision or vertigo.
- Any association with fatigue, insomnia, bright light.
- Any association with emotional stress or any specific trigger.
- Any association with motion sickness.
- Any association with cough, sneeze or valsalva maneuver.
- Any association with menstruation, weekends, food, season, alcohol intake and emotional situation.
- Any association with intake of drugs like alcohol, oral contraceptives and vasodilators.
- Any association with vomiting providing relief or increases it.
- Any history of hypertension, diabetes, epilepsy, psychiatric problem, allergy, trauma to head even a mild one and recent lumber puncture.
- Any recent history of flu, sinusitis or nose running.
- Ask especially about any pain in any teeth.

- Family history is common, affects all ages but common in children and adults. Among adults it is more common in females.
- In children it may manifest as recurrent abdominal pain and malaise.

CLINICAL EXAMINATION

Headache is one of the commonest symptomatic condition for which the patient seeks the advice of an ophthalmologist, a neurologist and a physician. Headache may be of benign origin or it may be due to life-threatening diseases. Therefore, it becomes necessary for a doctor to assess the case thoroughly by a careful history and thereafter a careful examination of a case including investigations before dispensing the case as an idiopathic. A large number of cases with headache first come to an ophthalmologist to get their eyes check up. In case, if one does not find any eye problem as the cause for headache then the case must be referred to a neurologist or any other specialty depending on the presenting history and normal ocular findings.

Visual Acuity

- Record the visual acuity carefully. Missing a word or reading it incorrectly indicates an astigmatic error though the vision appears to be normal. The most common error in reading the vision chart is noticed with the letter 'O' or the letter 'C'. He reads either the letter O as C or the letter C as O.

- Record the visual acuity for near vision. Repeated change in glasses with no comfort in reading or no improvement in the reading with varying the plus glasses indicate towards the patient being a case of glaucoma. He will be having all his complaint of headache related to his near work only. There is no other positive finding in favor of glaucoma. Record the pressure and invariably it shall be rewarding.

Cover, Uncover and Alternate Cover Test

Perform the test for distance and near. Make a note about the amount of heterophoria. Note about the recovery whether it is quick or slow or breaks in heterotropia. Heterophoria itself can be the cause for the headache and eye strain.

Refraction

Refraction is a must to assess the refractive state of the eyes. Correct the astigmatic refractive error if any how soever small error it may be. A minor degree of astigmatic refractive error is more likely to be the cause of headache and eye strain than the higher degree of refractive error.

Test Convergence and Accommodation

Any marked deviation between the two can be the cause for headache. There may be a convergence deficiency or poor accommodation power both conditions can be responsible for headache and eye strain. The power of convergence can be improved by exercise and the accommodation can be helped by suitable prescription of glasses.

Ocular Movements

Conduct the ocular movements in all the cardinal direction and make a note if there is any restriction of movement of the eyeball in any direction. Pay special attention to the convergence movement of the eyeball. A deficiency of convergence is an important cause for headache and eye strain.

Grades of Fusion

Examine the patient for the grades of fusion on a synoptophore. The poor amplitude of fusion may be the cause for headache and eye strain. The amplitude of fusion can be improved by exercise on synoptophore.

Ophthalmoscopy

Ophthalmoscopy should be a part of routine examination in all the cases attending eye clinic. The fundus finding may help to clinch the diagnosis of headache. Specially look for an early papilledema and early hypertensive retinopathy.

General Clinical Examination

On ophthalmic check-up, if one is not able to find any positive finding for headache and eye strain, then it shall be rewarding to perform the following simple clinical examination and then refer the case accordingly to the concerned specialty.

Record the Blood Pressure and Pulse

Record the pulse for full one minute with patient relaxed. Record the blood pressure in a lying down position with patient in a relaxed mood. If blood pressure is high or pulse is fast and irregular then refer the case to physician.

Tenderness in Temporal Arteries

Feel the temporal region for any tenderness in the temporal arteries. The temporal arteritis is one of the common factor for headache.

Cervicle Muscles

Examine the cervicle muscles for any spasm and tenderness.

Percussion over Sinuses

If the percussion over sinuses exhibits tenderness and exacerbates headache then refer the case to ENT specialist.

Laboratory Investigation

1. Complete blood picture.
2. Urine.

3. X-ray spine, sinuses.
4. Biopsy-temporal artery.
5. CT scan and MRI.

VARIOUS COMMON CAUSES OF HEADACHE

1. Headache due to migraine.
2. Headache due to eye strain.
3. Headache due to emotional stress.
4. Headache due to sinusitis.
5. Headache due to eye problem:
   - Glaucoma.
   - Iritis.
   - Temporal arteritis.
   - Refractive errors.
   - Muscle imbalance.
   - Convergence deficiency.
   - Poor accommodation power.
   - Dissociation of accommodation and convergence.
6. Headache due to improper body posture and illumination:
   - Improper illumination (dim or very bright).
   - Improper posture for near work-reading and writing.
7. Headache due to intake of drugs:
   - Vasodilators.
   - Oral contraceptives.
8. Headache due to systemic disease:
   - Dental problems.
   - Middle ear diseases.
   - Trigeminal neuralgia.
   - Spondylitis (cervical).
   - Hypertension.
   - Diabetes.
   - Hypoglycemia.
   - Constipation.
9. Headache due to life-threatening lesions:
   - Meningitis.
   - Subarchnoid hemorrhage.
   - Intracranial tumor.
   - Trauma to head.
   - Arteriovenous fistula (carotid-cavernous fistula).
10. Headache due to benign factors:
    - Seasonal.
    - Emotional stress.
    - Weekends stress.
    - Specific foods.
    - Psychiatric factors.
    - Allergy.
    - Alcohol intake.
    - Premenstrual.
    - Flu (common cold).
    - Fevers.
    - Recent lumbar puncture.
    - Epilepsy.
    - Hypertension.
11. Headache in children
    - Refractive error.
    - Excessive use of accommodation and convergence due to reading at a very close distance.
    - Heterophoria.
    - Sinusitis and adenoids.
    - Allergy.
    - Emotional problem at home, school, and with neighbors.
    - Excessive attention to a child.
    - Specific foods.

Clinical Features and Management

1. Migraine.
2. Emotional stress.
3. Sinusitis.
4. Temporal arteritis.
5. Increased intracranial pressure.
6. Meningitis.

MIGRAINE

Migraine or migrainous headache is periodic, unilateral, boring or throbbing headache usually in the frontotemporal region accompanied with nausea, vomiting, emotional disruption, fatigue and visual disturbances.

Etiology

Vascular Hypothesis

Migrainous headache was produced by extra-cranial vasodilatation due the fact that patients presented with prominent painful temporal artery pulsation neurological symptoms were due to intracranial vasoconstriction.

Migraine is Analogous to Epilepsy

The more recent concept is that the migraine is analogous to epilepsy and clinically apparent vascular phenomenon secondary to neurophysiological changes in the cerebral cortex.

Migraine is a hereditary perturbation of serotonergic neurotransmission.

Pathogenesis

Pathogenesis is in three phases. The first phase is brainstem generation. The second phase covers vasomotor activation in which arteries within and outside the brain may constrict or dilate. The third phase is activation of the trigeminal nucleus caudalis in the medulla which is the brain's pain processing center of the head and face.

Activation of any one phase is enough to precipitate migrainous headache and that phase is dominant in a particular migrainous syndrome.

Clinical Features

- It affects 10% of population and characterized by headache in the fronto-temporal region.
- Usually it is unilateral but can be bilateral. There is a tendency to change the side to other side of head in next episode.
- There is always some kind of precipitating factor: menstrual cycle, puberty, pills, foods, alcohol, fatigue, insomnia, bright lights and emotional stress of any kind.
- Visual disturbances: zigzagging flashing lights, photophobia, blurred vision or field defect lasting for about 30 minutes, usually preceding the headache.
- Neurological signs: hemiplegic migraine, ipsilateral paralysis of one or more extra-ocular muscles more in children, sudden monocular loss of vision without flashes, bilateral blurring of vision, diplopia, vertigo, visual hallucinations, etc.

Clinical Types of Migrainous Headache

Migraine is a disorder with varying symptoms. Many factors have been thought to play a part as a stimulus such as heredity, psychic factors, allergens, oral contraceptives and endocrine changes. Whatever may be the stimulus, the clinical signs and symptoms can be attributed to changes associated with vasoconstriction and vasodilatation. It is considered that vasoconstriction initiates the various neurological manifestations and vasodilation is the cause of pain which is felt as a headache.

Classic Migraine

In a classic migraine, there is a scintillating scotoma. The positive scotoma appears in the visual field obscuring vision with peculiar shimmering character. It covers one half of the visual field leaving the fixation point. In the dark field the patient sees bright spots and rays of different colors. Usually, it is a homonymous hemianopia covering both half fields. The vision clears within half an hour and is followed by severe throbbing headache associated with nausea and vomiting.

Ophthalmoplegic Migraine

It is associated with ocular motor nerve palsy. Other nerves may be involved. The involvement of nerves frequently occurs during headache or afterwards. The diagnosis of ophthalmoplegic migraine must be made only after a thorough neurological examination and after multiple episodes.

Cluster Headache

It is a variant of migraine. The headache is associated with ipsilateral watering, nasal congestion, conjunctival congestion, with miosis and ptosis. The headache may last for half an hour to several hours. The headache may occur at the same time each day. Headache may occur in a season, during the year, every year. It affects young adults usually males.

Common Migraine

In this there is headache associated with nausea, vomiting, dizziness, imbalance, depression and gastrointestinal upset. It may precede the headache or may be occurring with the headache. The headache usually lasts for few days.

Management

- Correct any refractive error.
- Avoid trigger by conscious effort.
- Sumatriptan 25 mg as a single dose provides relief in susceptible cases.
- Ergotamine preparation preferably sublingual for a quick action.
- A combination of analgesic, antidepressants and tranquilizers modify the episode.
- Attend to any psychic factor, allergic factor and chemical factor. Some people get headache after consumption of food preservatives like mono sodium glutamate or nitrates.
- Attend to emotional stress headache, headache due to cervical arthritis, hypertension, hypoglycemia and any other medical problems.
- Refer the case to neurologist for check up and management.

EMOTIONAL STRESS

- The most important diagnostic point is that the headache is bilateral and non-throbbing type. It is a constant headache which starts in the occipital area and spreads to frontal region.
- It is not affected by valsalva maneuver.
- It is worse in the evening.
- Emotional situation act as trigger. A leading question shall help to get the answer from the patient about his emotional problem either in family or with job.
- There may be associated spasm of cervical muscles.
- *Management:* Treat by assurance, psychotherapy along with some tranquilizers, non-narcotic analgesics and anti-depressant therapy. Patient may be advised to attend stress management courses if available. Look for cervical spine disorders and treat if there is any.

SINUSITIS

- Headache is usually frontal, non-throbbing type and may be unilateral or bilateral.

- Always associated with some predisposing nasal abnormality like deviated septum, polyp and allergy.
- It is usually seasonal.
- Allergy plays an important role.
- Percussion over sinuses exacerbates the headache or exhibits tenderness.
- *Management:* X-ray sinuses, CT scan or MRI shall show changes. Refer the case to ENT specialist. The common treatment is by antibiotics, decongestants, antihistamines, non-narcotic analgesics and surgical drainage of sinuses if necessary.

TEMPORAL ARTERITIS

- A unilateral headache in an elderly person should arouse suspicion of temporal arteritis, with no other obvious etiological factor.
- A swollen, tender and non-pulsatile temporal arteries in the temporal area further confirms the diagnosis. Its absence does not exclude temporal arteritis.
- An elevated erythrocyte sedimentation rate (ESR) greater than 40 mm/h favors the diagnosis.
- There may be associated generalized muscle aches and pains in the body.
- A case of temporal arteritis should be treated early as the arteritis may involve the ophthalmic or other intracranial arteries leading to blindness and other focal neurological changes.
- **Management:** Start steroids systemically with a high dose. Monitor the case with report of erythrocyte sedimentation rate. Reduce the steroids with fall in the ESR. Patient requires treatment at least for one year with small maintenance dose of steroids.
- A biopsy of the temporal artery shall help further. As the arteritis is focal a sufficient length of temporal artery must be obtained for biopsy. A negative biopsy report does not exclude temporal arteritis as the focal point may be missed in the biopsy.

INCREASED INTRACRANIAL PRESSURE

- Headache is bilateral and it is worse in the morning. Initially mild, increasing to severe headache gradually.
- Headache is a non-throbbing type.
- Headache becomes worse with cough or sneeze, i.e. with valsalva maneuver.
- Severe headache is associated with vomiting.
- There may be an early papilledema.
- There may be associated early focal neurological signs.
- *Management:* Patient should be hospitalized and subjected to thorough investigation and treat the underlying cause.

MENINGITIS

- Headache is generalized but more in the occipital region.
- Headache is associated with fever, stiff neck, nausea and vomiting.
- Patient is irritable and restless with pain in the neck.
- Headache increases with physical activity.
- There may be associated photophobia, squint, ptosis and unequal pupil.
- A lumbar puncture is a must for diagnosis and treatment.
- *Management:* Treat by broad spectrum antibiotics depending on the culture report. Patient should be hospitalized immediately with even suspicion about meningitis. Refer the case to neurologist.

49

A Case with Flat Anterior Chamber following Filtering Surgery

History

Record the history with reference to the following:

- Duration of glaucoma: A patient with advanced (late) stage of glaucoma is likely to develop a flat or a shallow chamber postoperatively.
- Refractive state of the eye prior to surgery: The anterior chamber is shallow in a hypermetropic eye, therefore, it is more likely to develop a flat or shallow chamber postoperatively.
- Any history of uveitis: In an eye with previous history of uveitis the blood-aqueous barrier is fragile and is susceptible to sudden aqueous shut down. The decreased aqueous inflow may result in a shallow or a flat chamber.
- Type of glaucoma: A case operated with an advanced stage of glaucoma, narrow angle glaucoma, neovascular glaucoma and lens induced glaucoma is more likely to develop a shallow or a flat chamber often due to aqueous misdirection syndrome.
- Postoperative medication: Use of carbonic anhydrase inhibitors, beta-blockers, mydriatic, cycloplegic drugs and topical steroids affect the dynamics of the chamber.
- Any history of reduced vision, pain in the eye and seeing a dark shadow in the field of vision are indicative of chamber problems.
- An increase in the myopia is indicative of a chamber problem.

CLINICAL EXAMINATION

Visual Acuity

Record the visual acuity and compare with the visual acuity recorded before surgery. It is usually reduced.

Slit Lamp Biomicroscopy

A thorough examination with a slit lamp is essential. Evaluate the condition of cornea, filtering bleb, conjunctival wound, conjunctival button hole, depth of the anterior chamber, any signs of uveitis and patency of iridectomy.

Examine the conjunctiva and the wound for any leak using a wetted fluorescein strip with cobalt blue light. An excessive flow of the aqueous will dilute the fluorescein dye and thus pinpoint a leak. Ask the patient to look towards the right and left and also use a digital compression to reveal an otherwise concealed leak.

Examine cornea for Descemet's folds and corneal decompensation.

Grade the anterior chamber depth by slit lamp examination to help assess the condition and management.

Gonioscopy should be performed to assess the chamber angle and the patency of the iridectomy hole.

Tonometry

A low pressure is suggestive of excessive outflow of the aqueous, shutdown of aqueous infusion and detachment of choroid. A high pressure is suggestive of misdirection of aqueous flow in the eye due to pupillary block, iridocapsular block and aqueous misdirection syndrome.

Binocular Indirect Ophthalmoscopy

It helps to diagnose the choroidal detachment and assess the condition of the posterior segment of the eye.

Ultrasonography

It helps to diagnose a choroidal detachment and change in the position of ciliary body-iris-lens diaphragm.

Grading of Shallow Chamber

Grade I

The central depth of the chamber is slightly reduced with iris touching the cornea in the peripheral third.

Grade II

There is only a thin zone of aqueous which separates the crystalline lens from the corneal endothelium. The peripheral two-thirds of the iris is in contact with the cornea.

Grade III

The chamber is flat. The crystalline lens is in contact with the endothelium of the cornea. A flat chamber requires an early treatment.

Clinical Features and Management

1. Excessive aqueous outflow.
2. Decreased aqueous inflow.
3. Abnormal direction of aqueous.
4. Change in the ocular anatomy.

The anterior chamber maintains its normal depth, size and volume by a constant infusion and drainage of aqueous. A filtering surgery can change this dynamics which results in a shallow or a flat chamber.

1. *Excessive aqueous outflow*
   - Full thickness filtering procedures.
   - A loose scleral flap.
   - A wound leak or conjunctival button hole.
   - Excessive escape of aqueous into the suprachoroidal space.

2. *Decreased aqueous inflow*
   - Late stage of glaucoma.
   - Neovascular glaucoma.
   - Uveitis.
   - Patients who have undergone cyclo-destructive surgery.
   - Systemic use of carbonic anhydrase inhibitors.
   - Topical use of beta-blockers even in the opposite eye.
   - Detachment of choroid.

3. *Abnormal direction of aqueous*
   - Pupillary block.
   - Iridocapsular block.
   - Aqueous misdirection syndrome.

4. *Change in the ocular anatomy*
   - A closed (narrow) angle eyes.
   - Lens induced glaucoma.
   - Choroidal detachment due to effusion or hemorrhage.
   - Anterior rotation of the ciliolenticular apparatus.

MANAGEMENT

Wound Leak and Button Hole in the Conjunctiva

The management of the wound or the conjunctival leak depends on the location, duration and size of the leak. It is the most common cause for a shallow or a flat chamber postoperatively.

A small microscopic leak may close with withdrawal of topical steroids and repair by a suture with atraumatic needle.

A conjunctival button hole needs a closure by suture. A small conjunctival button hole may be closed by applying a drop of cyanoacrylate adhesive after drying the conjunctiva. A button hole near the limbus requires a soft contact lens bandage.

Do not use topical steroids at least for four days after repair of the wound leak or button hole.

Over Filtration of Aqueous

The common cause for over filtration of aqueous is either the full thickness scleral procedures or leaving a loose scleral flap. The over filtration is suspected when there is no leak, no signs of uveitis, iridectomy hole is patent and the fundus is normal with no detachment of the choroid.

The management depends on the grade of the chamber shallowness.

Grade I chamber needs no treatment. Grade II chamber responds to pressure patch bandage for 24 hours. Grade III chamber needs early correction of over filtration to avoid firm anterior synechia.

Choroidal Detachment and Change in Ciliarybody-iris-lens Diaphragm

The choroidal detachment can occur with any degree of the intraocular pressure usually the low pressure often associated with inflammation. Large choroidal detachment causes the ciliary body-iris-lens diaphragm to move forward and thus results in a flat chamber. The chamber is grade III. Treat the malady as follows

- Control inflammation by steroids.
- Topical mydriatics and cycloplegics to relieve ciliary body spasm.
- Drain the choroidal fluid if there is no response in grade III chamber.

Decreased Aqueous Inflow

The most common cause for decreased aqueous production is the uveitis which disturbs the blood-aqueous barrier and may result in a sudden shut down of aqueous formation. Treat the condition by:
- Intensive use of steroids topically as well as systemically.
- Topical use of mydriatics and cycloplegics
- Increase fluid intake.

Misdirection of Aqueous Flow in the Eye

The most common causes for this condition are pupillary block, iridocapsular block and aqueous misdirection syndrome.
  Manage the malady
- Topical mydriatics and cycloplegics.
- Topical steroids.
- Carbonic anhydrase inhibitors.
- Hyperosmotics.
- If there is no response to above therapy then a pathway must be reestablished between the vitreous body and anterior segment.
It can be done by the following
- Vitrectomy with opening in the anterior hyaloid face.
- YAG laser can disrupt the anterior vitreous or posterior capsule.

50

Notes on Congenital Ocular Defects

Clinical Features and Management

Record the history with reference to the following:
1. Oxycephaly (acrocephaly or tower skull).
2. Crouzon's dysostosis (parrot head).
3. Epicanthus.
4. Anophthalmos.
5. Congenital cystic eyeball.
6. Congenital colobomatous cyst.
7. Congenital non-attachment of retina.
8. Microphthalmos.
9. Buphthalmos.
10. Typical coloboma of retina-choroid.
11. Coloboma of iris.
12. Persistence of hyaloid artery.
13. Persistent pupillary membrane.
14. Choroideremia.
15. Oguchi's disease.
16. Medullated nerve fibers.
17. Albinism.
18. Melanosis bulbi.
19. Congenital essential nightblindness.
20. Ectopia lentis.
21. Aniridia (irideremia).
22. Anisocoria.
23. Polycoria.
24. Dyscoria (slit-shaped pupil).
25. Corectopia (ectopia pupillae).
26. Pits in the optic disk.
27. Microphakia or spherophakia.

OXYCEPHALY (Acrocephaly or Tower Skull)

The skull is elongated in a vertical direction with short transverse and antero-posterior measurements. This is due to premature ossification of all the sutures of skull. The anomaly is evident at birth and develops during first four years of life. In its typical form, the vertex is dome-shaped, a vertical flat forehead, absent superciliary arches, a prominent nose, a small upper jaw and a heavy lower jaw and shallow orbits.

Clinical Features

- Proptosis.
- Divergent strabismus.
- Nystagmus.
- Restriction of ocular movements.
- Dim vision due to papilledema followed by optic atrophy. The optic foramens are small and there is an increased intracranial pressure. No other cranial nerve is involved.

Management

The prognosis of a case depends upon the time when the synostosis is complete. If the active growth of brain is ceased by the age of 7 or 8 then one can expect that patient will lead almost a normal life without any further deterioration of vision with his anomaly. If the patient develops early rise in the intracranial pressure then surgery is the only answer to reduce it.

CROUZON'S DYSOSTOSIS (Parrot Head)

The fully developed anomaly shows the following:
- Protruding frontal boss.

- Palpebral aperture show an antimongoloid obliquity.
- Tiny upper jaw.
- Narrow and highly arched palate.
- Irregular dentition.
- Prognathus lower jaw.

Ocular Features

- Proptosis.
- Divergent squint.
- Nystagmus may occur if vision fails early.
- Ophthalmoscopy may show papilledema or optic atrophy.

Management

A decompression of skull and/or orbit may be needed if there is an early rise in the intracranial pressure and proptosis is endangering the cornea. Most cases lead a normal life.

EPICANTHUS

Epicanthus is a condition wherein a semilunar fold of skin is seen running downwards at the side of the nose with its concavity directed towards the inner canthus. The fold of the skin arises in the upper lid and takes a crescentic course round the inner canthus and merges in the lower lid. It is bilateral. It tends to disappear at puberty with the full development of the bridge of the nose. It may persist in some cases. Most commonly the epicanthus occurs as an isolated anomaly, the eyes and adnexa being normal. It gives a characteristic appearance—the eyes appear to be separated, a broad flat nose, an apparent convergent squint. The epicanthus can be made to vanish temporarily by pinching up the skin over the bridge of the nose into a fold. Epicanthus can be associated with ptosis.

Management

It requires no treatment if it is of mild or moderate. It tends to disappear with age. An excision of a vertically elliptical area of skin over bridge of nose shall cure the malady if it persists after the age of puberty.

ANOPHTHALMOS

Clinical Feature

The external appearance of a child with Anophthalmos is normal. The lids are kept closed and may be normal or rudimentary. The palpebral aperture is small which makes examination difficult. It may be associated with epicanthus. The lids show normal lashes, tarsal glands and lacrimal punctum. But lashes and punctum may be absent. The orbit is very shallow and small but well formed as the palpebral tissue and orbital tissues are self determining and not dependent upon optic vesicle for their differentiation but the absence of the eye disturbs their balance of growth. The orbital cavity is lined by the conjunctiva. The function of the lacrimal gland is normal as the child shows tears when he cries. The extraocular muscles are present but not sharply differentiated and may be inserted in the subconjunctival tissue or in the rudimentary nodule. The optic canal is very narrow and optic nerve is absent. The lower optic pathways and primary centers may be rudimentary, aplasic or well developed. If the child survives then the intellectual capacity may be subnormal or may approach complete idiocy.

Heredity

Most cases occur sporadically without apparent hereditary tendency. It may show occasional familial incidence. A recessive genetic influence has been observed. A hereditary factor in some families is also suggested by occurrence of Anophthalmos in some members of family and rnicrophthalmos or coloboma in other members of same pedigree. Consanguinity may play a part.

Etiology

There is a primary involvement of the neural ectoderm. The occurrence of sporadic cases with an isolated anomaly of anophthalmos with no history of any disease or consanguinity is suggestive of environmental factor particularly in the primary type of Anophthalmos.

The factor could be physical, mechanical or chemical. A deficiency of folic acid, pantothenic disturbed carbohydrate metabolism and thyroidectomy has been implicated.

Management

The aim of treatment is cosmetic improvement. Due to small orbit and palpebral aperture it is difficult to provide an artificial eye. Plan to enlarge the palpebral aperture by plastic surgery and at the same time plan to enlarge the orbit by putting an acrylic prosthesis. If this is undertaken at an early age, the orbit can usually be enlarged to twice its original size in short time. This should be maintained during the growth of the child to provide him a good cosmetic appearance.

CONGENITAL CYSTIC EYEBALL

A congenital cystic eyeball is the result of a partial or complete failure in the involution of the primary optic vesicle. The primary optic vesicle has formed but instead of going through the process of involution it persists as a cyst. At birth, the eyeball is replaced by a small cyst giving an appearance of an Anophthalmos. On the other hand, the cyst may be large even larger than the normal eyeball. In a case with a large cyst it appears as a bluish thin-walled cyst in the orbit and usually causes bulge of the lids particularly the upper lid. In contrast to this, the more common colobomatous cyst causes bulge of the lower lid. The lids and the conjunctiva are normal and the orbit may be small in size. In some cases, optic stalk remains while in other cases, there may be no evidence of optic stalk. The cyst contains albuminous yellow fluid and is usually self-contained with no connection with the ventricular system of the brain. A partial involution of optic vesicle results in congenital non attachment of the retina. Environmental factor is the most likely etiological factor. There is no hereditary tendency.

CONGENITAL COLOBOMATOUS CYST

A colobomatous cyst arises due to protrusion of a portion of the proliferating retina into the surrounding tissue in the region of the embryonic cleft. The protruded knuckle of the retina may be small or may be so large that a cystic formation occurs. The eye itself may be small and grossly deformed with a cyst known as Microphthalmos with cyst. Clinically it may present as

 i. Normal eye with cyst which is not apparent.
 ii. Deformed eye with an obvious cyst.
 iii. Eye not visible with a large cyst.

In a typical case of a large cyst and apparent Anophthalmos it causes the bulge of the lower lid as the cyst is attached to the lower aspect of the eye.

There is a tendency for the cyst to grow after birth. As the eye is grossly mal-developed, it is advisable to excise it. Perform a paracentesis and excise the globe with the cyst.

CONGENITAL NON-ATTACHMENT OF RETINA

The congenital non-attachment of the retina is the result of incomplete involution of the primary optic vesicle thus instead of forming a cyst the two layers of retina remains separated. This condition is found as an incident in microphthalmic eyes showing other deformities such as persistent hyaloid artery or coloboma of retina and choroid. In this condition, unlike acquired detachment the retina shows separation beyond the oraserrata. The retina may come forward to touch the lens or there is marked glial proliferation giving an appearance of a tumor. There is white reflex from the pupil. There is no treatment for this.

MICROPHTHALMOS

Microphthalmos is a condition in which there is a small eye with many other associated defects. Once there is budding of the optic vesicle the eye is formed. It is rare to have a pure microphthalmos. Microphthalmos is usually associated with coloboma or other complications or syndromes.

A pure microphthalmic eye is due to arrested development of the globe in all dimensions after the embryonic fissure has closed. The eyeball is small without presence of other congenital anomalies. There is an association of hypermetropia and glaucoma. The vision is subnormal with nystagmus and strabismus.

BUPHTHALMOS

Buphthalmos is a condition wherein there is a raised intraocular pressure due to congenital abnormality at the angle of the anterior chamber thereby offering an obstruction to the drainage of intraocular fluid which results in congenital glaucoma.

Simple buphthalmos is caused by primary developmental anomaly at the angle of anterior chamber. It is transmitted as a recessive character.

Buphthalmic Eye

The most obvious feature is enlargement of the whole globe usually into an oval shape which gives an appearance of proptosis.

Clinical Features

- The horizontal diameter of the cornea is more than 12 mm.
- The cornea is hazy due to striae or edema.
- Presence of striae in the cornea is due to rupture of Descemet's membrane.
- Anterior chamber is deep.
- Corneal sensation is diminished.
- Bulbar conjunctiva may be congested.
- Gonioscopy shows abnormality in the angle of anterior chamber.
- Intraocular pressure is raised.
- Fundus examination may show cupping of the disk.

Clinical Symptoms

There is a triad of symptoms-photophobia, blepharospasm and epiphora most probably due to irritation caused by corneal edema. Any infant with these symptoms must be carefully examined to exclude buphthalmos. These symptoms increase with further development of buphthalmos.

Differential Diagnosis

- Megalocornea.

- High congenital myopia.
- Congenital staphylomata.
- Congenital hereditary dystrophies of cornea.
- Corneal edema may occur in cases with intraocular tumor with raised tension, inflammatory conditions and metabolic disorders like gargoylism, cystinosis or lipoidosis.

Management

Buphthalmos—the congenital glaucoma can be treated by Goniotomy with good results. A Goniopuncture may be combined with the goniotomy. The prognosis depends age at onset of symptoms, early diagnosis and prompt surgery. The results are better if the symptoms are delayed until about fourth to seventh month of age. The case needs a regular follow up for years. The prognosis is good if the structural anomaly at the angle is not unusually gross.

TYPICAL COLOBOMA OF RETINA-CHOROID

Coloboma is a term which indicates a condition of the eye wherein a portion of the structure of the eyeball is missing. This congenital defect found in the region of the embryonic cleft is labeled as "Typical Coloboma".

A typical coloboma occurs in the region of the embryonic cleft. It is due to disturbance of the mechanism in closure of the cleft. It occurs between the time of invagination of the optic vesicle and closure of the cleft that is between the 7 and 14 mm stage of development that is between fourth and fifth week. This defect in the closure of the cleft may be complete implicating all the structures, the optic disk, the retina, the choroid, the ciliary body, the iris, the lens and even resulting in formation of a colobomatous cyst. The defect in the closure of the cleft may be partial with only a small notch at the pupillary border the minimum evidence visible clinically. This anomaly of coloboma is common and usually bilateral.

Etiology

A typical coloboma is due to some interference with the normal closure of the embryonic cleft the aberration lying primarily in the epiblast of the optic cup. The cause seems to be genetic. The transmission is dominant through a relatively weak and labile gene. The environmental factor has been implicated. Many theories like mesoblastic theory, vascular theory, lenticular theory, and inflammation has been put forward but without any firm evidence. Hereditary factor is the most acceptable.

Clinical Occurrence

The most common is coloboma of iris, followed by coloboma of choroid and retina, coloboma of optic nerve and coloboma of lens.

On Ophthalmoscopy

It shows the following features:
- A white grey color of the fundus reflex.
- A glistening white sclera seen in the down and in quadrant of the fundus. It may be large or small area. It may involve the optic disk. It may be bridged or show several isolated defects. It is usually oval in shape with round and narrow end towards the disk.
- The edge of the coloboma may be sharp or fading gradually with pigmentation.
- The floor may be depressed or ectatic.
- The retinal vessels appear to dip down into the coloboma as they pass from the normal fundus.
- The choroidal vessels are lying at deeper level and are tortuous and broader in appearance.
- The macula appears normal.

Other Features

- The visual acuity is usually low.
- Strabismus and nystagmus is seen commonly.
- Field charting shows a scotoma.
- Other congenital defect like persistent pupillary membrane and hyaloid remnants are common.

COLOBOMA OF IRIS

A typical coloboma of iris is situated in downward and inward position. A coloboma of iris due to defect in the closure of embryonic fissure must be accompanied by the coloboma of choroid and retina. A coloboma of iris without involvement of choroid and retina cannot occur as iris develops long after the closure of fissure. Thus a coloboma involving only iris alone must be due to some other cause and this coloboma of iris alone is termed as simple coloboma of iris (Iridoschisma). A simple coloboma if involves the whole sector of iris up to the ciliary body then it is called as total coloboma. If it does not then it is called as partial coloboma. The simple coloboma can adopt various forms like a notch in the pupillary margin, a hole in the substance of iris, a defect at the ciliary border (iridodiastasis), a bridge across the defect in the iris. A simple coloboma of iris is one of the most common congenital defect of the eye affecting about 1 in 6000 of population. It affects both the sexes equally and is as often unilateral as bilateral (Fig. 50.1).

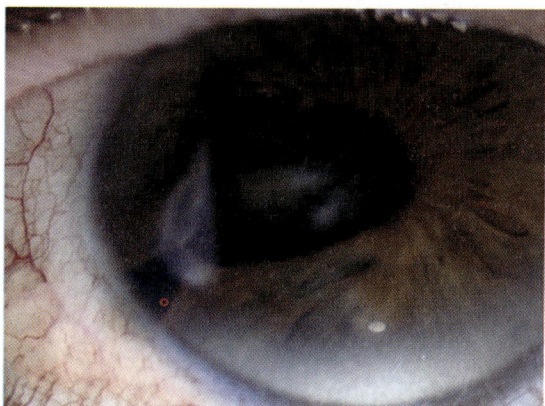

Fig. 50.1: Iris coloboma

Heredity

The deformity is transmitted as an autosomal dominant characteristic.

Etiology

The most accepted theory is that the growth of the iris is prevented by abnormally developed and persistent vascularized strands belonging to the fibrovascular sheath of the lens.

Treatment

It does not affect the vision or the cosmetic appearance of the individual. It may produce a glare. Advise use of sunglasses.

PERSISTENCE OF HYALOID ARTERY

The persistence of the hyaloid artery in a wide range of variation is one of the commonest developmental anomaly seen in a human eye.

Variations

i. *Persistence of entire artery from disk to lens:* The artery may take a form of a fine thread-like structure or a thick cord. It is thin in its central part where it first disappears in fetal life. Its shrinkage may cause a cataract and dislocation of lens.

ii. *Persistence of the artery attached to the optic disk:* It may appear as a white bud on the central retinal artery. More commonly it appears as a strand of fibrous tissue obviously an obliterated posterior end of the artery which may extend for some distance in the vitreous and may show movement upon the movement of the eye.

iii. *Prepapillary membrane or a cyst:* It may appear as a well-defined membrane stretching over the disk. Sometimes the hyaloid remnants at the disk are associated with cyst formation. The cyst is usually small, round and sessile upon the disk or as peduncle. These must be differentiated from juxtapapillary cysticercus. These are stationary and associated with other remnants of hyaloid artery with absence of inflammatory signs and no loss of vision.

iv. *Persistence of artery attached to lens:* On slit lamp examination it may appear as a delicate cord slightly coiled and attached to posterior capsule of the lens and hanging freely in the vitreous. It is attached at about 1.5 to 2 mm to the nasal side and slightly below the posterior pole of the lens.

PERSISTENT PUPILLARY MEMBRANE

It is an extremely common anomaly. The persistent pupillary membrane represents a failure of the normal process of the atrophy of the central arcades and their associated mesodermal tissue. The remnants of the pupillary membrane are always attached to the superficial mesodermal layer on the anterior surface of the iris usually at the lesser circle that is at the collarette or some times more peripherally towards the ciliary margin. It is this attachment away from the pupillary border helps to diagnose and differentiate these from the inflammatory synechia (Fig. 50.2).

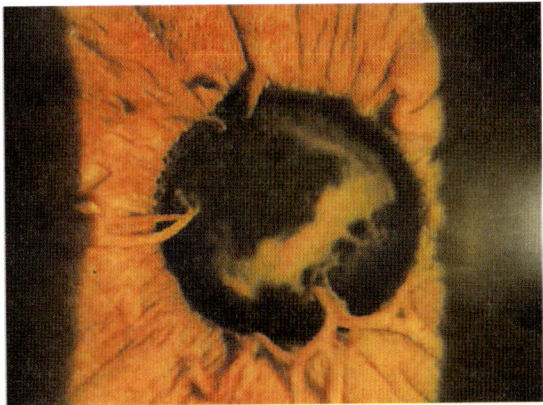

Fig. 50.2: Persistent pupillary membrane

Clinical Appearance

i. *The remnants are attached to the iris only:* One or more fibers run over the iris into the pupillary area, unite to form a loop, run across the pupillary aperture to opposite side or may unite to form a very thin membrane.

ii. *The remnants are attached to the lens:* The fibers run from the iris and get attached to the anterior lens capsule. There is usually a white plaque at the site of the attachment of fibers on the lens capsule.

iii. *Pigments on the anterior lens capsule:* On slit lamp examination and with dilated pupil the pigments over the lens can be seen. The pigments are minute or thick, arranged in a regular circular fashion. The iris moves freely over these. There is no synechia.

iv. *The remnants are adherent to cornea*: Fine fibers are seen arising from the lesser circle and run across the anterior chamber to get attached to the posterior surface of cornea. One can see small pigmented bodies floating freely in the anterior chamber also.

Management

As these fibers do not interfere with the vision therefore do not require any treatment. The pigments on the lens must be differentiated from the pigments left on the lens in a case of iridocyclitis. The pigments left after iridocyclitis are thick, irregular in arrangement and show synechia with other inflammatory signs of iritis like keratic precipitates, iris atrophy, anterior peripheral synechia and aqueous flare.

CHOROIDEREMIA

Choroideremia is inherited in an Intermediate Sex-Linked manner with minimal evidence in a female carrier.

Choroideremia is a condition wherein the choroid and the pigment epithelium of retina are completely absent except in a region around the macula. It is seen in its typical and fully developed form in males. In females the condition remains benign and does not progress, showing very little changes in the periphery of fundus.

Symptoms

- Night blindness is the most common and presenting symptom.
- Extreme concentric contraction of visual fields.
- Visual acuity is usually diminished and blindness is rule after the age of sixty.
- Electroretinogram shows absence of scotopic activity and progressive failure of photopic responses until it becomes extinguished.
- Females are asymptomatic with normal vision and dark adaptation.
  The condition remains stationary.

Clinical Features

On ophthalmoscopic examination the fundus shows:

- In early stage, there is a pepper and salt appearance in the periphery of fundus with small areas showing the choroidal vessels.
- With advance in age there is gradual loss of choroidal vessels exposing the white sclera.
- By the age of fifty the fundus appears uniformly glistening white and only central area shows a red reflex.
- The optic disk is normal.
- The retinal vessels are normal.
- The anterior segment of the eye is normal with clear media including the lens.

OGUCHI'S DISEASE

Oguchi's disease is characterized by the structural anomalies in the retina with night blindness. It is a congenital bilateral and stationary condition with hereditary in incidence. It is transmitted as an autosomal recessive without sex discrimination. Consanguinity has been observed in their antecedents.

Clinical Features on Ophthalmoscopy

- The fundus usually the posterior region appears grey or golden in color.
- The retinal vessels appear very clear with one side of the vessel showing a bright white edge and other side a dark shadow.
- **Mizuo's phenomenon:** The fundus takes up its normal color if the patient is kept in a dark room for about 2 to 8 hours.
- These changes are less marked in some cases.

Clinical Symptoms

- The visual acuity is normal in day light.
- There is night blindness in dim light. The vision slowly improves if the patient is kept in a dark room for few hours.
- Visual fields are normal.
- Electroretinogram shows a complete absence of the scotopic responses while the photopic responses are present.

- The change in the color of the fundus is due to anomalies of the visual purple or the pigment epithelium is not known.
- There is a lack of the activity of rods.

MEDULLATED NERVE FIBERS

The medullation of the optic nerve fibers starts centrally reaching the lamina cribrosa at the birth. The process ceases here. In some cases the fibers of retina may acquire a medullary sheath in the first month of postnatal life. Thus the condition is developmental and not found in the eyes of a newborn.

Symptoms

- Normal visual acuity unless the macula is involved.
- There is a scotoma corresponding to the area of medullated nerve fibers.
- Enlargement of the blind spot if it is in close relation to the optic disk.

Clinical Features on Ophthalmoscopy

- A feathery white patch in the fundus. It may be a small patch circular or irregular. Usually it is in close association of optic disk but may be seen away from it. There may be one or more patches. It may be unilateral or bilateral.
- The patch shows a striated fibrillar appearance (Fig. 50.3).

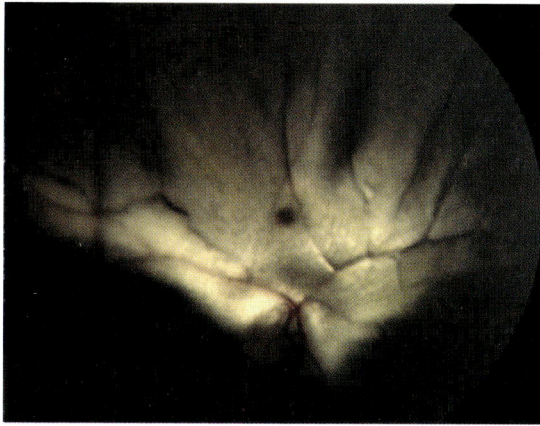

Fig. 50.3: Myelinated nerve fibers

- The retinal vessel may pass over it, dip in it or obscured by it.
- It is stationary throughout life. These may disappear if optic atrophy sets in due to any cause. The disappearance of fibers is late and gradual.

ALBINISM

Albinism is a congenital condition wherein pigment is deficient. The total albinism is due to an inborn error of metabolism, characterized by the lack of enzyme. Tyrosinase-which normally converts the dopa (3, 4-dihydroxyphenylalanine) into melanin. The partial type of albinism is due to some kind of insufficiency of this system or defective distribution of this enzyme.

Albinotic Eye

The criterion of ocular albinism is either lack or deficiency of pigment in the retinal pigment epithelium.

Clinical Features

- The eyebrows and lashes are usually white.
- There is red reflex from the pupil.
- The refractive error is usually myopia.
- Nystagmus is a constant feature due to defective macula.
- The visual acuity is subnormal.
- Photophobia due to entry of excess of light through the translucent ocular coats.
- Electroretinogram is normal.

Management

Except the absence of pigment there is no other defect. Patient lives a long useful life. Advise to use goggles to avoid photophobia.

General Total Albinism

There is no trace of melanotic pigmentation throughout the body. There is an albinotic eye, skin is white, the hairs, brows and lashes are fine, white or straw colored. It may be associated with other defects like small stature, hypogenitalism. The relatives of total albinotics may show signs of partial albinism (leucism).

MELANOSIS BULBI

Melanosis bulbi is a condition wherein there is great increase in the pigment of the uveal tract. The following three cardinal signs are universal for this condition.

i. *Pigmentation of the sclera:* There may be a few small flecks, exaggeration of perivascular and perineural deposits, large isolated patches, mottling of sclera or a pericorneal pigment ring.

ii. *Pigmentation of the iris:* The iris appears very deep brown in color. It may only show few isolated flecks or a sector gets involved.

iii. *Dark appearance of fundus:* The fundus appears chocolate color the pigmentation being marked at macula and posterior pole. There may be pigmentation around the disk.

CONGENITAL ESSENTIAL NIGHTBLINDNESS

Congenital essential nightblindness is a condition, wherein there is normal ophthalmoscopic appearance with symptom of night blindness. The nature of lesion is unknown. It is a hereditary condition showing three types of transmission, namely, autosomal dominant, a recessive sex-Linked form, and an autosomal recessive form.

Clinical Features

- The fundus is normal.
- The scotopic function of the retina is normal.
- Normal central visual acuity.
- Normal visual fields.
- Normal color sense.
- There may be some degree of blue blindness.
- Patient has no difficulty in the day.
- Patient is unable to work or see in night.
- The electroretinogram shows no scotopic components.
- The disease is stationary, permanent and no treatment.

Differential Diagnosis

- Oguchi's disease.

- Retinitis pigmentosa albicans.
- Retinitis pigmentosa.

In pigmentary retinopathy there is complete absence of b-wave in the electroretinogram while in essential nyctalopia and Oguchi's disease the photopic bl-wave is present.

ECTOPIA LENTIS

Ectopia lentis is a condition wherein the lens is displaced in the direction away from the poorly developed segment of zonule. There is a strong hereditary tendency with transmission by a dominant trait and an Autosomal Recessive with incidence of consanguinity. It can occur as

i. Isolated ectopia lentis

ii. Ectopia lentis with ectopia pupillae and other ocular anomalies;

iii. With systemic syndromes: Marfan's syndrome, Marchesani's syndrome and Ehlers-Danlos syndrome.

Clinical Features

- The edge of the lens may be seen in the pupillary area. The edge appears as a dark crescent on ophthalmoscopy owing to strong prismatic reflection.
- Iridodonesis is there.
- Anterior chamber is irregular.
- Slit lamp biomicroscopy may show zonular fibers.
- The lens is smaller than normal and more spherical.
- The lens remains clear but may be associated with coloboma or opacities.
- The lens is likely to subluxate or dislocate in the anterior chamber or the vitreous.
- Secondary glaucoma may occur.
- Detachment of retina is a rare complication.

Symptoms

- Uniocular diplopia.
- Binocular quadruplication.
- Dim vision due to myopic refraction in phakic part.
- The lens is usually displaced upwards and inwards.

Management

Remove the lens if there is diplopia and dim vision.

ANIRIDIA (Irideremia)

Aniridia is a rare condition in which the iris is extremely rudimentary.

Clinical Features

- Pupil is very large.
- On focal illumination and slit lamp examination the margin of the lens, the zonules and even ciliary process can be seen.
- Patient complains of low vision and photophobia.
- Patient may show nystagmus due to maldevelopment of macula.
- An early glaucoma may develop due to anomaly at the angle of anterior chamber.

Management

- Sunglasses.
- Remove the lens if it is opaque.
- Correct the refractive error.
- Keep a watch for glaucoma and treat early if detected.

ANISOCORIA

Anisocoria is a condition in which the size of the two pupils is unequal. Normally the two pupils are of same size and also react equally. The normal diameter of the pupil at rest is from 2.5 to 4 mm. Some inequality is common. A difference of more than 20% is taken as abnormal.

POLYCORIA

Polycoria is a condition in which there is more than one pupil. It is rare to have another true pupil with sphincter. Most pupils are holes in the iris or belong to the category of coloboma. These holes appear to react to light and drug but in fact the change in the size of the pseudo-pupil is due to sharing the movement of the iris. It is of no significance and does not require any treatment.

DYSCORIA (Slit-shaped Pupil)

Dyscoria is a condition in which the pupil takes the form of a slit as occurs normally in the contracted pupil of the cat. It may be unilateral or bilateral. In dark it may assume round, oval, hour glass or rectangular shape. The vision is good and requires no treatment.

CORECTOPIA (Ectopia Pupillae)

Corectopia is a condition in which the pupil is not at its normal position. The normal position of the pupil is slightly down and in from the center of the iris. The most common position of corectopia is up and out. It is usually bilateral. The eyes are myopic and vision is poor.

PITS IN THE OPTIC DISK

It is not uncommon to see holes, pits or crater like cavities in the optic disk. The ophthalmoscopic picture is characteristic. The pit is usually oval with long axis concentric with the margin of the disk. It may be circular, triangular or slit like. The floor is clearly seen. There may be a single pit or more. It may be unilateral or bilateral. No clinical symptoms. The field may show enlargement of blind spot or a sector defect.

MICROPHAKIA OR SPHEROPHAKIA

Microphakia (spherophakia) is a condition in which the lens is unusually small and spherical in shape. It is usually bilateral. Clinically under full mydriasis the entire lens is visible. The eye is myopic with defective accommodation. It is rare as an isolated anomaly. It is seen in Marfan's and Marchesani's syndrome. The patient is prone to develop glaucoma at an early age.

51

Notes on
Ocular Syndromes

Clinical Features and Management

1. van der Hoeve's syndrome
2. Marfan's syndrome
3. Marchesani's syndrome
4. Ehlers-Danlos syndrome (fibrodysplasia hyperplastica, dermo-ligamentorum)
5. Turner's syndrome (status Bonnevie-Ullrich syndrome)
6. Ullrich's syndrome
7. Conradi's syndrome
8. Sturge-Weber syndrome
9. Incontinentia pigment (Bloch-Sulzberger syndrome)
10. Laurence-Moon-Bardet-Biedl syndrome
11. Biemond's syndrome
12. Sorsby's syndrome
13. von Graefe's syndrome
14. Sjögren's syndrome
15. Mikulicz's syndrome
16. Mucus fishing syndrome
17. Floppy eyelid syndrome
18. Stevens-Johnson syndrome (erythema multiforme major)
19. Cogan's syndrome
20. Reiter's syndrome
21. Behcet's disease
22. Posner-Schlossman syndrome (glaucomato-cyclitic crisis)
23. Fuch's uveitis syndrome (Fuch's heterochromic cyclitis)
24. Parry-Romberg syndrome (progressive facial hemiatrophy)
25. Vogt-Koyanagi-Harada's syndrome (uveo-meningitis syndrome)
26. Presumed ocular histoplasmosis syndrome
27. Lowe's syndrome (oculo-cerebro-renal syndrome)
28. Down syndrome (mongolism)
29. Werner's syndrome
30. Rothmund's syndrome
31. Vitreous touch syndrome
32. Vitreous wick syndrome
33. "Ugh" syndrome
34. "Sunset" syndrome
35. Plateau iris syndrome
36. Iridocorneal endothelial syndromes
37. Refsum's syndrome (heredopathia atactica polyneuritiformis)
38. Bassen-Kornzweig syndrome (acanthocytosis)
39. Usher's syndrome
40. Favre-Goldmann syndrome
41. Mobius syndrome
42. Alport's syndrome
43. Empty sella syndrome

van der Hoeve's Syndrome

It is congenital and hereditary syndrome of genetic origin characterized by the blue sclera, brittle bones and deafness. It is relatively common and a well-known syndrome.

Blue sclera: Is a constant feature of the syndrome. The sclera is not colored blue but appears blue due to increased translucency of the sclera allowing the underlying uveal pigment to shine. The sclera is unusually thin.

Brittle bones (fragilitas ossium): An abnormal fragility of the bones has been noted in cases with blue sclera. An infant develops a fracture without any real substantial injury. The tendency to fracture persists throughout life and though the pain is less than usual the union is imperfect and fibrous resulting in development of deformities.

Deafness: The deafness usually sets in after the age of 20 and occurs in about 30% of cases. The cause of deafness is varied. In van der Hoeve's syndrome the cause of deafness is otosclerosis.

Marfan's Syndrome

It is due to a congenital mesodermal dystrophy. The features are opposite to Marchesani's syndrome. The common feature is the Ectopia lentis. The other features are due to hypoplasia. The arachnodactyly is the prominent feature.

Clinical Features

- **Ectopia lentis** is symmetrical, bilateral and displaced upwards. The lens is spheromicrophakic. There is iridodonesis, hypoplasia of iris and miosis with poor reaction to atropine. The poor reaction is due to defect in musculature of pupil. The lens may dislocate in the anterior chamber or the vitreous. Glaucoma can arise due to persistence of mesodermal tissue in the angle of anterior chamber.
- The affected individual is tall with elongated hands and feet. The face is long and thin. There is kyphoscoliosis.
- There is generalized muscular hypoplasia.
- The joints are lax with good mobility.
- There is lack of subcutaneous fat.
- The thorax is barrel shaped.
- The ear may show malformation.
- Patient may show various cardiac, renal and pulmonary lesions.

Most cases lead a normal life. Surgical interference is needed on dislocation of the lens and if there is a secondary glaucoma.

Marchesani's Syndrome

The features of this syndrome are opposite to the features of the Marfan's syndrome. The only common feature is the ectopia lentis. The Marfan's syndrome is a hypoplastic form of congenital mesodermal dystrophy. The Marchesani's syndrome is a hyperplastic form of the congenital mesodermal dystrophy.

Clinical Features

- Ectopia lentis with spheromicrophakia. There is a tendency for dislocation of the lens in the anterior chamber or the vitreous. There is also tendency for secondary glaucoma to develop due to spherophakia.
- The affected individual is of short height with short hands and feet. The hands are spade like. There is a brachycephaly well-developed musculature, abundance of subcutaneous fat, large thorax and reduced mobility of the joints.

Most people can lead a normal life. The lens can be removed if opaque or dislocates in the anterior chamber. Treat the glaucoma if present.

Ehlers-Danlos Syndrome (Fibrodysplasia Hyperplastica, Dermo-Ligamentorum)

It is due to dysplasia affecting the collagen fibers of the dermis, subcutaneous tissue and the articular ligaments. The malady is present at birth, becomes apparent in early infancy and remains stationary throughout life. It has two main features: hyperelastic skin and hypermobility of joints. An incomplete form may occur affecting either skin or joints.

Clinical Features

Cutis Hyperelastica (Dermatorrhexis, Rubber skin): The skin shows heperelasticity, hyperextensibility and extreme fragility. The skin is supple and elastic. It can be pulled away from the body and on releasing it returns to normal shape with an audible snap like a rubber band. The anomaly maybe generalized or limited to one part of the body usually face and lids. The skin is fragile. A slight trauma may cause gaping wound and hematoma.

Hypermobility of Joints: The fingers can be easily retroflexed on to the back of hand. Ruptures and luxations are common.

Turner's Syndrome (Status Bonnevie-Ullrich Syndrome)

- Lymphangiectatic edema of the hands and feet.

- Pterygium colli.
- Paralysis of 3rd, 6th, 7th, 12th nerve.
- Hypertelorism.
- Epicanthus.
- Malformation of ears.
- Digital deformation.
- Defect in pectoralis muscle.
- Infantilism.
- Webbing of the skin of the neck and cubitus valgus.

Ullrich's Syndrome

- Brady or acrocephaly.
- Broad nose.
- Small mandible.
- Associated skeletal, visceral and ocular deformities such as spina bifida, polydactyly, bilateral anophthalmos, extreme microphthalmos, degenerative and cystic changes in the viscera.

Conradi's Syndrome

- Cataract-bilateral and total is characteristic.
- Heterochromia iridum and optic atrophy is rare.
- Skeletal changes—a short limbed dwarf, immobile joints, flexion contractures and muscles becoming fibrosed.

Sturge-Weber Syndrome

- A cutaneous capillary angioma (nevus flammeus) of the upper part of the face and often of the associated mucous membranes. It is typically unilateral and is usually limited to the distribution of the first or second division of the trigeminal nerve or both. Its extension into the area of seventh nerve is common. In every case, there is involvement of forehead and upper lid. An angioma limited to below the level of the palpebral aperture does not embrace this syndrome. An angioma in the orbit may produce a reducible proptosis.
- A leptomeningeal angioma on the same side in the subarachnoid space, in the region of cerebrum particularly at the posterior pole.

- A choroidal angioma frequently near the optic disk is relatively a common occurrence. Glaucoma with deep cupping develops at an early age. Buphthalmos may develop.

Incontinentia Pigment (Bloch-Sulzberger Syndrome)

In this, there are two types—a **patchy** pigmentary dermatosis which is usually congenital and a **reticular form** which does not appear until the infant reaches the age of two.

The ocular anomalies are common: corneal opacities, congenital cataract, persistent hyperplastic primary vitreous, pseudoglioma, prenatal or postnatal uveitis, chorioretinitis, retinal folds, microphthalmos, nystagmus and strabismus.

Laurence-Moon-Bardet-Biedl Syndrome

It is an autosomal recessive genetic disorder. Its five classical features include polydactyly or syndactyly, retinitis pigmentosa, obesity, mental retardation, and hyogonadism. Some cases may also show brachycephaly, short stature, congenital heart disease, deafness and various neurological disorders. This syndrome can be confused with alstrom-hallgren syndrome in which there is retinitis pigmentosa, obesity, deafness and diabetes mellitus and no polydactyly, mental retardation and hypogonadism.

- Atypical pigmentary degeneration of the retina.
- Hypogenitalism.
- Mental deficiency.
- Obesity.
- Polydactyly.
- Microphthalmos and colobomata may be associated.

Biemond's Syndrome

- Hypophysial infantilism.
- Mental retardation.
- Polydactyly.
- Coloboma of iris.

Sorsby's Syndrome

- Apical dystrophy of the extremities.
- Bilateral coloboma of macula.

von Graefe's Syndrome

- Congenital deafness.
- Pigmentary degeneration of retina.

Sjögren's Syndrome

Sjögren's syndrome is an autoimmune disease. In a "**primary Sjögren's syndrome**" there is involvement of salivary glands with involvement of mucous membrane of bronchial tree and vagina. The involvement of salivary glands causes a dry mouth (xerostomia), therefore, there is a difficulty in mastication and thus patient requires liquid for mastication and swallowing. In a "**secondary Sjögren's syndrome**" there is an association of connective tissue disorder the most common being the seropositive rheumatoid arthritis. Other systemic diseases associated, include systemic lupus erythematosus, systemic sclerosis, psoriatic arthritis, juvenile chronic arthritis, and polymyositis.

Mikulicz's Syndrome

It is characterized by symmetrical enlargement of the lacrimal and salivary glands. It is of varied etiology but the swelling is of lymphomatous nature. In uveoparotitis (Heerfordt's disease), there is an enlargement of salivary (parotid) glands along with uveitis.

Mucus Fishing Syndrome

It is seen in any condition of the conjunctiva wherein there is excess mucus secretion commonly seen in keratoconjunctivitis sicca. While removing the mucus from the conjunctival sac, the patient produces trauma to the conjunctival epithelium, thereby further increases mucus secretion thus creating a vicious cycle.

Floppy Eyelid Syndrome

It is an uncommon condition, typically seen in obese persons in whom the upper eyelid everts during sleep exposing the upper tarsus and cornea. There is bilateral or unilateral chronic papillary conjunctivitis. Treat by shortening the lid by surgery.

Stevens-Johnson Syndrome
(Erythema Multiforme Major)

This is a type II hypersensitivity or immunological reaction to drugs; antibiotics, sulphonamides, acetazolamide, non-steroidal anti-inflammatory drugs, antimalarials, bacteria, virus and fungi. It is a muco-cutaneous-vesiculo-bullous disease.

Clinical Features

- *Systemic features:* There is fever, malaise, sore throat, cough and arthralgia. It is followed by symmetrical erythematous erruptions affecting any part of the body.
- *Ocular features:* There is mucopurulent conjunctivitis with papillae and focal fibrotic patches. There is cicatricial entropion, aberrant eyelashes and keratinization of conjunctiva and dry eye.

Management

- Enquire about any allergy to drugs before prescribing antibiotics and sulphonamides
- Topical steroids help to control vasculitis and prevents infarction of the conjunctiva.
- Surgery to correct entropion.

Cogan's Syndrome

Cogan's syndrome is characterized by a non-syphilitic interstitial keratitis associated with vestibulo-auditory symptoms first described by Cogan.

Ocular features: The interstitial keratitis is bilateral and presents with pain, photophobia, circumciliary congestion, dim vision, patchy infiltration of deep corneal stroma and mild uveitis.

Aural features: There is vertigo, tinnitus and nerve deafness. The aural symptoms may precede or follow the onset of ocular features.

The etiology is unknown. The syndrome appears to be a part of general hypersensitivity reaction affecting particularly the eye and ear due to many cause such as periarteritis nodosa, vasomotor disturbances, viral infection and also following intake of drugs and chemical poisons. It has been seen in association with diseases with infiltrative processes like sarcoidosis, Hodgkin's disease and mycosis fungoides.

Reiter's Syndrome

The traid of urethritis, arthritis and mucosal inflammation such as conjunctivitis, often with iritis, is known as Reiter's syndrome. It affects young men. About 70% of these are positive for HLA-B27. Other systemic features of this syndrome include keratoderma blennorrhagicum of palms or soles, circinate balanitis, nail dystrophy, painless mouth ulcer and plantar fasciitis.

The acute non-granulomatous iridocyclitis occurs independently of the conjunctivitis and is like seen with ankylosing spondylitis. It is of unknown etiology. Serologic evidence has confirmed its relationship with ankylosing spondylitis. Treat iritis with cycloplegics and steroids.

Behcet's Disease

It presents as a hypopyon due to iritis and is associated with ulcers in mouth, on tongue and genitalia. The ocular manifestations include acute iritis, hypopyon, vitreous haze, macular edema, retinal phlebitis and obliterative arteritis. The cause of the disease is unknown but the viral and immunologic factors have been proposed. Treat by steroids and immunosuppressives under supervision of a physician.

Posner-Schlossman Syndrome
(Glaucomatocyclitic Crisis)

The patient comes with pain, discomfort and blurring of vision usually in one eye. On clinical examination, there is mild congestion, corneal edema, few keratic percipitates, no posterior synechia, mild aqueous flare, heterochromia and raised intraocular pressure. The eye is normal between the attacks. Treat by steroids and carbonic anhydrase inhibitors.

Fuch's Uveitis Syndrome
(Fuch's Heterochromic Cyclitis)

The triad of syndrome consists of iris hetero-chromia, keratic precipitates and cataract. The following manifestations are seen:
  i. Iris stromal atrophy.
  ii. Diffusely scattered small white keratic precipitates.
  iii. Mild aqueous flare and cells.
  iv. Anterior vitreous show cells.
  v. Normal fundus.

It affects young people. There are less acute symptoms of iritis than those associated with the Parry-Romberg syndrome and glaucoma-tocyclitic crisis. The loss of vision is due to cataract and glaucoma. Patient must be watched for these. Treat by steroids. Response is good for cataract surgery. Glaucoma is an open angle type and difficult to manage.

Parry-Romberg Syndrome
(Progressive Facial Hemiatrophy)

The patient develops chronic iridocyclitis on the affected side. Clinical examination show atrophic iris, keratic precipitates and cataract. The clinical findings are like that of Fuch's heterochromic cyclitis. It is felt that the eye signs are part of the facial inflammatory-atrophic process.

Vogt-Koyanagi-Harada's Syndrome
(Uveomeningitis Syndrome)

The syndrome consists of uveitis, meningeal signs, vitiligo, poliosis, alopecia and auditary signs. There is exudative detachment which settles and leaves the characteristic mottled fundus appearance of Harada's disease. The common complications are macular pathology, cataract, posterior synechia and glaucoma. The syndrome resembles clinically and immunologically with sympathetic ophthalmia.

Presumed Ocular Histoplasmosis Syndrome

The syndrome has a triad of:
  i. Multifocal atrophic choroidal spots.
  ii. Peripapillary atrophy.
  iii. Hemorrhagic disciform maculopathy.

It is common among the age group of 20 to 50. It is twenty times more common in whites than in blacks. Patient complains of metamorphopsia and blurred vision due to involvement of the macula. Steroids have been found to be useful in aborting the attack of macular disease.

Lowe's Syndrome
(Oculocerebrorenal Syndrome)

It is a rare disease with inborn error of amino acid metabolism which predominantly affects boys. The lens is small and thin with lens opacities which may be capsular, lamellar, nuclear or total. Glaucoma is associated in 50% cases. Mother of the child may show multiple punctate lens opacities.

Down Syndrome (Mongolism)

Ocular features include lens opacity, strabismus, nystagmus, keratoconus and myopia. Systemic features are mental retardation, stunted growth, mongoloid facies and congenital heart defect.

Werner's Syndrome

Ocular features consist of bilateral cataract occurring between the ages of 20 and 40. Systemic features are premature senility, diabetes, hypogonadism and arrested growth.

Rothmund's Syndrome

Ocular features consist of bilateral cataract manifesting during 20 to 40 years of age. Systemic features are skin changes in form of atrophy, pigmentation and telangiectasia, bony defects, hypogonadism, disturbance of hair growth and saddle-shaped nose.

Vitreous Touch Syndrome

It occurs due to contact of formed vitreous with the corneal endothelium. It follows an intracapsular cataract extraction after several weeks or months of surgery. The cornea shows edema. The only treatment is to excise the vitreous with vitreous cutter.

Vitreous Wick Syndrome

It is a condition in which there is a bead of vitreous in the incision as if prolapsing through the incision. It causes ocular irritation. It can lead to bacterial endophthalmitis.

"Ugh" Syndrome

It is common with anterior chamber intraocular lens implant. There is a triad of uveitis, glaucoma and hyphema. Treat by topical steroids or by removal of implant.

"Sunset" Syndrome

It is a rare complication following posterior chamber implant. It is more frequent when the optic has been dialled into position. It is characterized by dislocation of implant in the vitreous months after surgery.

Plateau Iris Syndrome

It is a condition in which the iris is inserted anteriorly on the ciliary body. Gonioscopy shall help to diagnose it. Clinically the chamber depth is normal and iris plane appears flat. Treat by miotics and not by iridectomy.

Iridocorneal Endothelial Syndromes

It embraces following three conditions:
- The iris naevus (Cogan-Reese) syndrome.
- Chandler's syndrome.
- Essential iris atrophy.

In these conditions the glaucoma is secondary to endothelial overgrowth in the anterior chamber and formation of peripheral anterior synechia.

Refsum's Syndrome
(Heredopathia atactica polyneuritiformis)

It is an autosomal recessive inherited syndrome. Its main features include atypical retinitis pigmentosa, peripheral neuropathy and cerebellar ataxia. Sudden death can occur due to acute heart failure or respiratory paralysis.

Bassen-Kornzweig Syndrome
(Acanthocytosis)

It manifests with atypical retinitis pigmentosa, neuromuscular disease like Friedreich's ataxia, celiac disease and malformation of erythrocytes.

Usher's Syndrome

It is an autosomal recessive inherited syndrome. It is characterized by retinitis pigmentosa and congenital neurosensory deafness.

Favre-Goldmann Syndrome

There is vitreoretinal degeneration with poor night vision. It shows an autosomal recessive inheritance pattern. Its features include atypical retinitis pigmentosa, vitreous degeneration (liquefaction), retinoschisis, lens opacities and marked electroretinogram abnormalities.

Mobius Syndrome

It is caused by congenital aplasia of the sixth, seventh and sometimes of the ninth and twelfth cranial nerve nuclei. The lower facial muscles are spared. Clinically, there is difficulty in infantile feeding due to involvement of the ninth nerve. The patient presents with expressionless face, exposure keratitis, and fibrotic horizontal rectus muscles.

Alport's Syndrome

It is characterized by familial occurrence of progressive hematuric nephritis and sensoryneural deafness. It may be associated with ocular features like anterior lenticonus, lens opacities and retinal flecks in the macula.

Empty Sella Syndrome

The syndrome is defined as enlarged sella in the absence of an intrasellar tumor. A primary empty sella syndrome develops spontaneously. Its incidence is high in young obese females. Endocrine abnormalities are rare. Patient may complain of severe headache. The secondary empty sella syndrome occurs following surgical removal or radiotherapy of intrasellar tumors.

52

Notes on
Uncommon Ocular Topics

Clinical Features and Management

1. Orbit
2. The superior orbital (sphenoidal) fissure
3. The inferior orbital (spheno-maxillary) fissure
4. Canal and foramen of orbit
5. Paranasal sinuses
6. The angular vein
7. Cavernous sinuses
8. Acne rosacea conjunctivitis
9. Pemphigus
10. Conjunctival ecchymosis
11. White with pressure or white without pressure lesions
12. Choroidal detachment
13. Arterial pulse
14. Venous pulse
15. Strabismus fixus
16. Double elevator palsy
17. Adoption of abnormal head posture
18. Chin elevation or depression
19. Tilting of head towards the shoulder
20. Scotoma
21. Heteronymous hemianopia
22. Homonymous hemianopia
23. Altitudinal field defects
24. Arcuate defects
25. Diplopia
26. Metamorphopsia
27. Macropsia
28. Micropsia
29. Photopsia
30. Enlargement of blind spot
31. Hallucinations
32. Bonnet's sign
33. Gunn's sign
34. Dalrymple's sign
35. von Graefe's sign
36. Kocher's sign
37. Double ring sign
38. Fleischer's ring
39. Hudson-Stahli line
40. Ferry's line
41. Kayser-Fleischer ring
42. Krukenberg's spindle
43. Lenders' sign
44. Munson's sign
45. Arlt's line
46. Fuchs' ring
47. Fuchs' spot
48. Herbert's pits
49. Horner-Trantas spots
50. Mittendorf's dots
51. Port-wine stain
52. Purkinje images
53. Rathke's pouch
54. Roth's spots
55. Shagreen patches
56. Uhthoff's sign
57. Bandage contact lens
58. Intranasal spray in ocular allergy
59. Ophthalmic viscosurgical devices (OVDs)
60. Femtosecond laser
61. Aspheric vs spheric IOLs
62. Laser presbyopia reversal (LAPR)
63. Intracameral antibiotics
64. Foldable IOLs
65. Optical coherence tomography (OCT)
66. Vascular endothelial growth factors (VEGFs) inhibitors
67. Photodynamic therapy (PDT)
68. Steroids in neurophthalmic cases
69. Gene therapy in ocular disorders
70. USG and UMB imaging for vitreoretinal disorders
71. Belin/ambrosio enhanced ectasia display (BAD display)
72. Posterior capsule opacification (PCO)

ORBIT

The orbit is formed by seven bones namely:
- Superior maxilla
- Palate
- Frontal
- Sphenoid
- Malar or zygomatic
- Ethmoid
- Lacrimal

Relations of Orbit

- Above—Anterior cranial fossa
- Below—Maxillary antrum (antrum of highmore).
- Medially—Nasal cavity and air sinuses.
- Laterally—Middle cranial and temporal fossa.

Fissures, Canals and Foramen of Orbit

- The superior orbital (sphenoidal) fissure.
- The inferior orbital (spheno-maxillary) fissure.
- The anterior and posterior ethmoidal canals.
- The ethmoid foramen and optic foramen.

The Superior Orbital (Sphenoidal) Fissure

It lies between the roof and lateral wall of the orbit. It is a space between the small and great wings of the sphenoid. It is about 22 mm long and is the largest gap or communication between the orbit and the middle cranial fossa. The structures passing through this are fourth, frontal, lacrimal, both division of third nerve, nasociliary and sympathetic root of the ciliary ganglion, sixth nerve, superior ophthalmic vein, inferior ophthalmic vein and recurrent lacrimal artery.

The Inferior Orbital
(Sphenomaxillary) Fissure

It lies between the lateral wall and floor of the orbit. It allows communication between the orbit and pterygopalatine (sphenomaxillary) and infratemporal (zygomatic) fossae. Its anterior extremity reaches to about 2 cm from the inferior orbital margin. The structures passing through this are second division of fifth nerve, zygomatic nerve, branches to the orbital periosteum from the sphenopalatine ganglion and a communication between the inferior ophthalmic vein and the pterygoid plexus. The anterior extremity of the fissure plays an important landmark in the operation of lateral orbitotomy.

Canal and Foramen of Orbit

The anterior ethmoidal canal: It opens in the anterior cranial fossa at the side of the cribriform plate of the ethmoid. It transmits the nasal nerve and artery.

The posterior ethmoidal canal: It opens in the anterior cranial fossa. It transmits the posterior ethmoidal artery and sometimes the small spheno-ethmoidal nerve of Luschka.

The ethmoidal foramen: These are the opening of the ethmoidal canals.

The optic foramen and canal: It is formed by the two roots of the lesser wing of the sphenoid. It is a communication from the middle cranial fossa to apex of the orbit. It is in close relation to the sphenoidal air sinus and sometimes to posterior ethmoidal air sinus. It transmits the optic nerve with its coverings, ophthalmic artery which is embedded in the dural sheath of the optic nerve and few twigs from the sympathetic which accompany the artery. The optic canal is about 5 to 7 mm long.

Paranasal Sinuses

There are four paranasal sinuses, namely the maxillary, the frontal, the ethmoidal and the sphenoidal.

The maxillary sinus (Antrum): At birth the maxillary antrum is a groove in the lateral nasal wall. It grows rapidly with second dentition reaching nearly to the adult size by the age of twelve.

The maxillary antrum is a pyramidal cavity situated in the superior maxilla. Its base forms the part of the lateral wall of nose. Its apex lies under the malar bone. There is a small opening situated near the roof of the antrum in the lateral wall therefore the drainage of the antrum is improper. It opens in the middle meatus of the nose in the hiatus semilunaris.

The frontal sinus: All the sinuses arise as a bud from the nasal mucosa. The bud which is to develop as a frontal sinus passes up through the ethmoid bone and at the birth it is just present in the frontal bone. The stalk remains as the frontonasal duct. The frontal sinus is about the size of a pea at the age of seven and attains full size at about the age of twenty-five.

The frontal sinuses are situated anteriorly between the two plates of the frontal bone on either side and have a septum separating these. The frontal sinus is about 3 cm in height, 2.5 cm in breadth and about 2 cm in depth. The frontal sinus opens by an infundibulum into the hiatus semilunaris in the middle meatus near the openings of the anterior ethmoid and maxillary sinus.

The ethmoidal sinuses (Air cells): At birth, the ethmoidal air cells are present as small depressions and grow rapidly after the age of seven. The ethmoidal air cells are situated in the lateral mass of ethmoid and completed by the frontal, palate, sphenoid, superior maxilla and lacrimal bone. The air cells are separated by the surrounding structures by very thin bones which are not good barriers to check the spread of infection. Thus ethmoiditis is one of the common cause for orbital cellulitis.

The anterior ethmoid opens into the hiatus semilunaris in the middle meatus of nose.

The middle ethmoid opens on the bulla ethmoidalis in the middle meatus of the nose.

The posterior ethmoid opens into the superior meatus.

The sphenoidal air sinus: The sphenoidal air sinus starts to grow at the age of about eight.

The sphenoidal air sinus lies in the body of the sphenoid bone. Above the sphenoidal sinus are the pituitary body and the optic nerve. A sinusitis may result in retrobulbar neuritis. Laterally, it is in relation with the cavernous sinus containing the internal carotid artery and the sixth nerve.

The sphenoidal sinus opens into the sphenoethmoidal recess.

The Angular Vein

The angular vein is the most important vessel to be taken care of during surgery on the lacrimal sac. It is a subcutaneous vessel visible through the skin about 8 mm from the inner canthus.

It is formed by the union of the supraorbital and frontal veins and runs down at the side of nose, lateral to angular artery passing across the nasal edge of the medial palpebral ligament, piercing the orbicularis, below the ligament. It has communication with the superior ophthalmic vein and facial vein. The facial vein runs obliquely downwards and backwards across the face. It crosses the mandible and joins the posterior facial vein to form a common facial vein which opens into the internal jugular vein. The facial vein communicates with the nasal veins and pterygoid plexus of veins and inferior ophthalmic vein. This explains that any septic lesion on the face can result in cavernous sinus thrombosis. Tributaries of angular vein are:

- Supraorbital vein
- Frontal vein
- Superficial nasal veins
- Facial vein

Cavernous Sinuses

The cavernous sinuses are venous channels formed by the splitting of the dura mater. These sinuses extend on each side of the pituitary body and the body of the sphenoid. Each sinus is traversed by the following structures

- Internal carotid artery
- Sixth nerve
- Filaments of sympathetic and a venous plexus
- In the lateral wall, from above downwards:
  - Third nerve
  - Fourth nerve
  - First and second division of fifth nerve.

Tributaries of Cavernous Sinuses

- Ophthalmic veins
- Emissary veins

- Superior petrosal sinus
- Inferior petrosal sinus
- Circular sinus

Ophthalmic veins: These communicate with the angular vein on the face. Through this infection spreads to cavernous sinus from any acute septic lesion on the face, nose and lips.

Emissary veins: These communicate with the pterygoid plexus. This explain how a thrombosis of cavernous sinus may spread to the pterygoid plexus.

Superior petrosal sinus: It crosses above the fifth and sixth nerve and joins the cavernous sinus with transverse sinus.

Inferior petrosal sinus: It receives the veins from the internal ear. It unites the cavernous sinus with the internal jugular vein below the base of skull.

Through the petrosal sinuses, the thrombosis of cavernous sinus may spread to the lateral sinus.

The swelling behind the ear, in a case of cavernous sinus thrombosis is due to spread of infection through the mastoid emissary vein.

Circular sinus: It connects the two cavernous sinuses and surrounds the sella turcica of the pituitary body. It explains how the thrombosis of cavernous sinus becomes bilateral in most cases, if not treated early.

CONJUNCTIVA

Acne Rosacea Conjunctivitis

Acne rosacea is a skin disease of unknown etiology which affects females in the age group of 30 to 50. The skin lesions consist of a chronic hyperemia of face usually involving the nose, central forehead and upper cheeks. Pustules may form but resolve without scarring. The ocular lesions include conjunctivitis, pannus, punctate epithelial keratopathy, chronic blepharitis and meibomitis. If untreated then there is corneal stromal scarring.

Management

- Topical steroids
- Systemic tetracycline –1 gm, in four divided doses for a month
- Good diet. No alcohol and condiments.
- Dark goggles
- Vitamins

Pemphigus

It is characterized by the presence of bullae on the mucus membrane and on the skin. It may be localized to the conjunctiva causing submucus fibrosis thereby thickening and contraction of the conjunctiva. It is also known as essential shrinkage of the conjunctiva. Steroids help. Bandage Contact Lens may help to prevent adhesions of lids to eyeball.

Conjunctival Ecchymosis

Conjunctival ecchymosis is common and vary in degree from a minute petechial to extensive spread in the exposed part of the bulbar conjunctiva.

Causes

- Local trauma to the conjunctiva by foreign body, hand or postoperative.
- Injury to orbital structures.
- In fracture of roof of orbit, the blood tracks along the levator muscle to upper fornix and lids.
- In fracture of floor of orbit, the blood tracks along in lower fornix and lids.
- In fracture of apex of orbit, the blood tracks along the lateral rectus muscle.
- In fracture of orbital plate of sphenoid, the blood tracks along the temporal aspect of the globe.
- In fracture of base of skull, the blood tracks along the floor of orbit then fornix and then to conjunctiva.
  Usually it takes 12–24 hours for the blood to reach the sub-conjunctival tissue.
- Petechial hemorrhage in pneumococcal conjunctivitis.
- Sudden severe venous congestion of head as in whooping cough, vomiting, blowing

the trumpet, fits, strangulation, violent compression of thorax in stampede or accidents.

- Systemic vascular diseases, like arteriosclerosis, hypertension, nephritis or diabetes. A patient with a small tiny hemorrhage should be subjected to a thorough check up of cardiovascular system.
- Blood dyscrasias, as purpura, thrombocytopenia, leukemia.

Investigation: Angiography, platelet count, RBC, Hb, total and differential count, complete systemic check up specially CV system.

Treatment: Assurance, cold packs, vitamin C and evacuate.

RETINA

White with Pressure or White without Pressure Lesions

A region in the fundus which appears iridescent white over the depression during scleral depression on binocular ophthalmoscopy is known as white with pressure lesion. A similar appearance if seen without pressure by scleral depressure is known as white without pressure lesion. It is seen in conditions like flat retinal detachment, retinoschisis, peripheral cystoid degeneration and peripheral preretinal membrane.

Choroidal Detachment

It is common after a cataract operation. It appears as a large elevation solid with normal colour of retina. The intraocular pressure is low and anterior chamber is either flat or very shallow.

Arterial Pulse

There are two types of retinal arterial pulsation the expansile and serpentine. Both are due to the rhythmic variations of pressure within the artery-expansile pulsation is seen as a variation in the calibre of the vessel while serpentine pulsation is seen as lateral movement of the part of the artery. It is the expansile pulsation which we see on

Ophthalmoscopy. It is due to transmission of a pressure pulse from the heart through the large arteries to the retinal vessels. The pressure within the retina artery is counter balanced by two factors:

- Tension in the vascular wall and
- Intraocular pressure.

The variations of intraocular pressure in the normal eye are seen by the familiar rhythmic movement of the pointer of the Schiötz tonometer.

The arterial pulsation can be seen ophthalmoscopically in 36% of normal individuals. The arterial pulsation is seen in the following conditions:

  (i) Increased distensibility of the coats of eye:
- High myopia.
- Keratoconus.
- Corneal ulcer threatening to perforate.

 (ii) High systemic pulse pressure:
- Graves' disease.
- Aortic aneurysm.
- Aortic incompetence.

(iii) Intraocular pressure is high:
- Glaucoma.

(iv) Arterial pressure is low:
- Anemia.

Venous Pulse

It occurs at the optic disk seen clearly by ophthalmoscope in large number of normal persons. The venous pulsation can be elicited in non-spontaneous pulse or increased in its amplitude by applying slight external pressure on the eye by a finger. Its presence or absence has no clinical significance.

SQUINT

Strabismus Fixus

It is a condition of the eyes in which both the eyes are fixed in the convergent position due to fibrous tightening of the medial rectii.

Double Elevator Palsy

There is a paresis of both the superior rectus muscle and inferior oblique muscle of the same eye. It may be associated with ptosis and occasionally with Marcus Gunn jaw-winking phenomenon. It is a congenital lesion of third nerve nuclei.

Adoption of Abnormal Head Posture

The purpose of abnormal head posture is to turn the eyes as far away as possible from the field of action of the paralyzed muscle. For this the head is turned in the direction of the field of action of paralyzed muscle so that the eyes are automatically turned in the opposite direction.

Chin Elevation or Depression

It occurs in cases with vertical deviation of the eye. If one elevator is weak then the patient will elevate the chin so that the eyes become depressed.

Tilting of Head towards the Shoulder

It is tilted to make up for the tortional deviation, e.g. if one intortor muscle such as right superior oblique is paralyzed then the eye will become extorted. In order to compensate for this to make the right eye to intort, the head will have to be tilted to the left shoulder.

VISUAL SYMPTOMS

Scotoma

A scotoma is an area of total or partial loss of visual function.

Absolute scotoma: There is total loss of vision, i.e. there is no light perception also.

Relative scotoma: There is some vision. Quite often an absolute scotoma may be surrounded by a relative scotoma.

Positive scotoma: There is an obstruction of visual field. It appears as a dark area in the field of vision. It is usually present in cases with macular lesions.

Negative scotoma: There is a blind area in the field of vision. One can say that it produces a hole in the visual field. A negative scotoma is usually seen in optic nerve lesions.

Central scotoma: Central scotoma involves fixation area. It can be relative or absolute. It occurs in cases with cptic neuritis.

Centrocaecal scotoma: In this the scotoma extends from the fixation to blind spot. It is seen in cases with toxic neuritis, Leber's optic neuropathy and congenital optic disk pits.

Heteronymous Hemianopia

There is an involvement of opposite sides of visual fields such as bitemporal hemianopia and binasal hemianopia. These are usually associated with lesions at optic chiasma.

Homonymous Hemianopia

There is an involvement of the same side of visual fields in each eye, i.e. right field of each eye or left field of each eye. These are seen in lesions of optic tract, optic radiations and visual cortex.

Altitudinal Field Defects

There is an involvement of two quadrants either superior or inferior visual field. It is seen in ischemic optic neuropathy.

Arcuate Defects

There is damage to superior or inferior retinal nerve fiber bundles seen typically in glaucoma.

Diplopia

There is a double vision. It is usually due to misalignment of the visual axis thereby stimulating non-corresponding retinal points. In convergent squint there is uncrossed or homonymous diplopia. In divergent squint there is a crossed or heteronymous diplopia.

Metamorphopsia

In this the straight lines appear to be wavy. It is due to swelling or edema of the macular area, thereby the contour of the retina is altered and thus the objects appear wavy.

Macropsia

The objects appear larger than the normal size. It is due to crowding of rods and cones in any inflammatory condition of macula.

Micropsia

The objects appear smaller than the normal size. It is due to separation of rods and cones in any inflammatory condition of the macula.

Photopsia

The patient complains of seeing a flash of light. It is due to irritability of the retina.

Enlargement of Blind Spot

It is a field defect due to optic nerve which does not produce any visual sensation. This can enlarge and known as enlargement of blind spot occurring typically in a case of papilledema due to separation of retina around the disk by edema.

Hallucinations

Hallucinations are the important visual symptom of an occipital and temporal lobe tumor. Visual hallucinations of unformed images such as moving lights, circles, flashes and flickering lights are diagnostic for occipital tumor. Visual hallucinations of formed images such as people, animals, objects, etc. are diagnostic for temporal lobe tumor.

MISCELLANEOUS

Bonnet's Sign

In Bonnet's sign, there is banking of the vein where it appears dilated distal to the arterio-venous crossing seen in the Grade III of arteriosclerotic changes in fundus.

Gunn's Sign

There is a tapering of the vein on either side of the crossing.

Dalrymple's Sign

There is lid retraction in a case of thyroid ophthalmopathy.

von Graefe's Sign

There is lid lag of the upper lid in the down gaze seen in thyroid orbitopathy.

Kocher's Sign

Patient with thyroid orbitopathy presents with staring and frightened look of the eyes.

Double Ring Sign

In a case of optic nerve hypoplasia, ophthalmoscopy shows a small grey optic disk surrounded by a yellow halo of hypo-pigmentation due to a concentric choroidal and retinal pigment epithelial atrophy. This appearance is known as "Double ring sign".

Fleischer's Ring

It develops in the epithelium and seen in case of keratoconus surrounding the base of the cone of cornea. It is due to deposition of iron.

Hudson-Stahli Line

It is common in elderly people. It is located at the junction of upper two-thirds with lower two-thirds of the corneal epithelium. There is deposition of iron.

Ferry's Line

It is seen in the epithelium just anterior to the filtering bleb.

Kayser-Fleischer Ring

It is seen in Wilson's disease-hepatolenticular degeneration. It is due to deposition of copper.

Krukenberg's Spindle

It is seen in pigment dispersion syndrome. The melanin pigment gets deposited in a shape of a spindle on the endothelium of cornea. It is common in myopes, diabetics and pigmentary glaucoma.

Lenders' Sign

In sarcoidosis appearance of preretinal nodules which are discrete, grey-white and located inferiorly and anterior to the equator of fundus.

Munson's Sign

In keratoconus there is a bulging of the lower lid when the patient looks down.

Arlt's Line

It is a linear line of tarsal conjunctival scarring seen about 2 mm from the margin of the upper eyelid in third stage of trachoma.

Fuchs' Ring

It is seen in posterior vitreous detachment. On examination, there is condensed vitreous behind the lens and an optically empty space behind the detached posterior hyaloid membrane. Some cases may show a ring like opacity (Fuchs' ring) on the detached hyaloid membrane anterior to the optic disk corresponding to the torn glial attachment of this membrane to the optic disk.

Fuchs' Spot

It is seen in high myopes. Retinal pigment epithelial hyperplasia and pigmented products of hemorrhage at the macula produces a well-known pigmented macular lesion in high myopes-"fuchs spot".

Herbert's Pits

Herbert's pits are small depressions in the connective tissue of the limbocorneal junction. They are filled with epithelium and look like small lucid circles or semi-circles in a semi-opaque limbus. These are seen in the third stage of trachoma.

Horner-Trantas Spots

In limbal form of vernal catarrh, there is limbal hypertrophy which occurs in the superior limbus or around entire cornea. In addition to limbal hyperplasia, there may be nodular whitish Horner-Trantas spots at any stage.

Mittendorf's Dots

The remnants of the vascular sheath of the lens are commonly seen as light gray opacities or dots at or near the posterior pole of the lens. These dots are known as "Mittendorf's dots".

Port-Wine Stain

The Sturge-Weber syndrome is congenital and is characterized by two lesions: angiomatosis of face and ipsilateral leptomeningeal angiomatosis. The facial angiomatosis is called as port-wine stain or nevus flammeus present at birth. It consists of one or several red patches of irregular outline. Because of its color, the name has been given as port-wine stain.

Purkinje Images

The Purkinje images are reflections from the optical media the cornea and the lens of the eye. There are four Purkinje images: from the anterior surface of the cornea, the posterior surface of the cornea, the anterior surface of the lens and posterior surface of the lens. The brightest image is from the anterior surface of the cornea. In keratometer—the first Purkinje image is utilized to measure the radius of the curvature of the anterior surface of the cornea.

Rathke's Pouch

Craniopharyngiomas are congenital tumors which arise from the squamous epithelial cell rests which are the remnants of Rathke's pouch.

Roth's Spots

The white-centered hemorrhages seen on ophthalmoscopy are known as Roth's spots. These are suggestive of leukemia but are also seen in bacterial endocarditis, sepsis, trauma, anemia, and hypertension.

Shagreen Patches

Shagreen patches are seen in case of tuberous sclerosis. Shagreen patches appear as leathery thick plaques on skin of lower thoracic and lumbosacral region of the back.

Uhthoff's Sign

There is temporary exacerbation of visual symptoms, ataxia and weakness of extremities by the heat and exercise in a case of multiple sclerosis. This is known as Uhthoff's sign. This phenomenon may be caused by transient edema the result of venous congestion induced by heat and exercise.

RECENT ADVANCES

Bandage Contact Lens

Bandage contact lenses are to prevent pain, infection and promote healing. The present lenses are thinner, more oxygen permeable and function better as bandage lenses and available in various sizes also to customize patients. These are useful in severe diseases like Stevens-Johnson syndrome, after stem cell transplantation, in refractory vernal ulcers, postoperative corneal transplant and phototherapeutic keratectomy patients especially when patients have persistent epithelial problems.

Intranasal Spray in Ocular Allergy

Ocular allergy can be a separate entity or accompanying allergic rhinitis.

In such cases intranasal sprays shall help to treat both at the same time.

Ophthalmic Viscosurgical Devices (OVDs)

Ophthalmic viscosurgical devices are used extensively in cataract surgery and have played a very important role in intraocular lens implant. The results have improved tremendously due to better OVDs rather than better phaco or foldable IOLs. Viscoat (Sodium chondroitin sulphate 4%-sodium hyaluronate 3%) based OVDs play a role in maintaining the anterior chamber depth, protect corneal endothelium and easy wash out. These provide low viscosity and dispersion. This dispersive nature results in better adherence of OVDs to the corneal endothelium, therefore better protection of corneal endothelium against fluid turbulence and lens fragments during phacoemulsification. It presents good visual acuity postoperatively because of corneal clarity. OVDs if not washed out properly may lead to **capsular block syndrome**—rise of intraocular pressure.

Femtosecond Laser

Femtosecond laser is a breakthrough in ultrafast laser science. This laser uses an infrared beam of light to precisely separate tissue by a process called photo disruption. The laser pulse divides material at molecular level without transfer of heat or impact to the surrounding tissue. The intralase femtosecond laser is used to create corneal flap in the LASIK procedure eliminating the use of microkeratome and blade. It cuts the flap with precision, accuracy and safety. The surgeon lifts the flap to allow treatment by excimer laser. The femtosecond laser has eliminated the risk of blade related flap complications such as free caps, button-hole, incomplete or decentered flaps. It has reduced postoperative complication of dry eye syndrome and the incidence of induced postoperative astigmatism.

The femtosecond laser does not depend on the inherent wavelength of the absorption of corneal tissue. This property allows the surgeon to cut very precise corneal incisions for various types of corneal surgical procedures. Femtosecond laser is used to treat astigmatic keratotomy. It is more effective in treating naturally occurring astigmatism rather than post operative astigmatism.

Femtosecond laser technique results in faster visual recovery and better uncorrected visual acuity with lower intraoperative and postoperative complications.

Femtosecond Laser in Cataract Surgery

The most crucial point of phacoemulsification is the capsulorhexis which should be central, curvilinear and continuous. Femtosecond laser technique is being used for incisions, capsulorhexis and nucleus softening. Thus, the entire lens can be aspirated with little or no ultrasound energy. The laser surgery is performed before surgical entry thereby reducing open eye time increasing safety and surgical efficiency. There shall be much less damage to endothelial cells. The femtosecond laser are precise down to micron level instead of millimeters in capsulorhexis.

It can be concluded that femtosecond laser cataract surgery offers precise and reproducible capsulorhexis, easier emulsification of cataract

Aspheric Vs Spheric IOLs

Aspheric IOLs provide better visual acuity than spheric IOLs. Asherical IOLs provide better photopic contrast sensitivity, spatial frequencies and less myopic shift.

Laser Presbyopia Reversal (LAPR)

Presbyopia is the age-related relentless regression of near vision due to progressive weakness of accommodation. Helmholtz theory stipulates that there is lenticular sclerosis thereby the increase in the lens anterior surface curvature and power is affected. Schachar theory stipulates that accommodation fails due to weaker action of the ciliary muscle on the lens and its capsule as a result of increased equatorial lens diameter coupled with decrease in the ciliary body-lens equator distance.

Presbyopia can be corrected by near work glasses, presbylasik or multifocal intraocular lens.

Another method to correct presbyopia has been suggested by Laser Presbyopic Reversal (LAPR) by Erbium YAG laser to ablate sclera tissue in eight radial lines over ciliary body. The ablation starts 0.5 mm from limbus and extends for 4.5 mm to weaken the sclera. The ablation heals by fibrinoid tissue rather than fibrous tissue. This widens the ciliary body ring up to 10 mm. This result in stretching of the zonules thereby increases its contractile power. The weakening of the sclera also results in lowering the intraocular pressure. It helps to protect vulnerable ocular hypertensive patients from manifesting open angle glaucoma in due course of time. After this treatment, patient must be under corrected for presbyopic glasses so as to help the ciliary muscles to act.

Intracameral Antibiotics

Intracameral antibiotic at the end of phacoemulsification surgery before closing the wound is mandatory.

Following antibiotics are in use
1. Vancomycin
2. Cefuroxime
3. Gentamicin
4. Moxifloxacin 0.5% topical eyedrops

Moxifloxacin has become the first choice of intracameral use.

Moxifloxacin is a fourth-generation fluoroquinolone antibiotic that is active against broad spectrum of gram-positive, gram-negative, atypical microorganisms and anaerobes.

Moxifloxacin maintains high concentration in the anterior chamber for six hours.

Moxifloxacin is safe and non-toxic for intravitreal use also.

Moxifloxacin can be just withdrawn from the newly opened moxifloxacin 0.5% topical eyedrop bottle. Just withdraw 0.3 to 0.5 ml and inject 0.1 ml of this in the capsular bag as the last step of surgery.

Follow strict and scrupulous preoperative and postoperative regime.

Moxifloxacin is an adjunct to these measures.

Foldable IOLs

The foldable IOLs have helped to evolve microincision phacoemulsification surgery even with topical anesthesia. The microincision surgery denotes a small incision 2.2 to 3.2 mm for emulsification and insertion of foldable IOLs. Aspheric IOLs provide good vision, better contrast sensitivity and also improves night vision.

Single piece IOLs are considered as best design.

AcrySof IQ foldable IOLs are preferred as first choice.

Optical Coherence Tomography (OCT)

Optical coherence tomography is non-invasive diagnostic method. It performs a cross sectional imaging of retina and optic nerve with a resolution of 5–10 micron. There are two types of machines—Time domain and Spectral OCT. Spectral OCT is faster with better resolution (3–5u).

It is an invaluable non-invasive technique to study retinal changes in maculopathies especially in age-related macular degeneration when used along with fundus fluorescein angiography.

Optical coherence tomography has found wide applications in neuroophthalmology. All the neuroophthalmic diseases of afferent visual system involve damage to retinal nerve fiber layer which coalesce to form the optic nerve. Therefore OCT becomes valuable diagnostic tool for the multiple sclerosis, parachiasmal lesions, Alzheimer's disease and tumors compressing anterior visual pathways.

It is very useful in cases with

- Vitreomacular traction
- Epiretinal membrane
- Macular hole
- Vascular blocks
- Diabetic maculopathy
- Age-related macular degeneration
- Central serous retinopathy
- Any lesion in retina or optic disk especially macula.

Vascular Endothelial Growth Factors (VEGFs) Inhibitors

Anti-vascular endothelial growth factors (VEGFs) helps to control neovascularization. Intravitreal injections of VEGFs are helpful to control neovascularization. Bevacizumab (avastin) is VEGFs inhibitor to control wet age-related macular degeneration. Bevacizumab is a full-length humanized monoclonal anti-human VEGFs. It is useful in maculopathies with edema.

Photodynamic Therapy (PDT)

Choroidal neovascularization is a leading cause for blindness. Photodynamic therapy has been used in the cases of choroidal neovascularization with wet type of age-related macular degeneration. It helps in stabilization of the malady therefore the vision.

In photodynamic therapy, the photosensitive dye *Verteporfin (Visudyne)* is administered intravenously diluted in 5% dextrose over a period of 10 minutes. The diode laser 810 nm light with power of 50 mj is suitable for exciting the photosensitizer dye in retina after 5 minutes of infusion. It causes thrombosis of the low flow vessels within the choroidal neovascularization lesion. An inflammatory response ensues coupled with fibrosis and regression of the choroidal neovascularization. The photodynamic therapy produces thrombosis in small vessels but induces inflammatory response by release of vascular endothelial growth factors (VEGFs). Therefore, intravitreal anti-VEGF agents should be given to negate the effect of VEGFs. Addition of intravitreal steroids shall help to reduce inflammation, fibrosis and edema.

Steroids in Neuroophthalmic Cases

Optic neuritis
Multiple sclerosis
Arteric or non-arteric anterior ischemic optic neuropathy
Thyroid ophthalmopathy
Papilledema
Maculopathies.

In fact there is no contraindication if it is used judiciously to save the life or vision.

Gene Therapy in Ocular Disorders

Gene therapy is the gift of the nature to the humanity. Gene therapy is the best contribution of the biotechnology and bio-scientist to the humanity. In Gene therapy-the Gene is transferred by vectors. The vector encapsulates therapeutic genes for delivery to cells. The vector can be viral or non-viral in origin. The success of gene therapy depends and limited by the host immune response to foreign antigens in the transgene and/or vector. Fortunately, the immunological response of the eye is unique. It has contributed to rapid progress in ocular gene therapy. The immune-privileged status of the eye has been well demonstrated by clinical success in corneal transplants and tissue grafts. Presently, the gene therapy is being explored in; retinitis pigmentosa, leber congenital amaurosis, gyrate atrophy, age-related macular degeneration and retinoblastoma.

USG and UMB Imaging for Vitreoretinal Disorders

Ultrasound is essential for ocular examination in cases with opaque media and inadequate pupil dilation.

Ultrasound is based on the principle that the sound is reflected when it encounters any interface with different tissue densities resulting in an echo whose strength relates to difference in tissue density.

B-Scan Ultrasonography (USG)

USG aids in differentiating asteroid hyalosis from vitreous hemorrhage, tumors, choroidal detachment, and also localizing intraocular foreign body, etc.

Ultrasound Biomicroscopy (UBM)

Ultrasound biomicroscopy provides high resolution imaging of the eye anterior to the equator.

Interpretation of imaging should always be correlated with clinical evaluation.

Belin/Ambrosio Enhanced Ectasia Display (BAD display)

Belin/ambrisio enhanced ectasia display is the first comprehensive refractive surgical screening technique that is fully elevation-based. It shall provide greater specificity and sensitivity for detecting early ecstatic diseases of cornea.

Posterior Capsule Opacification (PCO)

Posterior capsule opacification is the most common postoperative problem that results in decrease of visual acuity and preferably treated by Nd:YAG laser posterior capsulotomy.

The transformation and the proliferation of lens epithelial cells (LECs) is the process that leads to posterior capsule opacification. The lens epithelial cells are composed of two cell types: anterior cells located under anterior capsule and equatorial cells located on equatorial capsule. The equatorial lens epithelial cells are unabatedly proliferating and transforming in lens fiber cells. The presence of telomerese in lens epithelial cells indicate that lens epithelial cells are stem cells. It is easy to remove cells or polish anterior capsule but not equatorial capsule. The ARC Nd:YAG laser is efficient and safe for detaching and polishing capsular bag. Thus the ARC Nd:YAG laser dodick photolysis shock wave system is promising for prevention of posterior capsule opacification.

53

Ocular Cryo and Laser Therapies

CRYOTHERAPY

Cryotherapy is given by application of a cryoprobe to the tissue. To achieve the desired effect on the tissue, the tip of the cryoprobe must attain a temperature much below the freezing point. Three factors play an important role in achieving the desired effect on various tissues: the size of the cryo tip, the temperature of the cryo tip and the duration of the freezing process. The size of the tip varies from 1 to 4 mm. The temperature of the cryo tip varies with the coolant used; feron gives minus 40 to 70° C, carbon dioxide gives minus 78° C, and nitrous oxide gives minus 89° C. The duration of the freezing process depends upon the tissue to be treated. A longer duration of freezing process gives a larger size of ice ball at the cryo tip. With the popularity of cryotherapy, many types of cryo units are available. A cryo unit with defrosting device is better. Disposable cryo units are available for the cataract extraction using feron to cool the tip.

Effect of Cryotherapy on Tissue

I. **Necrosis-of Tissue**
This effect of cryotherapy is used in the treatment of retinal tumors, retino-blastoma and hemangioma.

II. **Adhesion-for Repair**
This effect of adhesion produced by cryotherapy has been used in treating retinal detachment.

III. **Vascular occlusion**
This effect of vascular occlusion has been used in treating condition which require vascular occlusion, as in Coats disease and Eales' disease.

IV. **Adhesion of cryoprobe**
The cryosurgery became popular when it was used to deliver cataract.

Ocular Lesions for Cryopexy

Lids
- Warts, molluscum contagiosum, xanthe-lasma, basal cell carcinoma, palpebral angioma are amenable to cryopexy. There is a minimal scarring.
- Papillary hypertrophy in a case of vernal conjunctivitis responds well to cryo application, about six to eight applications, given on alternate day.

Conjunctiva
- An excessive filtering bleb is made to shrink by cryo application for about 30 seconds.
- Iris prolapse can be treated with cryo. A single application causes necrosis.

Cornea
It can be used in a case of herpes involving stroma. Take care not to damage the endo-thelium.

Ciliary Body

Cyclo-cryopexy has been used in cases of raised intraocular pressure due to rubeosis, and absolute glaucoma. It is safe to use in a case of glaucoma following keratoplasty. A 4 mm cryo tip with nitrous oxide as a coolant, applied at about 4 mm from the limbus, covering half circle, shall be sufficient. If there is still a rise of pressure, the process can cover remaining half circle to destroy the ciliary processes. It helps to lower the pressure. As the sensory nerves to cornea are damaged, the patient is comfortable, as there is no pain in spite of raised pressure. The complications of cyclo-cryopexy include hyphema, iris atrophy, uveitis, phthisis bulbi and anterior segment ischemia.

Cataract

Extraction of lens is very popular. The cryo tip is placed at the junction of middle and superior third of lens and thereafter as the ice ball is firmly adhered to the lens capsule, the lens can be slowly glided, out of the section, using slight support interiorly. Defrost the tip if in any case the ice ball adheres to iris or cornea.

Retinal Lesion

Retinal breaks: The effect of cryo to cause adhesion for repair has been used to seal the retinal breaks in the retina with or without retinal detachment. It has become a part of the surgical treatment of detachment.

Retinal Tumors

The effect of necrosis has been utilized to treat the retinal tumors. All living tissue frozen to minus 20° C or below, for one minute, would get necrotic. Small retinoblastoma and small retinal capillary angioma responds well to this therapy. Use nitrous oxide with a large tip of 4 mm, to treat. Observe the freezing with indirect ophthalmoscope. Allow the ice ball to grow until it completely covers the tumor mass. Repeat the cycle three times, at each site covering the tumor all around. The complications include exudative retinal detachment, vitreous haze and late vitreous traction.

Retino-vitreal Neovascularization

Peripheral retinal neovascularization occurs in many condition such as diabetic retinopathy, occlusion of central retinal vein, Eales' disease and leukemia. The cryotherapy is useful in the cases where the fundus is hazy. Cover the area of neovascularization with ice ball and let it grow until it covers the entire area.

Technique for Transconjunctival Cryopexy

Anesthetize the conjunctival sac. Infiltrate the subconjunctival area of the quadrant to be treated. Use Desmares retractor to retract the lid. Apply a cryoprobe and look for a mound on the retina with binocular indirect ophthalmoscope, and start freezing, as desired, light, medium or heavy cryopexy. The light cryopexy is seen as yellow sub-retinal glow with indistinct edges. The medium cryopexy is seen as white glow with sharp edges. The heavy cryopexy is seen as white glow with ice ball growing for few seconds or more as desired to cover the treating area. If there is a fluid then cryopexy will not produce adhesion. In such cases the cryopexy should be done at the edges of the sub-retinal fluid. If the ice ball is not visible in few seconds then check the pressure in coolant and re-apply the cryo tip properly.

LASER THERAPY

The term LASER is an acronym for "**Light Amplification by Stimulated Emission of Radiation**". Laser is the brightest light in existence.

Types of Laser

1. Argon—Its effect is photocoagulation.
2. Krypton—Its effect is photocoagulation.
3. Diode—Its effect is photocoagulation.
4. Diode-pumped frequency doubled. Nd:YAG—Its effect is photocoagulation.
5. Nd:YAG—Its effect is photodisruption.
6. Excimer—Its effect is photoablation.

Mechanism of LASER Effects

1. Photocoagulation
2. Photodisruption
3. Photoablation

PHOTOCOAGULATION THERAPY

Meyer-Schwickerath, in 1949, was the first to use and publish details about photocoagulation therapy of the retina. Meyer-Schwickerath's first instrument used the sun light. Thereafter came, the Beck arc and later xenon arc. The commercial use of xenon arc came in 1958. The use of xenon arc is limited as it cannot be used to treat a lesion smaller than 1.5° and exposure time cannot be reduced less than 0.2 second. In 1963 ruby laser came with short exposure of about one millisecond and red color to which hemoglobin is transparent. It limited its use in occlusion of blood vessels. The argon laser with green continue wave permitted direct coagulation of blood vessels. It has an advantage of selection of duration of exposure and slit lamp delivery which provided a well-illuminated stereoscopic view of the site to be coagulated. New modes of therapy such as krypton laser and tunable dye laser are available. Most photocoagulation treatment is performed with xenon arc photocoagulator or argon laser coagulator.

Xenon Arc Coagulator

In xenon arc the light is delivered to the patient's eye through a rotatable mirror. The surgeon observes the retina through a pin hole in the mirror, and directs the beam. The image is in sharp focus on the retina only in emmetropic eyes. In xenon arc, the optical system of the eye is used to focus the light rays to produce an image of the arc on the retina. A contact lens or plus or minus lens from a trial set can be used to focus the light in an ametropic eye. In xenon arc the light is absorbed by the pigment epithelium for conversion to heat or shock wave and affect the retina and choroid.

Argon Laser Coagulator

In argon laser the light is delivered through the slit lamp adapter. The adapter helps to focus the light on the tissue to be coagulated. In this system the optic of the eye does not play any part. In the treatment of the retina a contact lens with three mirrors is used. In argon laser the light is absorbed by the pigment epithelium and hemoglobin for conversion to heat or shock wave and affect the retina and choroid.

Effect of Photocoagulation on Tissue

Treatment with photocoagulation can achieve the following effects.

- Necrosis of the tissue by burning.
- Contraction of collagen by heating.
- Coagulation of blood vessels and blood within by heating.
- A tear of tissue due to explosion.
- Repair of tissue by adhesion.

The surgeon decides what he wants to achieve and thereby accordingly adjust the power, exposure time and size of the spot.

Ocular Lesions for Photocoagulation

Hemangioma Lid

Xenon arc photocoagulation is effective for treating hemangioma of lids.

Corneal Lesions

Argon laser therapy has been used for pterygium, corneal vascularization, disrupting the corneal nylon sutures and for deep vessels in the corneal wound responsible for repeated hyphema.

Cyclophotocoagulation

The ciliary body can be destroyed by cyclophotocoagulation like diathermy and cryopexy.

Iridotomy

A laser iridotomy by argon laser creates an opening in the iris in a case of angle closure glaucoma, aphakic pupillary block glaucoma, and any condition needing a hole in iris.

Goniotomy

A case of open angle glaucoma which is not controlled by medical therapy can be considered for laser goniotomy. The laser goniotomy creates holes in the trabecular meshwork thereby allowing the aqueous to reach the canal of Schlemm. It is helpful in few cases. In most cases the lowering of the pressure is for few weeks only. A recurrent bleeding from the site of trabecular tear is one of the complications of laser goniotomy. The bleeding vessel may be coagulated by argon laser using a large spot with long duration exposure.

Sub-retinal Neovascularization

It is the retinal pigment epithelium which plays a part in the conversion of light of xenon arc or argon laser to heat or shock wave which is conducted in all the direction from the pigment epithelium and affects the choroid and retina. This phenomenon is used to treat the lesions of choroid and retina. The sub-retinal neovascularization occurs in any condition in which there is a stimulus for choriocapillaries to proliferate through a break in the Bruch's membrane, e.g. senile macular degeneration, presumed ocular histoplasmosis syndrome, angoid streak and choroidal tear. Sub-retinal neovascularization causes loss of vision, bleeding, exudative retinal detachment and fibrous scar tissue. Involvement of fovea causes marked loss of central vision. It is best treated with argon laser therapy in which the light is absorbed by both pigment epithelium and hemoglobin giving a better effect than xenon arc coagulation.

Panretinal Photocoagulation

Panretinal photocoagulation is indicated in proliferative diabetic retinopathy and retinal vein occlusion with neovasculatization. It causes regression or attenuation of neovascularization. This effect is due to ischemic retina with decreased release of an angiogenic substance responsible for neovascularization. In a case of Eales' disease occlude the feeding arteries and their veins by direct treatment. It is useful in retinal angioma, leukemia, Coats' disease, and micro-aneurysms of diabetic retinopathy or central retinal vein branch occlusion (Fig. 53.1).

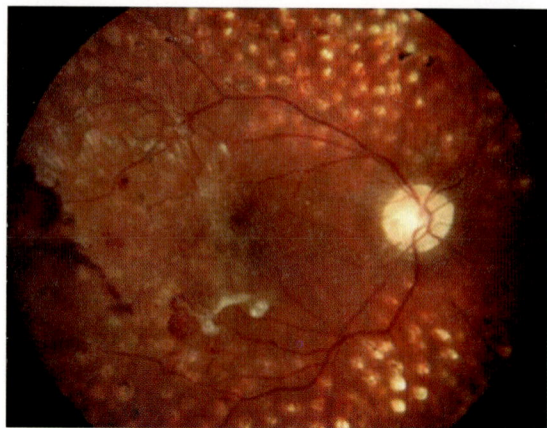

Fig. 53.1: Panretinal photocoagulation

Central Serous Retinopathy

A localized area of leakage in the retinal pigment epithelium can be treated with photocoagulation. The leakage stops after leaking site is covered by new proliferative epithelium.

Retinoblastoma

Retinoblastoma up to four disk diameters and posterior to equator may be destroyed by large spots with longer exposure of high intensity xenon arc coagulator, anterior lesions are treated with cryopexy.

Malignant Melanoma

A small pigmented, choroidal melanoma, anterior to the vascular arcades and about 6 disk diameters can be treated with photo-coagulation.

Rentinal Breaks and Lattice

Photocogulation is indicated in retinal breaks which are likely to result in a detachment. A lattice degeneration can be treated prophy-lacitically.

PHOTODISRUPTION THERAPY

Laser based on this mechanism ionize the electrons of the tissue resulting in a physical state known as *Plasma.* This plasma expands with momentary pressure exerting incisional effect upon the tissue.

Nd:YAG laser is based on this mechanism of photodisruption. Its therapeutic uses are posterior capsulotomy, pupillary membranectomy and have been tried for phacolysis.

PHOTOABLATION THERAPY

Laser based on this mechanism produce ultraviolet light that breaks chemical bonds of biologic materials into small molecules which diffuses. Such types of lasers are known as *Excimer lasers.* These are used for Photorefractive keratectomy, keratomileusis (LASIK) and for phototherapeutic keratectomy.

54

Fundus Fluorescein and Indocyanine Green Angiography

FUNDUS FLUORESCEIN ANGIOGRAPHY

Fundus fluorescein angiography is non-invasive established technique for examining the circulation of retina. An angiogram is obtained by photographing the fluorescein dye emitted from the retina after intravenous injection. Digital imaging, easy storage and retrieval of large data has made it very popular.

Technique

Intravenous Fluorescein Angiography

In the technique of fluorescein angiography, the fluorescence is visualized in intravascular and extracellular spaces. The low molecular weight and high solubility in water of sodium fluorescein allows rapid diffusion. For angiography-usual dose is 3 ml of 20% sodium fluorescein solution for adults and 0.04 ml/kg of sodium fluorescein in children. The solution is injected intravenously and very fast through a wide bore 19 gauge needle. Inject the dye after the patient has been adjusted to slit lamp for angioscopy and photography.

Modifications of Fluorescein Angiography

1. *Oral fluorescein angiography:* It is useful for patients who are psychologically or technically unsuitable for intravenous injection. Mix 5 ml of 20% dye in 200 ml of cola or juice and give orally to the patients up to 40 kg body weight. Photographs are taken at the 0, 5, 10, 15, 30, 45, and 60 minutes interval.

2. *Scanning laser ophthalmoscopy:* HRA-II provides better resolution and can be combined with Indocyanine Green Angiography (ICG angiography).

Normal Angiogram

The normal angiogram has four overlapping phases. The arm to retina circulation time is interval between injection and appearance at the disk which is about 10 seconds.

Phase I: Choroidal Phase

It is prearterial phase in which the dye has reached the choroidal circulation but has not reached the retinal arteries. The dye enters the choroidal circulation through the short posterior ciliary arteries and retinal circulation through the central retinal artery. As the route to the retinal circulation is longer so the dye reaches the choroidal circulation one second earlier than retinal circulation. No details are seen in this phase.

Phase II: Arterial Phase

It is the arterial phase which follows one second after the phase I. The dye has filled the retinal arteries.

Phase III: Early Arteriovenous Phase

It is the capillary phase (arteriovenous phase) in which there is complete filling of retinal arteries and capillaries with early lamellar flow in the retinal veins. The choroidal filling shows a flush. The choroidal fluorescence increases as more fluorescein leaks from the choriocapillaries into the extravascular spaces. The flush is more marked in less pigmented eyes.

Phase IV: Mid and Late Venous Phase

It is the venous phase in which there is complete filling of retinal arteries, capillaries and veins with beginning of arterial emptying. The late phase of the angiogram shows effect of continuous recirculation, dilution and elimination of the dye. The circulation of the dye occurs within 3–5 minutes. There is late staining of the optic disk. The fovea appears dark due to blockage of the choroidal fluorescence by increased amount of xanthophyll pigment melanin content of pigment epithelium and avascularity.

Abnormal Angiogram

The term used to describe an abnormal fluorescein angiogram includes hyperfluorescence, hypofluorescence, retrofluorescence, fluorescein leakage, fluorescein pooling and fluorescein staining.

Hyperfluorescence

It is an increased fluorescence as compared to the normal. It is seen in vascular tumors and neovascularization. Any defect in the pigment epithelium of the retina allows the normal background choroidal fluorescence which appears as hyperfluorescence.

Hypofluorescence

It is decreased fluorescence as compared to the normal. It is seen in conditions like retinal vascular occlusion, atrophy of choriocapillaries, hemorrhages, pigmentation, and abnormal tissue proliferation, hard exudates, choroideremia and myopic degeneration.

Retrofluorescence

Retrofluorescence occurs when non- fluorescent structures are silhouetted against a background fluorescence.

Fluorescein Leakage and Pooling

It is a passage of the dye beyond the physiological barriers of the retinal vessels and the pigment epithelium of the retina into spaces between cells and tissue layers. It occurs from the neovascularization of retinal vessels and seen as leakage in macular lesions.

Fluorescein Staining

It occurs due to attachment of the dye to the tissue. It is seen in both, abnormal tissue like drusen, fibrous scar tissue and normal tissue like optic disk and sclera. It is a late phenomenon and seen in late pictures after 5 to 15 to 30 minutes.

Clinical Indication

- Diabetic retinopathy—detects macular edema, ischemia and neovascularization.
- Choroidal lesions—detects choroiditis, neovascular membrane, etc.
- Tumors—melanoma and hemangioma.
- Retinal vasculitis—leakage, etc.
- Central serous retinopathy.
- Maculopathies.
- Optic nerve lesions-papillitis, papilledema, anterior ischemic optic neuropathy.

Contraindications

It is contraindicated in patients with history of reaction to fluorescein dye and in patients with severe renal and liver dysfunction.

Side Effects

The common side effects of fluorescein are nausea and vomiting. The other less common side effects are urticaria, hypotension or shock. Even myocardial infarction and cardiac arrests have been reported. It is advisable to have an emergency tray ready in the department. No sensitization by prior injection has been reported. All the patients have a slightly yellow skin discoloration for about 12–24 hours after fluorescein injection. The patient may also have a dyschromatopsia-yellow or blue purple hue of the visual field. This is due to presence of fluorescein in the vitreous and aqueous and also due to pooling of fluorescein in the macula. Extravasation of the dye in the skin while giving intravenous injection can cause severe skin reaction. The fluorescein is mainly excreted in the urine and small amount in the bile. Avoid the test in pregnancy.

Disadvantages

It cannot be performed in patients with hazy media.

Lesions under preretinal and subretinal hemorrhage cannot be detected.

INDOCYANINE GREEN ANGIOGRAPHY

Digital indocyanine green angiography is useful in imaging the choroid and its associated pathological lesions while **fluorescein angiography** is useful for retinal lesions.

Indocyanine green—a tricarbocyanine dye is better and safe dye due to its properties for ophthalmic imaging. Its molecular weight is 775 daltons. It is excreted via bile by liver.

- Age-related macular degeneration
- Retinal angiomatous proliferation
- Polypoidal choroidal vasculopathy
- Central serous chorioretinopathy.